Surgical Anatomy of the Heart

Benson R. Wilcox
Professor of Surgery
University of North Carolina
Chapel Hill, NC
USA

Andrew C. Cook
British Heart Foundation Lecturer
Cardiac Unit
Institute of Child Health
University College London
London, UK

Robert H. Anderson
Professor of Paediatric Cardiac Morphology, Cardiac Unit
Institute of Child Health
University College London
London, UK

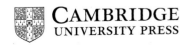

CAMBRIDGE
UNIVERSITY PRESS

CAMBRIDGE UNIVERSITY PRESS
Cambridge, New York, Melbourne, Madrid, Cape Town, Singapore, São Paulo

Cambridge University Press
The Edinburgh Building, Cambridge CB2 2RU, UK

Published in the United States of America by Cambridge University Press, New York

www.cambridge.org
Information on this title: www.cambridge.org/9780521861410

First published 2004
Third printing 2006

Printed in the United Kingdom at the University Press, Cambridge

A catalog record for this book is available from the British Library

Library of Congress Cataloging in Publication data

ISBN-13 978-0-521-86141-0 hardback
ISBN-10 0-521-86141-1 hardback

Every effort has been made in preparing this book to provide accurate and
up-to-date information that is in accord with accepted standards and
practice at the time of publication. Nevertheless, the authors, editors and
publisher can make no warranties that the information contained herein is
totally free from error, not least because clinical standards are constantly
changing through research and regulation. The authors, editors and
publisher therefore disclaim all liability for direct or consequential
damages resulting from the use of material contained in this book. Readers
are strongly advised to pay careful attention to information provided by the
manufacturer of any drugs or equipment that they plan to use.

Contents

Preface

The books and articles devoted to technique in cardiac surgery are legion. This is most appropriate, since the success of cardiac surgery is greatly dependent upon excellent operative technique. But excellence of technique can be dissipated without a firm knowledge of the underlying cardiac morphology. This is as true for the 'normal heart' as for those hearts with complex congenital lesions. It is the feasibility of operating upon such complex malformations that has highlighted the need for a more detailed understanding of the basic anatomy in itself. Thus, in recent years surgeons have come to appreciate the necessity of avoiding damage to the coronary vessels, often invisible when working within the cardiac chambers, and particularly to avoid the vital conduction tissues, invisible at all times. Although detailed and accurate descriptions of the conduction system have been available since the time of their discovery, only rarely has its position been described with the cardiac surgeon in mind. At the time the first edition of this volume was published, to the best of our knowledge, there had been no other books that specifically displayed the anatomy of normal and abnormal hearts as perceived at the time of operation. We tried to satisfy this need in the first volume by combining the experience of a practicing cardiac surgeon with that of a professional cardiac anatomist. We added significantly to the illustrations in the second edition, whilst seeking to retain the overall concept, since feedback from those who had used the first edition was very positive.

This third edition now seeks to expand and improve still further on the changes we made in the second edition. In our second edition, we added an entirely new chapter on cardiac valvar anatomy, and greatly expanded our treatment of coronary vascular anatomy. We have retained the format adopted in that edition, since we were gratified that, as hoped, readers were able to find a particular subject more easily. This third edition now contains still more new illustrations. We have retained our approach of orientating these illustrations, where appropriate, as seen by the surgeon working in the operating room, albeit that for most of the pictures of specimens we have reverted to anatomical orientation. So as to clarify the various orientations of each individual illustration, we have continued to include a set of axes showing the directions of superior (S), inferior (I), anterior (A), posterior (P), left (L), right (R), apex (a) and base (b). All our accounts are based on the anatomy as it is observed and, except in the case of malformations involving the aortic arch and its branches, they owe nothing to speculative embryology. As with the first two editions, it is our hope that the third edition will continue to be of interest not only to the surgeon, but also to the cardiologist, anaesthesiologist and surgical pathologist. All of these practitioners ideally should have some knowledge of cardiac structures and their exquisite intricacies, particularly those cardiologists who increasingly treat lesions that previously were the province of the surgeon. The major change in this third edition, nonetheless, is the addition of Andrew Cook to the editorial team. In the time that has passed since we produced the second edition, the senior author has retired from active surgery, whilst the time grows ever closer that the other initial author will be hanging up his morphological "shooting boots". We are confident that Andrew Cook will ensure that, if supply demands, the book will pass through still further editions, hopefully improving with each version.

Benson R. Wilcox, Andrew C. Cook &
Robert H. Anderson
London and Chapel Hill
May 2004

Acknowledgments

A good deal of the material displayed in these pages, and the concepts espoused, are due in no small part to the help of our friends and collaborators. A major change since we produced the second edition has been the translocation of Robert H. Anderson from Royal Brompton Hospital in London to Great Ormond Street Children's Hospital. This has enabled many new hearts to be specifically photographed for this new edition. We continue, nonetheless, to owe a particular debt to Anton Becker of the University of Amsterdam, and Bob Zuberbuhler of Pittsburgh Children's Hospital, Pennsylvania, United States of America, both of whom permitted us to use material from the extensive collections of normal and pathological specimens held in their centres. We have acknowledged our other friends at the appropriate point in the text, but here we would like to thank particularly Siew Yen Ho, of the National Heart and Lung Institute, now part of Imperial College in London. Yen produced many of the original drawings from which we prepared our artwork. The photographs and surgical artwork could not have been produced without the considerable help given by the Department of Medical Illustrations and Photography, University of North Carolina. For this edition, however, we have prepared a completely new series of cartoons. These have been expertly produced by Gemma Price, and we thank her sincerely for her hard work over and above the call of duty. We also thank Vi Hue Tran, who helped photograph the new hearts from Great Ormond Street, and took great care in labelling the numerous illustrations. We are again indebted to Christine Anderson and Peacelyn Jeyaratnam for their help during the preparation of the manuscript.

Finally, it is a pleasure to acknowledge the support of Greenwich Medical Media, now incorporated as part of Cambridge University Press, who have taken over as our new publishers, and have ensured that all the good parts of the previous editions were retained. In particular, we thank Gavin Smith for all his help during the preparation of the book for publication.

1

Surgical approaches to the heart

When the heart is described in this and in subsequent chapters, we account for the organ in its anatomical position[1]. Whenever possible, however, the heart will be illustrated as it would be viewed by the surgeon during an operative procedure, irrespective of whether the pictures are taken in the operating room, or are photographs of autopsied hearts. Where an illustration is in a non-surgical orientation, this is clearly stated.

In the normal individual, the heart lies in the mediastinum with two-thirds of its bulk to the left of the midline (Fig. 1.1). The surgeon, therefore, can approach the heart and great vessels either laterally through the thoracic cavity, or directly through the mediastinum anteriorly. To make such approaches safely, knowledge is required of the salient anatomical features of the chest wall, and of the vessels and the nerves that course through the

mediastinum. The approach used most frequently is a complete median sternotomy, although increasingly the trend is to use more limited incisions. The incision in the soft tissues is made in the midline between the suprasternal notch and the xiphoid process. Inferiorly, the white line, or linea alba, is incised between the two rectus sheaths, taking care to avoid entry to the peritoneal cavity, or damage to an enlarged liver, if present. Reflection of the origin of

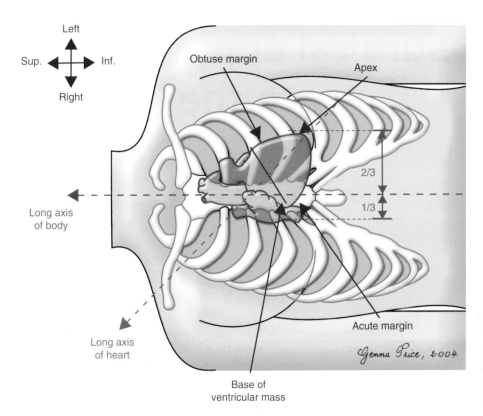

Fig. 1.1 This cartoon shows the usual position of the heart within the thorax, illustrating the vital landmarks and areas seen with the patient supine on the operating table, as viewed from the perspective of the surgeon.

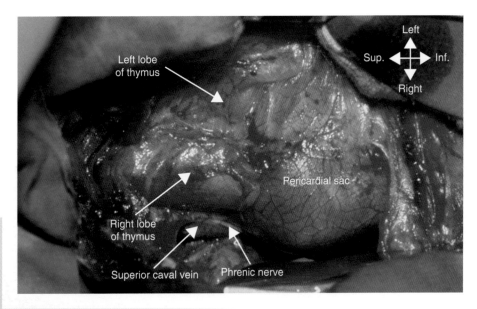

Fig. 1.2 This operative view, taken through a median sternotomy in an infant, shows the extent of the thymus gland.

the rectus muscles in this area reveals the xiphoid process, which is then incised to provide inferior access to the anterior mediastinum. Superiorly, a vertical incision is made between the sternal insertions of the sternocleidomastoid muscles. This exposes the relatively bloodless midline raphe between the right and left sternohyoid and sternothyroid muscles. An incision through this raphe then gives access to the superior aspect of the anterior mediastinum. The anterior mediastinum immediately behind the sternum is devoid of vital structures, so that the superior and inferior incisions into the mediastinum can safely be joined by blunt dissection in the retrosternal space. When the sternum has been split, retraction will reveal the pericardial sac, lying between the pleural cavities. Superiorly, the thymus gland wraps itself over the anterior and lateral aspects of the pericardium in the area of exit of the great arteries, the gland being a particularly prominent structure in the infant (Fig. 1.2).

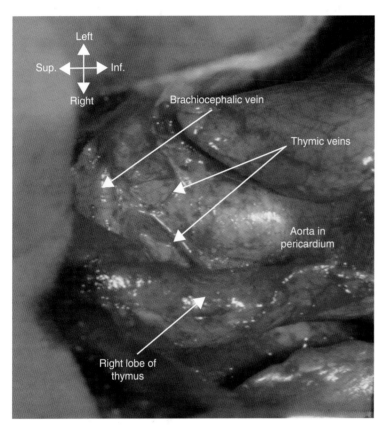

Left

Sup. ◄────► Inf.

Right

Brachiocephalic vein

Thymic veins

Aorta in pericardium

Right lobe of thymus

Fig. 1.3 This operative view, again taken through a median sternotomy, shows the delicate veins that drain from the thymus gland to the left brachiocephalic veins.

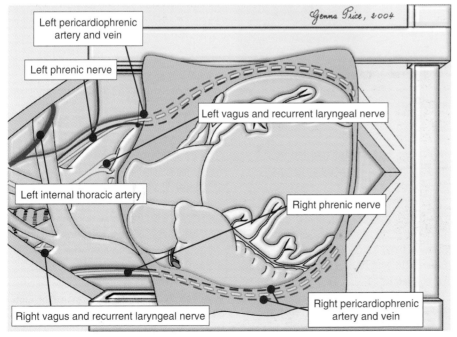

Genma Price, 2004

Left pericardiophrenic artery and vein

Left phrenic nerve

Left vagus and recurrent laryngeal nerve

Left internal thoracic artery

Right phrenic nerve

Right vagus and recurrent laryngeal nerve

Right pericardiophrenic artery and vein

Fig. 1.4 As shown in this cartoon of a median sternotomy, the pericardium can be opened so that the phrenic and vagus nerves stay well clear of the operating field.

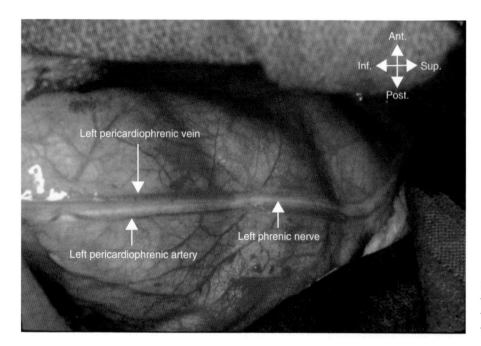

Fig. 1.5 This operative view, taken through a left lateral thoracotomy, shows the course of the left phrenic nerve over the pericardium.

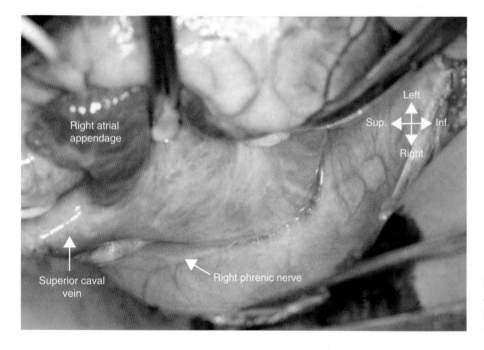

Fig. 1.6 This operative view, taken through a median sternotomy, shows the right phrenic nerve as seen through the reflected pericardium.

It has two lateral lobes, joined more or less in the midline. Sometimes this junction must be divided, or partially excised, to provide adequate exposure. The arterial supply to the thymus is from the internal thoracic, or mammary, and inferior thyroid arteries. If divided, these arteries tend to retreat into the surrounding soft tissues, and can produce troublesome bleeding. The veins are fragile, often emptying into the left brachiocephalic, or innominate, vein via a common

trunk (Fig. 1.3). Undue traction on the gland can lead to damage to this major vessel.

When the pericardial sac is exposed within the mediastinum, the surgeon should have no problems in gaining access to the heart. The vagus and phrenic nerves traverse the length of the pericardium, but are well lateral (Fig. 1.4). The phrenic nerve on each side passes anteriorly, and the vagus nerve posteriorly, to the hilum of the lung.

The course of the phrenic nerve is seen most readily through a lateral thoracotomy (Fig. 1.5). It is when the heart is approached through a median sternotomy, therefore, with the nerve not immediately evident, that it is most liable to injury. Although it can sometimes be seen through the reflected pericardium (Fig. 1.6), its proximity to the caval veins (Figs. 1.7, 1.8) is not always easily appreciated when these vessels are dissected from the anterior approach. Near the thoracic inlet, it passes

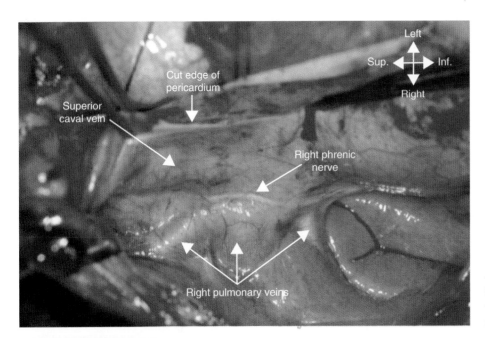

Fig. 1.7 This operative view, taken through a median sternotomy having pulled back the edge of the pericardial sac, shows the right phrenic nerve in relation to the right pulmonary veins.

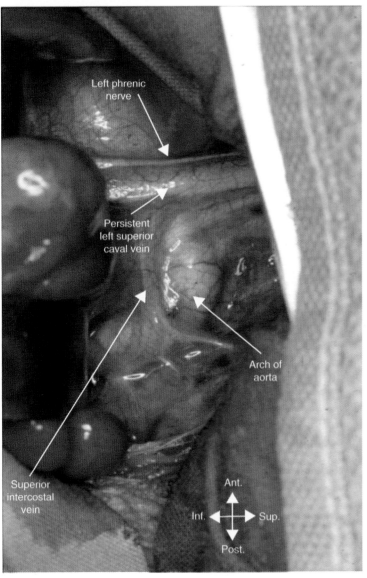

Fig. 1.8 This operative view, taken through a left thoracotomy, shows the relationship of the left phrenic nerve to a persistent left superior caval vein. Note also the course of the superior intercostal vein.

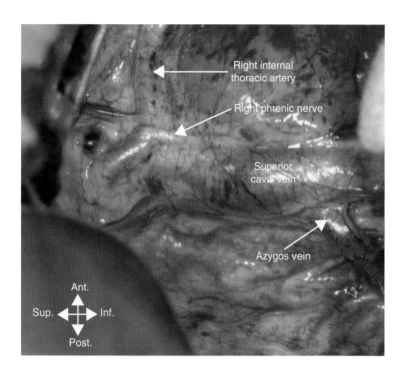

Right internal thoracic artery

Right phrenic nerve

Superior caval vein

Azygos vein

Ant.
Sup. ⟷ Inf.
Post.

Fig. 1.9 This operative view, taken through a right thoracotomy, shows the relationship of the right phrenic nerve to the right internal thoracic artery and the superior caval vein.

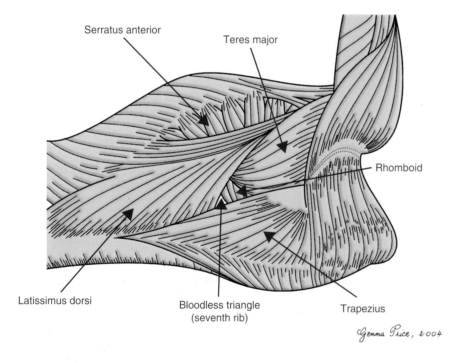

Serratus anterior

Teres major

Rhomboid

Latissimus dorsi

Bloodless triangle (seventh rib)

Trapezius

Gemma Price, 2004

Fig. 1.10 This cartoon shows the location of the bloodless area overlying the posterior extent of the sixth intercostal space.

close to the internal thoracic artery (Fig. 1.9), exposing it to injury either directly during takedown of that vessel, or by avulsing the pericardiophrenic artery with excessive traction on the chest wall. The internal thoracic arteries themselves are most vulnerable to injury during closure of the sternum. The phrenic nerve may be injured when removing the pericardium to use as a cardiac patch, or when performing a pericardiectomy.

Injudicious use of cooling agents within the pericardial cavity may also lead to phrenic paralysis or paresis.

A standard lateral thoracotomy provides access to the heart and great vessels via the pleural space. Left-sided incisions provide ready access to the great arteries, left pulmonary veins, and the chambers of the left side of the heart. Most frequently, the incision is made in the fourth intercostal space. The

posterior extent is through the triangular, relatively bloodless, space between the edges of the latissimus dorsi, trapezius, and teres major muscles (Fig. 1.10). The floor of this triangle is the sixth intercostal space. Division of the latissimus dorsi, and a portion of trapezius posteriorly, together with serratus anteriorly, frees the scapula so that the fourth intercostal space can be identified. Its precise identity

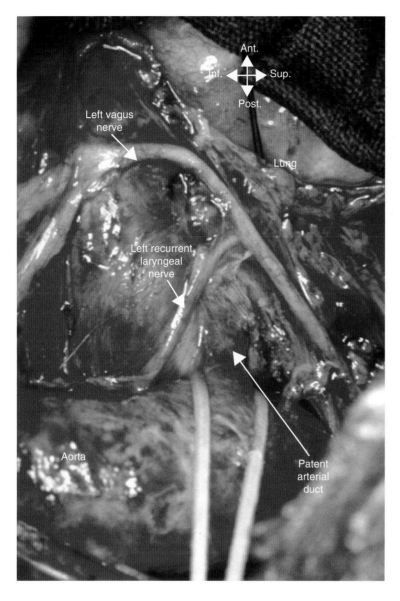

Ant.

Inf. — Sup.

Post.

Left vagus nerve

Lung

Left recurrent laryngeal nerve

Aorta

Patent arterial duct

Fig. 1.11 This operative view, taken through a left lateral thoracotomy in an adult, shows the left recurrent laryngeal nerve passing round the arterial duct.

should be confirmed by counting down from above. The intercostal muscles are then divided equidistant between the fourth and fifth ribs. The incision is carried forward beyond the midclavicular line in a submammary position, being careful to avoid damage to the nipple and the tissue of the breast. The intercostal neurovascular bundle is well protected beneath the lower margin of the fourth rib. Having divided the musculature as far as the pleura, the pleural space is entered, and the lung permitted to collapse away from the chest wall. Posterior retraction of the lung reveals the middle mediastinum, in which the left lateral lobe of the thymus, with its associated nerves and vessels, is seen overlying

the pericardial sac and the aortic arch. Intrapericardial access is usually gained anterior to the phrenic nerve. On occasion, the thymus gland may require elevation when the incision is extended superiorly. The same precautions should then be taken as discussed above. The lung is retracted anteriorly to approach the aortic isthmus and descending thoracic aorta, and the parietal pleura is divided on its mediastinal aspect. This is usually done posterior to the vagus nerve. In this area, the vagus nerve gives off its left recurrent laryngeal branch, which then passes round the inferior border of the arterial ligament, or duct (Fig. 1.11). It then ascends towards the larynx on the medial aspect of the posterior wall of

the aorta. Excessive traction of the vagus nerve as it courses into the thorax along the left subclavian artery can cause injury to the recurrent laryngeal nerve just as readily as can direct trauma to the nerve in the environs of the ligament. The superior intercostal vein is seen crossing the aorta and insinuating itself between the phrenic and vagus nerves (Fig. 1.12). This structure, however, is rarely of surgical significance. The thoracic duct (Fig. 1.13) ascends through this area, draining into the junction of the left subclavian and internal jugular veins. Accessory lymph channels draining into the duct can be troublesome when dissecting the origin of the left subclavian artery.

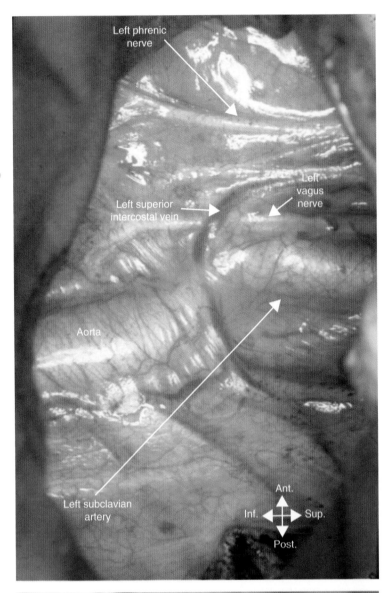

Left phrenic nerve

Left vagus nerve

Left superior intercostal vein

Aorta

Left subclavian artery

Ant.

Inf. ⟷ Sup.

Post.

Fig. 1.12 This operative view, again taken through a left lateral thoracotomy, shows the left superior intercostal vein.

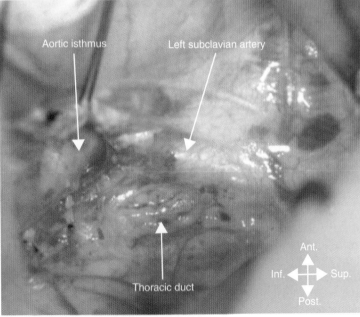

Aortic isthmus

Left subclavian artery

Thoracic duct

Ant.

Inf. ⟷ Sup.

Post.

Fig. 1.13 In this operative view, taken through a left thoracotomy, the thoracic duct is seen coursing below the left subclavian artery to its termination in the brachiocephalic vein.

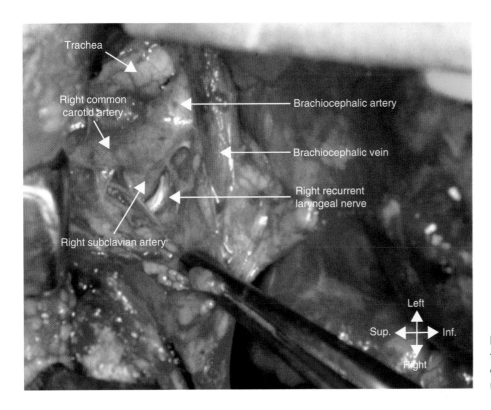

Trachea

Right common
carotid artery

Brachiocephalic artery

Brachiocephalic vein

Right recurrent
laryngeal nerve

Right subclavian artery

Left

Sup. ← → Inf.

Right

Fig. 1.14 This operative view, taken through a median sternotomy, shows the course of the right recurrent laryngeal nerve relative to the right subclavian artery.

A right thoracotomy in either the fourth or fifth interspace is made through an incision similar to that for a left one. The fifth interspace is used when approaching the heart, while the fourth permits access to the right-sided great vessels. Access to the pericardium is gained by incising anterior to the phrenic nerve, this approach often necessitating retraction of the right lobe of the thymus. To reach the right pulmonary artery and its adjacent mediastinal structures, it is sometimes useful to divide the azygos vein near its junction with the superior caval vein. Extension of this incision superiorly exposes the origin of the right subclavian branch of the brachiocephalic trunk. Laterally, this artery is crossed by the right vagus nerve, the right recurrent laryngeal nerve taking origin from the vagus and curling round the posteroinferior wall of the artery before ascending into the neck (Fig. 1.14). Also encircling the subclavian origin on this right side is the subclavian sympathetic loop, the so-called ansa subclavia, a branch of the sympathetic trunk that runs up into the neck. Damage to this structure can produce Horner's syndrome.

An anterior right or left thoracotomy is occasionally used in treating congenital malformations. Once the chest is opened, the same basic anatomical rules apply as described above. Thus far, our account has presumed the presence of normal anatomy. In many instances, the disposition of the thoracic structures will be altered by a congenital malformation. These alterations will be described in the appropriate sections.

Reference

1. Cook AC, Anderson RH. Attitudinally correct nomenclature. *Heart* 2002; 87: 503–506

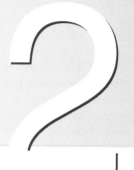

Anatomy of the cardiac chambers

Regardless of the surgical approach, once having entered the mediastinum, the surgeon will be confronted by the heart enclosed in its pericardial sac. Although, in the strict sense, this sac has two layers (fibrous and serous), from a practical point of view it is made up of the tough fibrous pericardium. This fibrous sac encloses the mass of the heart and, by virtue of its own attachments to the diaphragm, helps support the heart within the mediastinum. Free-standing around the atrial chambers and the ventricles, the sac becomes adherent to the adventitial coverings of the great arteries and veins at their entrances to and exits from it, these attachments closing the pericardial cavity. The pericardial cavity itself is contained between the two layers of the serous pericardium, this being a second thin-walled sac folded on itself. The infolding produces a double-layered arrangement, with the outer, or parietal, layer of the serous membrane being densely adherent to the fibrous pericardium. The inner serous, or visceral, layer is firmly attached to the myocardium, and is called the epicardium (Fig. 2.1). The pericardial cavity, therefore, is the space between the inner parietal serous lining of the fibrous pericardium and the surface of the heart (Fig. 2.2). By virtue of the shape of the cardiac chambers and great arteries, there are two recesses within this cavity that are lined by serous pericardium. The first is the transverse sinus, which occupies the inner curvature of the heart (Fig. 2.3). Anteriorly, it is bounded by the posterior surface of the great arteries. Posteriorly,

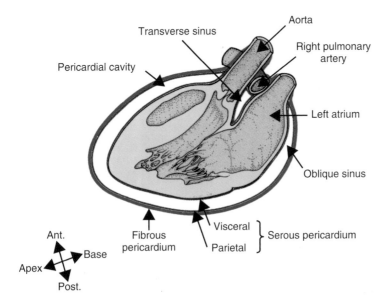

Fig. 2.1 The cartoon shows the arrangement of the pericardial cavity as seen in parasternal long axis view.

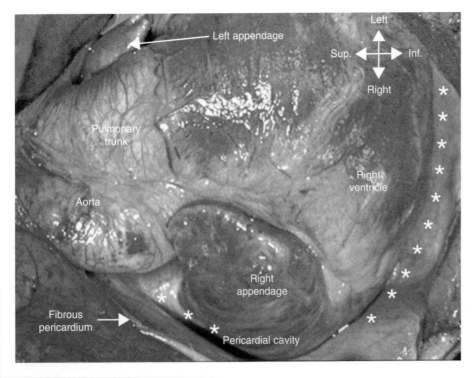

Fig. 2.2 The operative view, through a median sternotomy, shows the anterior surface of the heart following a pericardial incision. The asterisks show the extent of the pericardial cavity.

it is limited by the right pulmonary artery and the roof of the left atrium. There is a recess from the transverse sinus that extends between the superior caval and the right upper pulmonary veins, with its right lateral border being a pericardial fold between these vessels (Fig. 2.4). When exposing the mitral valve through a left atriotomy, incisions through this fold provide good access to the superior aspect of the left atrium and the right pulmonary artery. This fold is also incised when a snare is placed around the superior caval vein. Laterally, on each side, the ends of the transverse sinus are in free communication with the rest of the pericardial cavity. The second pericardial recess is the oblique sinus. This is a blind-ending cavity behind the left atrium, the upper boundary being formed by the reflection of serous pericardium between the upper pulmonary veins at their entrance to the left atrium (Figs. 2.5, 2.6). The right border is the reflection of

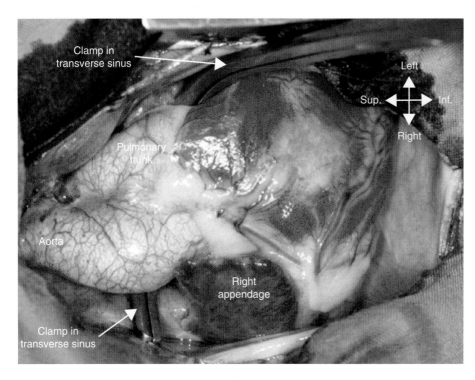

Fig. 2.3 Operative view through a median sternotomy. The clamp has been passed through the transverse sinus.

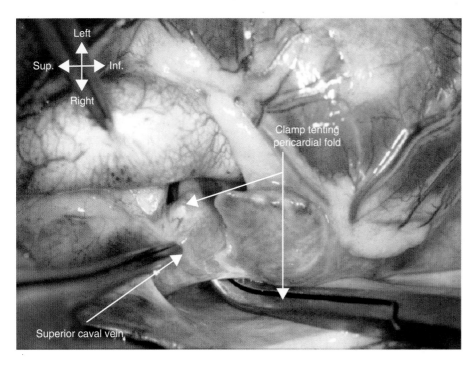

Fig. 2.4 Operative view through a median sternotomy showing the posterior recess of the transverse sinus limited by a pericardial fold around the superior caval vein. In this picture, the fold is being tented by a right-angled clamp passed behind the superior caval vein.

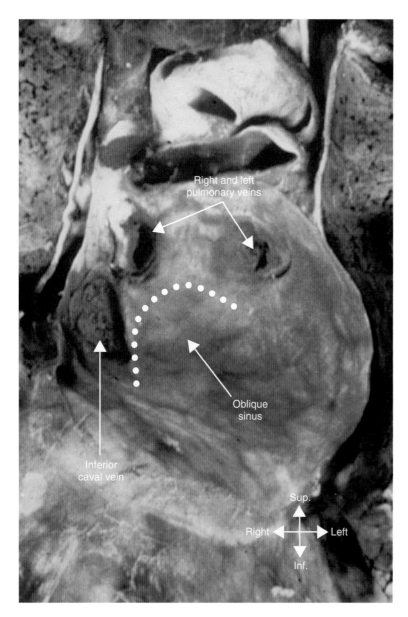

Right and left
pulmonary veins

Oblique
sinus

Inferior
caval vein

Sup.

Right ← → Left

Inf.

Fig. 2.5 Anatomical view showing the oblique sinus of the pericardial cavity (dotted line). The space behind the heart is limited by the attachments of the great veins. The heart has been removed.

pericardium around the right pulmonary veins and the inferior caval vein. To the left is found the reflection of pericardium around the left pulmonary veins.

With the usual surgical approach through a median sternotomy, the fibrous pericardium is opened more-or-less in the midline and retracted laterally, exposing the anterior sternocostal surface of the heart and great vessels. The pulmonary trunk and aorta are then seen leaving the base of the heart and extending in a superior direction, with the aortic root in posterior and rightward position (Fig. 2.2). Should the aortic root not be in this 'normal' relationship, then almost always the ventriculo–arterial connections will be

abnormal (see Chapter 8). The atrial appendages are usually seen one to either side of the prominent arterial pedicle. The morphologically right appendage is more prominent. It has a blunt triangular shape, and possesses a broad junction with the atrial cavity (Fig. 2.7). The morphologically left appendage may not be seen immediately. When found at the left border of the pulmonary trunk, it is seen to be a tubular structure, having a narrow junction with the rest of the atrium (Fig. 2.8). Presence of the two appendages on the same side of the arterial pedicle is an anomaly in itself, called juxtaposition, which is almost always associated with additional

malformations within the heart (see Chapter 8). Inspection of the left border of the heart should always include a search for a persistent left superior caval vein. When present, this venous channel enters the pericardial cavity between the left atrial appendage anteriorly and the left pulmonary veins posteriorly. Within the pericardial cavity, it lies between the left appendage and the left pulmonary artery, running down the posterior aspect of the left atrium to enter the inferior left atrioventricular groove.

The ventricular mass extends from the atrioventricular grooves to the apex. Its axis usually extends into the left hemithorax. An anomalous position of

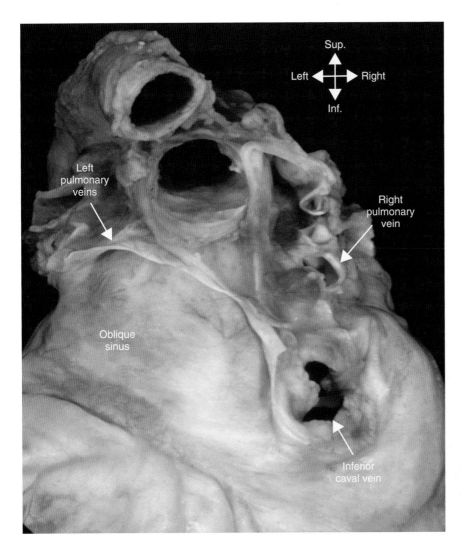

Fig. 2.6 This view of the posterior surface of an excised heart, shown in anatomical orientation, is the reciprocal of the situation shown in Fig. 2.5. The pericardial reflections around the pulmonary and inferior caval veins are seen to bound the oblique sinus of the pericardial cavity.

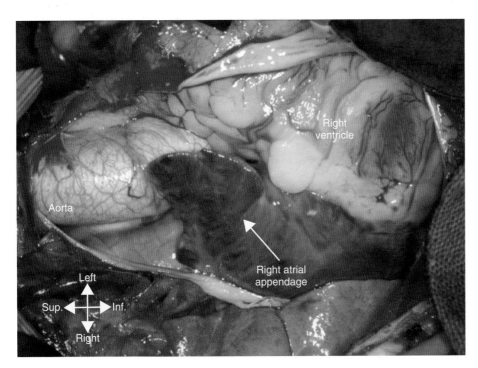

Fig. 2.7 Operative view through a median sternotomy showing the typical triangular shape of the morphologically right atrial appendage.

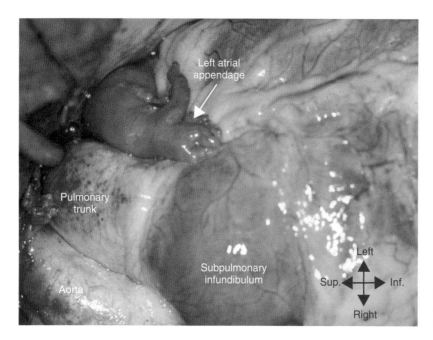

Fig. 2.8 Operative view through a median sternotomy showing the tubular morphologically left atrial appendage.

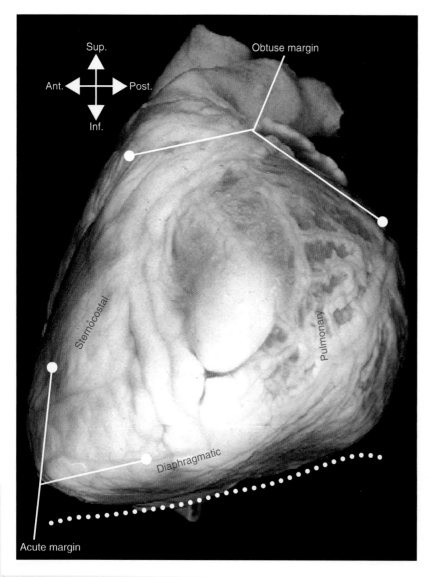

Fig. 2.9 Anatomical view of the surfaces and margins of the heart. The heart has been removed from the chest and is viewed from its apex.

either the ventricular mass or the apex is again highly suggestive of the presence of congenital cardiac malformations (see Chapter 10). In shape, the ventricular mass is a three-sided pyramid, having inferior diaphragmatic, anterior sternocostal, and posterior pulmonary surfaces (Fig. 2.9). The margin between the first two surfaces is sharp, hence its description as the acute margin. The margins between the pulmonary and the sternocostal surfaces anteriorly, and the pulmonary and diaphragmatic surfaces posteriorly, form more obtuse angles. The surgeon encounters these obtuse marginal areas when the apex of the heart is tipped out of the pericardium. The areas are irrigated by the obtuse marginal branches

of the circumflex coronary artery. The greater part of the anterior surface of the ventricular mass is occupied by the morphologically right ventricle. Its left border is marked by the anterior interventricular, or descending, branch of the left coronary artery, which curves onto the ventricular surface between the left atrial appendage and the basal origin of the pulmonary trunk. The right border of the morphologically right ventricle is marked by the right coronary artery, which runs obliquely in the atrioventricular groove. Unusually prominent coronary arteries coursing on the ventricular surface should always raise the suspicion of significant cardiac malformations.

The surface anatomy of the heart is helpful in determining the most appropriate site for an incision to gain access to a given cardiac chamber. For example, the relatively bloodless outlet portion of the right ventricle just beneath the origin of the pulmonary trunk affords ready access to the cavity of the subpulmonary infundibulum (Fig. 2.8). The important landmark for the right atrium is the terminal groove, or sulcus terminalis, marking the junction between the appendage and the systemic venous component of the right atrium (Fig. 2.10). The sinus node is located within this groove, usually laterally within the superior cavoatrial junction (Fig. 2.11), but occasionally extending over the crest

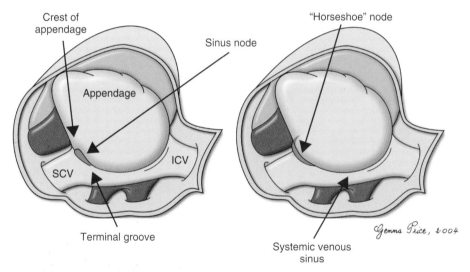

Fig. 2.10 The cartoon shows the usual site of the sinus node within the terminal groove (left hand panel). The right hand panel shows the horseshoe arrangement found in about one-tenth of cases. SCV – superior caval vein; ICV – inferior caval vein.

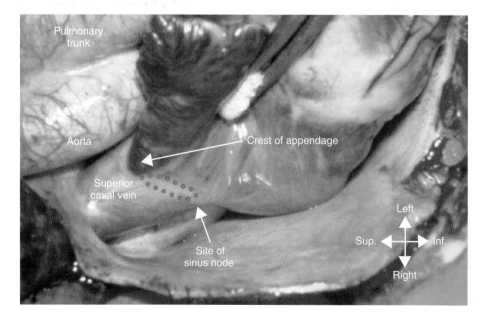

Fig. 2.11 Operative view through a median sternotomy demonstrating the usual site of the sinus node. The node can often be seen as a pale cigar-shaped area located anterolaterally in the terminal groove. This anticipated site is highlighted in the photograph by the green dotted outline.

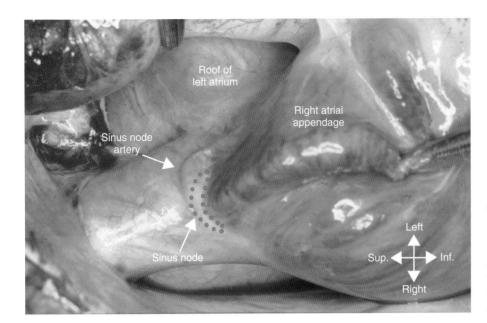

Fig. 2.12 Operative view through a median sternotomy showing a sinus node arranged in horseshoe fashion across the crest of the right atrial appendage, with one limb in the terminal groove and the other extending towards the interatrial groove. The nodal location is again highlighted by the green dots. Note the course of the artery to the node.

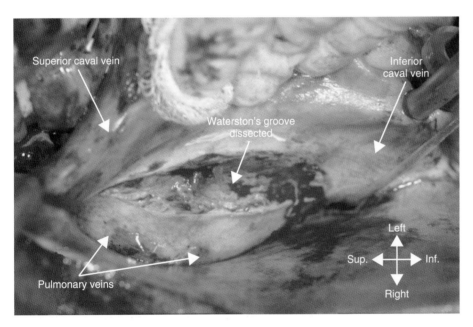

Fig. 2.13 Waterston's groove seen through a median sternotomy. The tissue plane between the atrial chambers has been partially dissected.

of the appendage (Fig. 2.12). The important artery to the sinus node can also be seen on occasion, either as it crosses the crest of the right appendage, or as it courses behind the superior caval vein to enter the terminal groove between the orifices of the caval veins. Posterior to, and parallel with, the terminal groove is a second, deeper, groove between the right atrium and the right pulmonary veins. This interatrial groove, known as Waterston's or Sondergaard's groove, is a guide for surgical incisions into the left atrium (Fig. 2.13). Access can be gained

directly to the left atrium through an incision between this groove and the right pulmonary veins, and also through its roof. The roof of the left atrium is seen behind the aorta to the left of the superior cavoatrial junction (Fig. 2.12).

MORPHOLOGICALLY RIGHT ATRIUM

The right atrium has three basic parts, the appendage, the venous component, receiving the systemic venous return, and the vestibule of the tricuspid valve. It also

has a small body, but the boundaries of this part cannot be distinguished from the venous sinus. It is then separated from the left atrium by the septum. The junction of the appendage and the systemic venous sinus is identified externally by the prominent terminal groove (Fig. 2.10). Internally, the groove corresponds with the terminal crest, which gives origin to the pectinate muscles of the appendage (Fig. 2.14). The morphologically right appendage is an extensive blunt, triangular structure that has a wide junction with the venous sinus across the terminal groove.

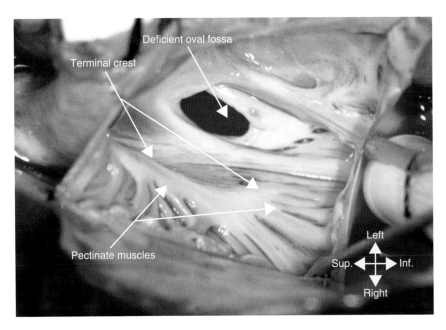

Fig. 2.14 Operative view through a median sternotomy having opened the right atrium. The terminal crest is seen giving rise to the pectinate muscles of the right atrial appendage. Note that, in this patient, the floor of the oval fossa is deficient, producing an atrial septal defect.

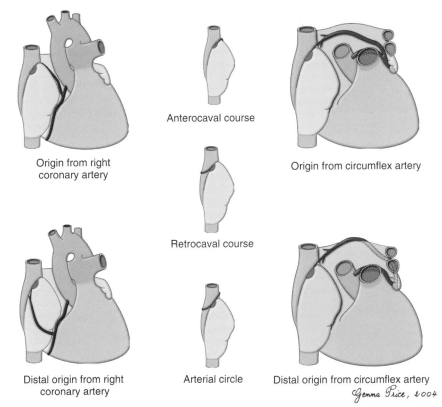

Fig. 2.15 The cartoon, drawn in anatomical orientation, shows the variations in the origin of the artery to the sinus node, and the variability relative to the cavoatrial junction. The left hand panels show the usual arrangement with origin from the right coronary artery, found in 55% of the population, with the rare variant of distal origin with coursing across the appendage (lower left hand panel). The right hand panels show proximal origin from the circumflex artery, found in around 45% of the population, with the rare variant of distal origin with coursing across the dome of the left atrium. The middle panels show the variation relative to the superior cavoatrial junction. The sinus node is shown in green.

The venous sinus is much smaller when viewed externally, with only that part extending between the terminal and Waterston's grooves being visible to the surgeon. It receives the superior and inferior caval veins at its extremities. Superiorly and anteriorly, the appendage has a particularly important relation with the superior caval vein. Here, the appendage terminates in a prominent crest (Fig. 2.11). This forms the summit of the terminal groove, and is continuous in the transverse sinus behind the aorta with the interatrial groove (Fig. 2.12). Absence of such a right-sided crest should alert the surgeon to the presence of isomerism of the left atrial appendages (see Chapter 6). As discussed, almost always the sinus node lies within the terminal groove in an immediately subepicardial position. It is a spindle-shaped structure that usually lies to the right of the crest, that is, lateral to the superior cavoatrial junction (Fig. 2.11). In about one-tenth of cases, nonetheless, the node extends across the crest into the interatrial groove, draping itself across the cavoatrial junction in horseshoe fashion[1] (Fig. 2.12).

Also of significance is the course of the artery to the sinus node (Fig. 2.15). This artery is a branch of the right coronary artery in about 55 percent of individuals, and a branch of the circumflex artery in the remainder[2]. Irrespective of its origin, it usually courses through the anterior interatrial groove towards the superior cavoatrial junction (Fig. 2.16), frequently running within the atrial myocardium.

The artery usually takes its origin from the proximal segment of its parent coronary artery (Fig. 2.17). A significant variant is found, however, when the artery

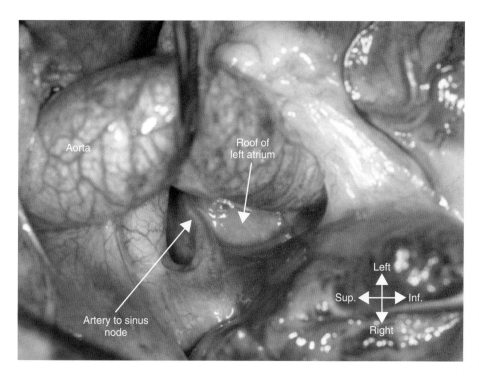

Fig. 2.16 Operative view through a median sternotomy showing the artery to the sinus node, which in this case originates from the circumflex coronary artery and extends across the dome of the left atrium.

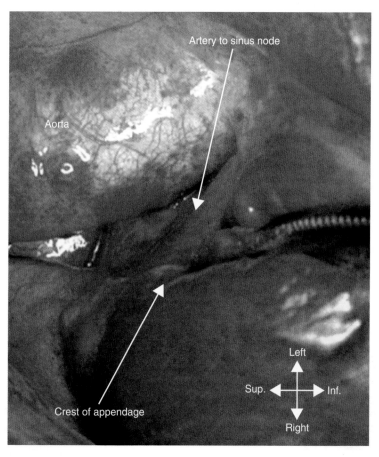

Fig. 2.17 Operative view through a median sternotomy showing the artery to the sinus node originating proximally from the right coronary artery.

originates from either coronary artery some distance from the aorta. Then, if taking origin from the right coronary artery, it courses over the lateral surface of the appendage to reach the terminal groove (Fig. 2.18). If originating from the circumflex artery, it crosses the roof of the left atrium (Fig. 2.19). Such lateral origin is rare in normal hearts[3,4], but more frequent in association with congenital malformations[5]. Irrespective of its origin, as it enters the sinus node, the artery

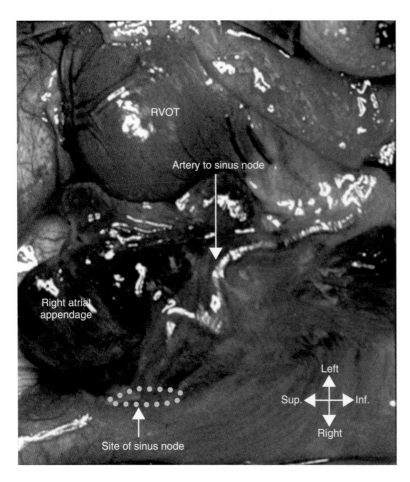

Fig. 2.18 Operative view through a median sternotomy showing the artery to the sinus node originating distally from the right coronary artery and coursing over the lateral surface of the right atrial appendage. The site of the sinus node is shown by the green dots.

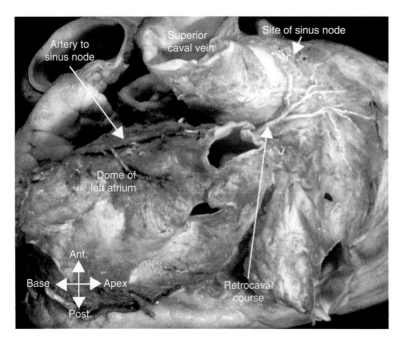

Fig. 2.19 In this specimen, seen in anatomic orientation, the artery to the sinus node originates laterally from the circumflex coronary artery and courses over the dome of the left atrium. The site of the sinus node is shown by the white cross-hatched area.

may cross the crest of the appendage, course retrocavally (Fig. 2.20), or even divide to form an arterial circle round the junction (Fig. 2.21). All these variations should be taken into account when planning the safest right atrial incision, particularly when the nodal artery crosses the lateral margin of the right appendage, or courses over the roof of the left atrium.

Opening the atrium through the most appropriate incision shows that the terminal groove is the external marking of a prominent muscle bundle, the terminal crest. This separates the pectinate muscles of the appendage from the smooth walls of the systemic venous sinus (Fig. 2.14). Anteriorly, the crest curves in front of the orifice of the superior caval vein, with its medial extension forming the border between the appendage and the superior rim of the oval fossa. On first sight, when inspecting the right atrium through this incision, there appears to be an extensive septal surface between the openings of the caval veins and the orifice of the tricuspid valve (Fig. 2.22). The apparent extent of this septum is spurious[6,7]. Opening into, and from, this 'septal' surface are the oval fossa and the orifice of the coronary sinus. The true septum between the right and left atrial chambers[7,8] is confined to the floor and the anteroinferior margin of the oval fossa, as shown by the dissections in Figures 2.23 and 2.24. The extensive superior rim of the fossa is produced by folding of the interatrial groove between the mouth of the superior caval vein and the entrance of the pulmonary veins to

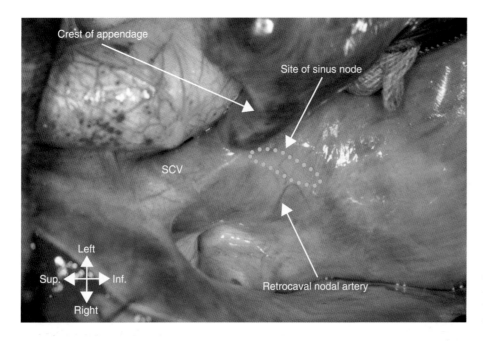

Fig. 2.20 Operative view through a median sternotomy showing a retrocaval course of the artery to the sinus node, the site of the node itself being emphasised by the green dots.

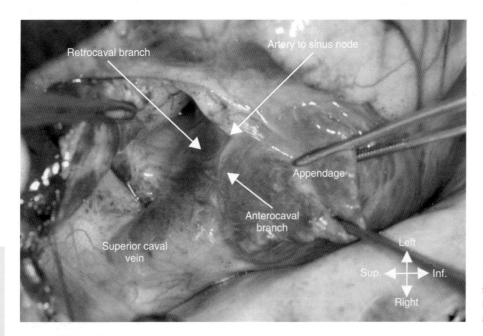

Fig. 2.21 Operative view through a median sternotomy showing the artery to the sinus node dividing to form an arterial circle around the cavoatrial junction.

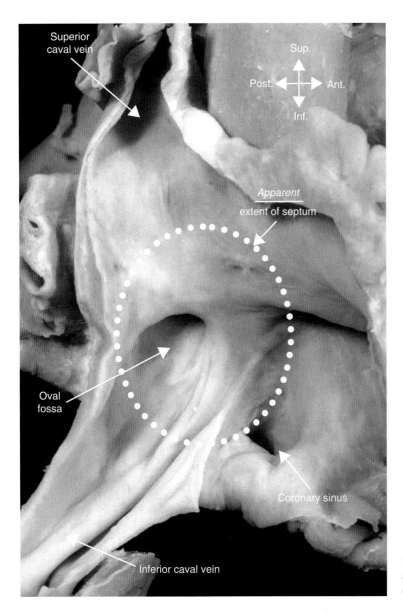

Superior
caval vein

Sup.

Post. ←→ Ant.

Inf.

Apparent
extent of septum

Oval
fossa

Coronary sinus

Inferior caval vein

Fig. 2.22 In this specimen, viewed in anatomical, the white dotted circle shows the apparently extensive 'septal surface' within the right atrium.

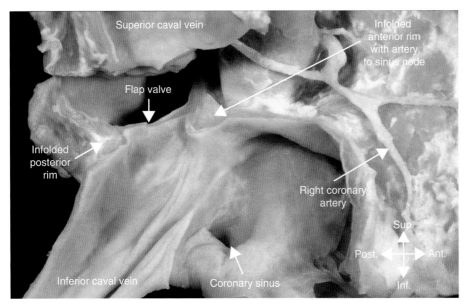

Superior caval vein

Infolded
anterior rim
with artery
to sinus node

Flap valve

Infolded
posterior
rim

Right coronary
artery

Sup.

Post. ←→ Ant.

Inf.

Inferior caval vein

Coronary sinus

Fig. 2.23 The same specimen as seen in Fig. 2.22 has been transected through the oval fossa. The section shows that the rims of the oval fossa are infoldings of the atrial walls. Note the relationship of the anterior fold to the aortic root, the right coronary artery, and the artery to the sinus node.

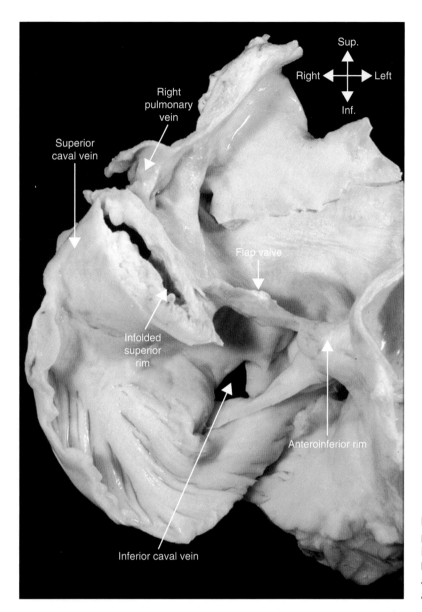

Sup.

Right ←→ Left

Inf.

Right pulmonary vein

Superior caval vein

Flap valve

Infolded superior rim

Anteroinferior rim

Inferior caval vein

Fig. 2.24 This heart has been sectioned in four chamber plane, confirming that the superior rim of the oval fossa is a deep infolding producing the interatrial groove between the systemic venous sinus of the right atrium and the entry of the pulmonary veins into the left atrium.

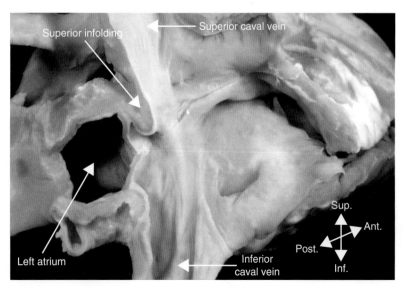

Superior infolding

Superior caval vein

Left atrium

Inferior caval vein

Sup.

Ant.

Post.

Inf.

Fig. 2.25 The heart shown in Figs. 2.22 & 2.23 has been sectioned in the long axis of the venous sinus, again showing that the superior rim of the oval fossa is an infolding of the interatrial groove. The heart is viewed in anatomical orientation from the back.

the left atrium (Figs. 2.24, 2.25). The posteroinferior rim of the oval fossa is another important muscular fold formed by reflection of the musculatures forming the mouth of the coronary sinus and the orifice of the inferior caval vein (Fig. 2.22). The fold continues anteriorly as the so-called Eustachian ridge. This is seen to advantage when the floor of the oval fossa is itself deficient (Fig. 2.26). The limited septal extent of the oval fossa is of major surgical importance, since it is an easy

matter to pass outside the heart when attempting to gain access to the left atrium through a right atrial approach.

In addition to the position of the sinus node, and the extent of the atrial septum, the other major area of surgical significance within the right atrium is the site of the atrioventricular node. This is contained within the triangle of Koch. This important landmark is bounded by the tendon of Todaro, the attachment of the septal leaflet of the tricuspid valve,

and the orifice of the coronary sinus (Fig. 2.27). The tendon of Todaro[9] is a fibrous structure formed by the junction of the Eustachian valve, the valve of the inferior caval vein, and the Thebesian valve, the valve of the coronary sinus. The fibrous continuation of these two valvar structures buries itself in the anterior continuation of the Eustachian ridge, this being the musculature between the coronary sinus and the inferior caval vein. It then runs medially as the tendon of Todaro to insert

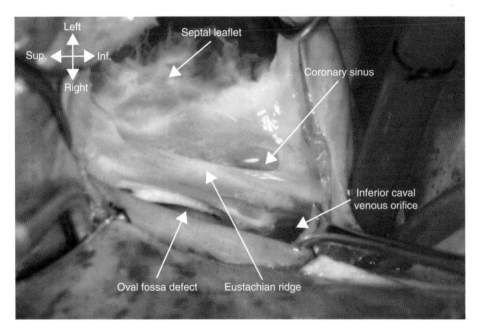

Fig. 2.26 The heart has been opened through an atriotomy, and the interior surface of the right atrium is shown in surgical orientation. Note the Eustachian ridge separating the mouth of the coronary sinus from the orifice of the inferior caval vein. The floor of the oval fossa is deficient, producing an atrial septal defect.

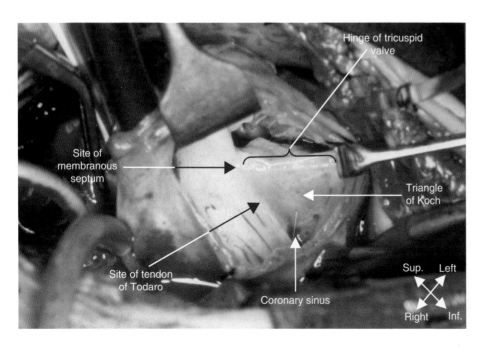

Fig. 2.27 This operative view through a right atriotomy shows the location of the triangle of Koch.

into the atrioventricular part of the membranous septum (Fig. 2.28). The entire atrial component of the axis of atrioventricular conduction tissues is contained within the confines of the triangle of Koch[10]. If, in hearts with normal segmental connections, this area is scrupulously avoided during surgical procedures, the atrioventricular conduction tissues will not be damaged. Should the node need to be precisely identified, it should be remembered that the attachment of the tricuspid valve is some way down the surface of the septum relative to that of the mitral valve (Fig. 2.29). The relationship between the atrial and ventricular muscular walls within the triangle of Koch is complex. At first sight, because of the off-setting of the attachments of the mitral and tricuspid valves, the entire muscular area seems to

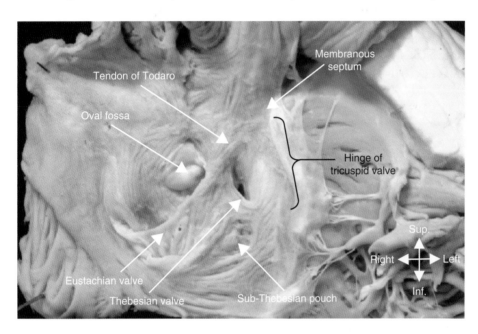

Fig. 2.28 The endocardium has been removed from this heart, viewed in anatomical orientation, to demonstrate the boundaries of the triangle of Koch. Note the non-uniform anisotropic arrangement of the myocardial fibres.

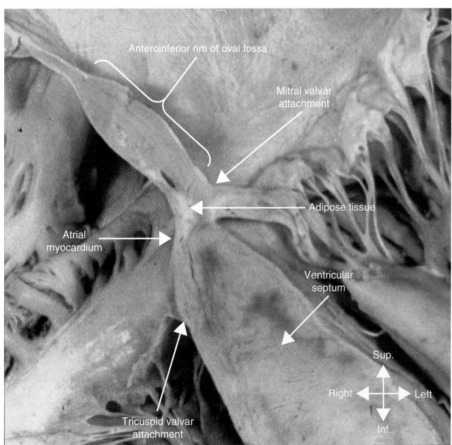

Fig. 2.29 This four-chamber section of a normal heart, shown in anatomical orientation, illustrates the differential attachments of the atrioventricular valves. Note the adipose tissue interposing between the right atrial wall and the crest of the ventricular septum.

interpose between the cavities of the right atrium and the left ventricle. Indeed, in the previous editions of the book, we described this area as the "atrioventricular muscular septum". It remains the case that, in the section illustrated in Fig. 2.29, part of the muscular septum is an atrioventricular septum. This is because the atrial musculature does not extend into the vestibule as far as the hinge of the tricuspid valve, so that the musculature interposed between the cavities of the right atrium and left ventricle is now itself an atrioventricular septum. In that area of the triangle containing atrial myocardium, however, the atrial musculature is separated from the underlying ventricular

myocardium by an extension of the inferior atrioventricular groove, the fibrofatty tissue insulating the atrial from the ventricular muscular layers[10]. The extent of this insulating layer can be demonstrated by dissecting away the superficial atrial musculature, revealing at the same time the location of the artery supplying the atrioventricular node (Fig. 2.30). In reality, therefore, the larger part of Koch's triangle as seen by the surgeon is formed by the atrial layer of an atrioventricular muscular sandwich, rather than a true muscular atrioventricular septum.

Much was written in the latter part of the twentieth century concerning the role

of 'specialised' pathways of myocardium in conduction of the sinus impulse to the atrioventricular node[11,12]. Indeed, some suggested that surgical operations should be specially modified to avoid these presumed tracts[13]. The paradigm of tracts of myocardium modified for conduction in the heart, however, is the ventricular conduction system[14]. There are no such insulated and isolated tracts of specialised atrial myocardium extending between the nodes in the right atrium that can be avoided in the way that it is possible, indeed essential, to avoid the penetrating and branching atrioventricular bundles[15,16]. The major muscle bundles of the atrial chambers certainly serve as

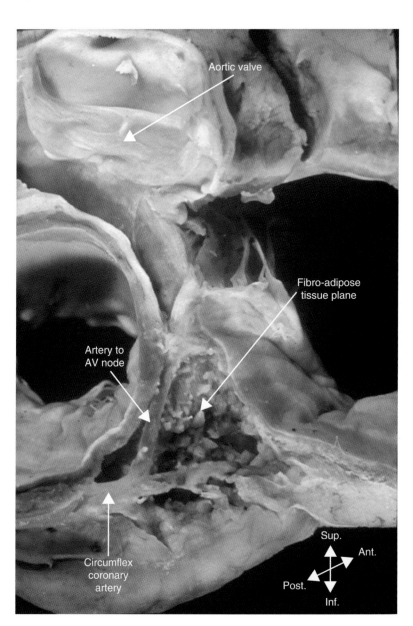

Fig. 2.30 This dissection, in anatomic orientation having removed the non-coronary sinus of the aortic valve, shows the fibrofatty tissue interposed between the atrial and ventricular muscular layers of the atrioventricular muscular sandwich. Note the artery to the atrioventricular node.

preferential pathways of conduction, but the course of these preferential pathways is dictated by the overall geometry of the chambers (Fig. 2.31). Ideally, prominent muscle bundles, such as the terminal crest, the superior rim of the oval fossa, or the myocardium of the Eustachian ridge, should be preserved during atrial surgery. But, even if they cannot be preserved, the surgeon can rest assured that internodal conduction will continue as long as some strand of atrial myocardium connects the nodes, providing that the arterial supply to the nodes, or the nodes themselves, are not traumatised. The key to avoiding postoperative atrial arrhythmias, therefore, is the fastidious preservation of the sinus and atrioventricular nodes and their arteries, rather than concern about non-existent insulated tracts of 'specialised atrial myocardium'.

The central fibrous body touches on three of the four cardiac chambers, but it is in the right atrium that it becomes first and, perhaps most clearly, evident to the surgeon (Fig. 2.32). Rather than being considered as a specific body, it is better

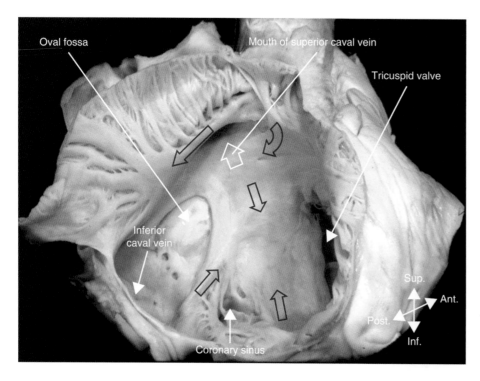

Fig. 2.31 The right atrium, seen in anatomical orientation, has been opened through a window in the appendage. The muscular walls surround several orifices, producing preferential routes of conduction (arrows).

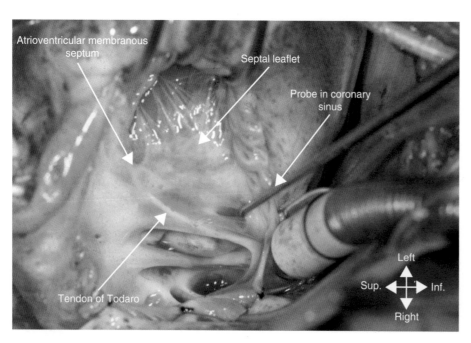

Fig. 2.32 Operative view through a right atriotomy, showing the tendon of Todaro inserting into the atrioventricular component of the membranous septum, which forms the right margin of the central fibrous body.

conceptualised as an area within the heart where the membranous septum, the atrioventricular valves, and the aortic valve join in fibrous continuity. It is best seen from the left side (Fig. 2.33). This view shows how the rightward margin of the area of continuity between the leaflets of the aortic and mitral valves, the right fibrous trigone, joins with the membranous septum to form the basis of the fibrous body (Fig. 2.34). This view also emphasises its intimate relationship to many important structures within the heart, particularly the fibrous triangle between the hinges of the right and non-coronary leaflets of the aortic valve. The central fibrous body, therefore, acts as an anatomical focal point for the cardiac surgeon. Operations involving valvar replacement or repair, closure of septal defects, and/or control of arrhythmias, all require the surgeon to understand implicitly its anatomical relationships from both the obvious right (Fig. 2.32) but usually invisible left (Fig. 2.34) sides.

The vestibule to the right ventricle, surrounding the orifice of the tricuspid valve, is contiguous with both the systemic venous component and the appendage of the right atrium. The anterior junction of

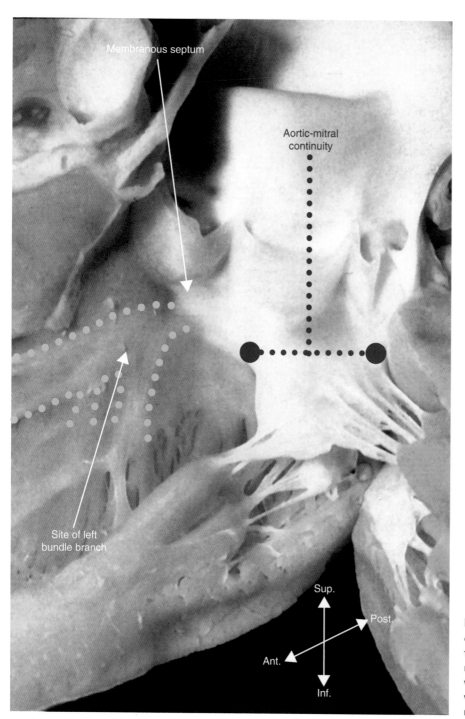

Membranous septum

Aortic-mitral continuity

Site of left bundle branch

Sup.

Post.

Ant.

Inf.

Fig. 2.33 This specimen, viewed in anatomic orientation, is opened to show the origin of the aorta from the left ventricle, with the membranous septum in fibrous continuity with the leaflets of the aortic and mitral valves. Note the site of the left bundle branch, marked by the green dots.

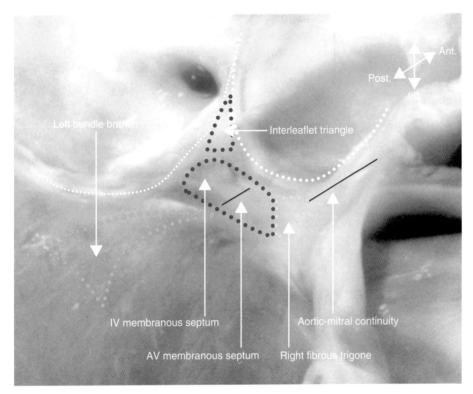

Fig. 2.34 This close-up, in anatomic orientation, shows the relationships between the membranous septum and the aortic valve having removed the leaflets of the valve itself. The red dotted area shows the membranous septum, in continuity superiorly with the interleaflet triangle between the right and non-coronary leaflets of the aortic valve, shown by the blue dots. The yellow dots show the thickened right end of the fibrous continuity between the leaflets of the aortic and mitral valve, known as the right fibrous trigone. The location of the left bundle branch is again shown by the green dots.

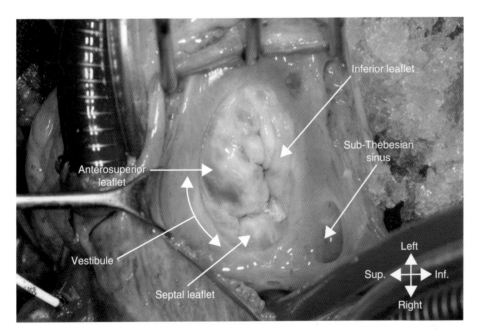

Fig. 2.35 This operative view through a right atriotomy, seen in surgical orientation, shows the vestibule of the atrium and the three leaflets of the tricuspid valve.

these two parts of the atrium overlies the peripheral attachment of the anteroseptal commissure of the tricuspid valve and the supraventricular crest of the right ventricle (Fig. 2.35). The posterior junction is at the orifice of the coronary sinus, where there is usually an extensive trabeculated diverticulum found inferior to the sinus. Although usually called the post-Eustachian sinus, it is sub–Thebesian when the heart is viewed in surgical position (Fig. 2.28).

MORPHOLOGICALLY LEFT ATRIUM

As with the right atrium, the left atrium possesses an appendage, an extensive venous component, and a vestibule. Unlike the right atrium, however, it is also possible to recognise the extensive body of the left atrium (Fig. 2.36). And the chamber is, of course, separated from its neighbour by the septum. Only the appendage of the atrium may be immediately evident to a surgeon on exposing the heart. The body of the

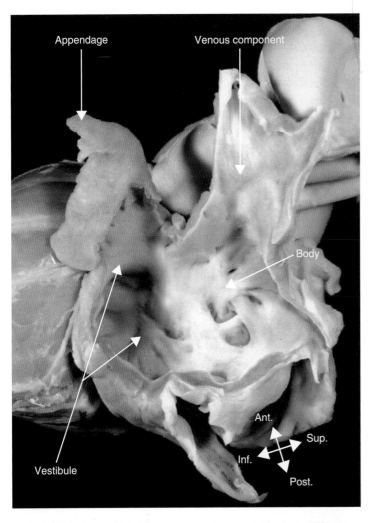

Fig. 2.36 In this heart, shown in anatomic orientation the left atrium is opened to show its components. Note the extensive body.

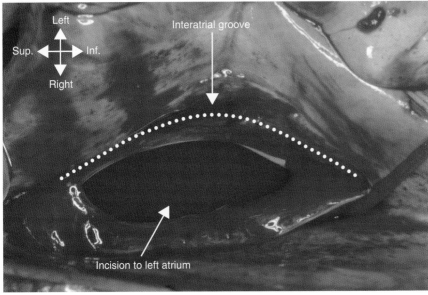

Fig. 2.37 This operative view, through a median sternotomy, shows how an incision through the bottom of Waterston's groove (white dotted line) takes the surgeon into the left atrium.

atrium is confluent with the venous component, and the narrow junction between this part and the appendage is unmarked by either a terminal groove or crest (Fig. 2.36). Because of its posterior position, and its firm anchorage by the four pulmonary veins, direct access to the left atrium can be difficult, so the surgeon must use his knowledge of anatomy to gain best exposure of the cavity. Probably the most popular route is an incision made just posterior to the right lateral aspect of the interatrial groove (Fig. 2.37). As has been described above, this extensive infolding between the right pulmonary veins and the venous sinus of the right atrium produces the superior rim of the oval fossa (Fig. 2.24). A posteriorly directed incision along this groove takes the surgeon directly into the left atrium. If necessary, the incision can be extended to the superior aspect of the left atrium by incising the pericardial fold between the superior caval vein and the right pulmonary artery (Fig. 2.4). Because the infolding of the interatrial groove also forms the superior border of the oval fossa, much the same access can be gained by approaching through the right atrium, and incising just superiorly within the fossa. It must then be remembered that an extensive incision may take the surgeon out of the confines of the atrial chambers and into the pericardial space. Perhaps more importantly, it should be noted that such an incision may damage the artery to the sinus node, either in the interatrial groove or on the roof of the left atrium. A further approach to the left atrium is the so-called superior approach, incising directly through the roof. If the aorta is pulled anteriorly and to the left, it can be shown that there is an extensive trough between the two atrial appendages (Fig. 2.38). An incision through the floor of this trough enters the roof of the left atrium. When making such an incision to enter the left atrium, it must be remembered that the artery to the sinus node may be coursing through this area when it takes origin from the circumflex artery (Fig. 2.38). In some instances, this artery may pass through the infolding of the interatrial groove to reach the terminal groove.

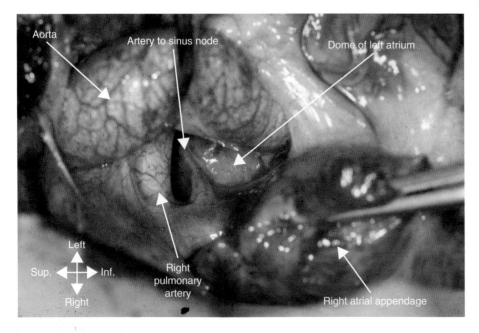

Fig. 2.38 This operative view through a median sternotomy shows how retraction of the aorta to the left reveals the deep trough inferior to the right pulmonary artery and between the atrial appendages. Note that, in this heart, the artery to the sinus node courses through this trough.

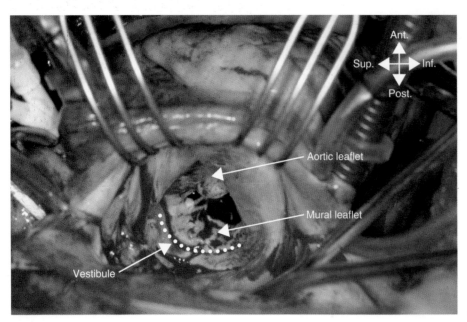

Fig. 2.39 On gaining access through a right-sided left atriotomy, the vestibule of the mitral orifice (dotted line) dominates the surgical picture. Note the leaflets of the mitral valve.

Once access is gained to the left atrium, the small size of the opening of the appendage is apparent, lying to the left of the mitral orifice as viewed by the surgeon. The greater part of the pulmonary venous sinus, confluent with the smooth-walled atrial body, will usually be located inferiorly, away from the operative field. It is the vestibule of the mitral orifice which dominates the picture (Fig. 2.39). The septal aspect will be anterior, exhibiting the typically roughened flap-valve aspect of its left side. The large sweep of tissue between the flap-valve of the septum and the opening of the appendage is the internal aspect of the deep anterior interatrial groove.

MORPHOLOGICALLY RIGHT VENTRICLE

The musculature of the right ventricle extends from the atrioventricular to the ventriculo-arterial junctions. Understanding of ventricular morphology in general is greatly aided by considering the ventricles in terms of three components[17], rather than the traditional 'sinus' and 'conus' parts. The three portions are the inlet, apical trabecular, and outlet parts, respectively (Fig. 2.40). The inlet portion of the right ventricle

contains, and is limited by, the tricuspid valve and its tension apparatus. Although not always easy, it is generally possible to distinguish three leaflets in the valvar orifice. They lie in anterosuperior, septal, and inferior or mural locations. When seen in closed position (Fig. 2.35), their boundaries are clearly marked by their zones of apposition, which extend to the centre of the valvar orifice. It is the apexes of these zones that are usually called the commissures, although in reality the entirety of the zones of apposition should, logically, be defined as the commissures. The peripheral ends of the zones of apposition are usually tethered by fan-shaped cords arising atop the prominent papillary muscles of the valve. The details of this valvar and commissural anatomy are discussed in the next chapter.

The most constant distinguishing morphological feature of the tricuspid valve is the direct attachments to the septum of the cords tethering its septal leaflet (Figs. 2.40, 2.41). The trabecular component of the right ventricle extends to the apex, where its wall is particularly thin, and is especially vulnerable to perforation by cardiac catheters and pacemaker electrodes. The apical trabeculations are uniformly coarse. The outlet component of the right ventricle is a complete muscular structure, the

infundibulum, which extends from the ventricular base as a muscular sleeve that supports the leaflets of the pulmonary valve. These leaflets are attached to the infundibular musculature in semilunar fashion, their hinges crossing the circular anatomic ventriculo-arterial junction to incorporate triangles of arterial wall within the ventricle, and crescents of ventricular muscle in the bases of the pulmonary valvar sinuses (Fig. 2.42). Another distinguishing morphological feature of the right ventricle is the prominent muscular shelf that interposes between the tricuspid and pulmonary valvar orifices, the supraventricular crest. Although at first sight (Fig. 2.43) it has the appearance of a large muscle bundle, much of the crest is no more than the infolded inner heart curve (Fig. 2.44). Incisions, or deep sutures, through this part run into the transverse sinus and right atrioventricular groove, and can jeopardise the right coronary artery[18]. Only a small part of the most medial part of the crest can be removed as a true septal structure, creating a hole between the subpulmonary and subaortic outflow tracts (Fig. 2.45). The distal part of the infundibulum is a free-standing muscular sleeve (Fig. 2.46). It is the presence of this sleeve which permits the valve itself to be removed as an autograft for use in the

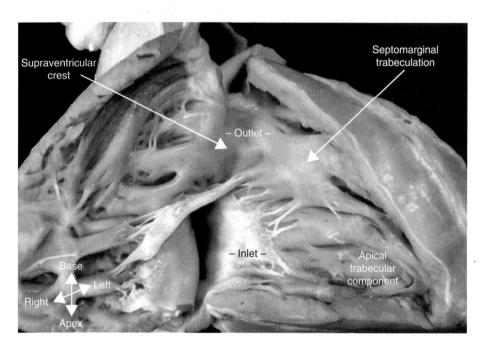

Fig. 2.40 This specimen, viewed in anatomical orientation, shows the three components of the morphologically right ventricle.

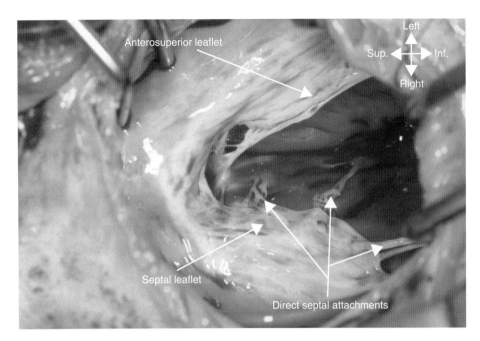

Anterosuperior leaflet

Left
Sup. ← → Inf.
Right

Septal leaflet

Direct septal attachments

Fig. 2.41 Operative view through a right atriotomy showing the direct cordal attachments to the septum of the septal leaflet of the tricuspid valve.

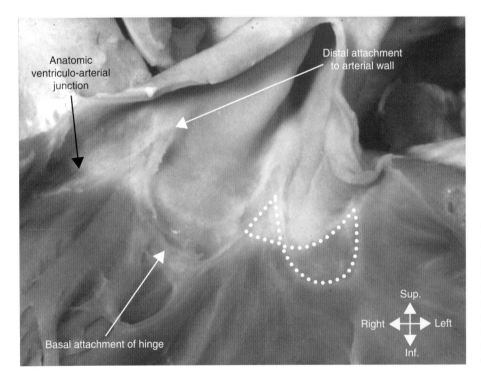

Anatomic ventriculo-arterial junction

Distal attachment to arterial wall

Sup.
Right ← → Left
Inf.

Basal attachment of hinge

Fig. 2.42 In this heart, shown in anatomical orientation, the leaflets of the pulmonary valve have been removed. Note how the semilunar attachment of the pulmonary valvar leaflets crosses the anatomic ventriculo-arterial junction, the dotted lines emphasising the crescents of ventricular muscle incorporated in the valvar sinus and the triangles of arterial wall within the ventricle.

Ross procedure (Fig. 2.47). Taken as a whole, the supraventricular crest inserts between the limbs of a prominent and important right ventricular septal trabeculation. This structure, which we term the septomarginal trabeculation, has anterosuperior and posteroinferior limbs that clasp the crest (Fig. 2.44). The anterosuperior limb runs up to the attachment of the leaflets of the pulmonary valve, overlying the outlet part of the muscular ventricular septum, while the posteroinferior limb extends backwards inferior to the interventricular component of the membranous septum, again reinforcing the muscular septum. The medial papillary muscle (Fig. 2.43) usually arises from this posteroinferior limb. The body of the septomarginal trabeculation itself runs to the apex of the ventricle, breaking up into a sheath of smaller trabeculations. Some of these mingle into the apical trabecular portion, and some support tension apparatus of the tricuspid valve. Several of these smaller trabeculations are often particularly prominent. One becomes the anterior

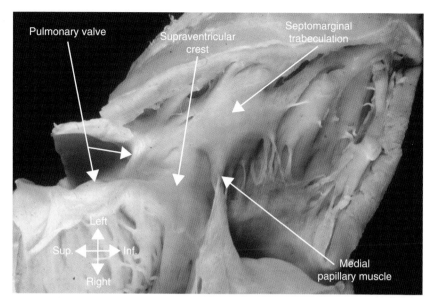

Pulmonary valve
Supraventricular crest
Septomarginal trabeculation

Left
Sup. — Inf.
Right

Medial papillary muscle

Fig. 2.43 In this anatomic specimen, viewed in surgical orientation, the prominent muscular supraventricular crest is seen between the leaflets of the tricuspid and pulmonary valves. Note the medial papillary muscle arising from the septomarginal trabeculation.

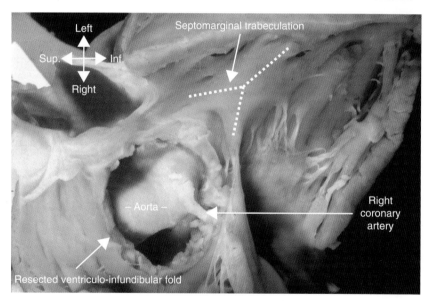

Left
Sup. — Inf.
Right

Septomarginal trabeculation

Right coronary artery

– Aorta –

Resected ventriculo-infundibular fold

Fig. 2.44 Dissection of the specimen shown in Fig. 2.43 shows that most of the supraventricular crest is the inner curvature of the heart, or the ventriculo-infundibular fold. Note the location of the right coronary artery. The white dotted lines show the limbs and body of the septomarginal trabeculation (septal band).

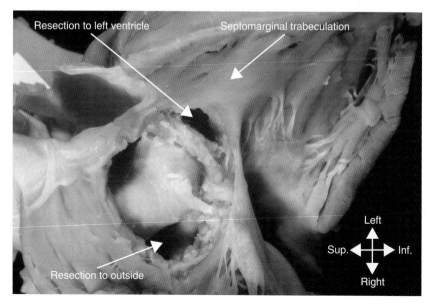

Resection to left ventricle
Septomarginal trabeculation

Left
Sup. — Inf.
Right

Resection to outside

Fig. 2.45 Further dissection of the specimen shown in Fig. 2.44 reveals that a small part of the muscle of the supraventricular crest inserting between the limbs of the septomarginal trabeculation can be removed as a true septal structure.

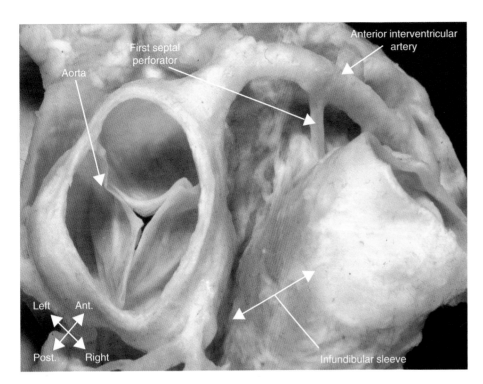

Fig. 2.46 In this heart, viewed from above and from the right, the space between the aorta and the pulmonary trunk has been cleaned. Turning the pulmonary trunk forward reveals the free-standing muscular infundibular sleeve. Note the location of the anterior interventricular artery and its first septal perforating branch.

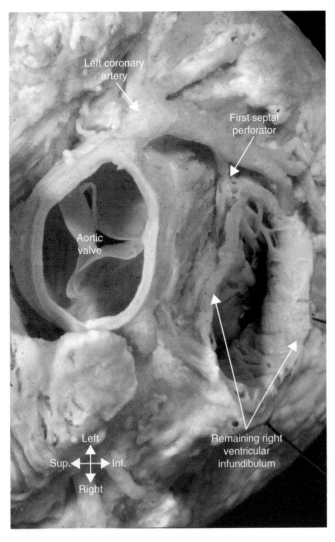

Fig. 2.47 In this heart, again viewed from above and from the right, the pulmonary infundibulum has been removed from the base of the heart, revealing the free-standing myocardial sleeve that 'lifts' the valvar leaflets away from the left ventricle. Note the site of the first septal perforating artery.

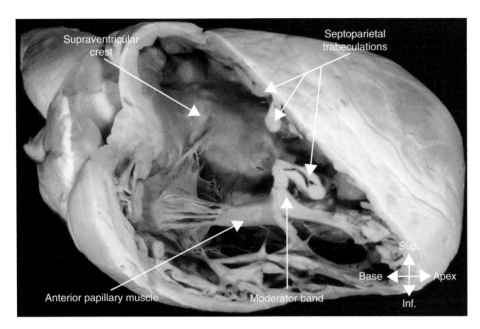

Fig. 2.48 The right ventricle has been opened from the front, with the heart orientated anatomically, to show the septoparietal trabeculations and the moderator band.

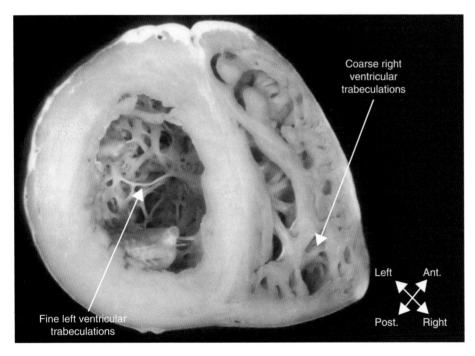

Fig. 2.49 The apical component of the ventricular mass has been transected, and is photographed from above to show the different patterns of the apical trabeculations of the two ventricles.

papillary muscle, while another extends from the septomarginal trabeculation to the papillary muscle, being termed the moderator band (Fig. 2.48). Additional significant right ventricular trabeculations are usually found arising from the anterior margin of the septomarginal trabeculation. Variable in number, these are the septoparietal trabeculations (Fig. 2.48).

The uniformly coarse apical trabeculations serve as the most constant anatomic feature of the morphologically right ventricle. In the normal heart,

there are a number of morphological differences between the two ventricles, including the arrangement of the leaflets of the atrioventricular valves and their tension apparatus, ventricular shape, the thickness of the ventricular walls, and the configuration of the outflow tracts. These features, however, can be altered or lacking in the congenitally abnormal heart. In final arbitration of ventricular morphology, therefore, the morphologist relies on the contrast between the coarse trabeculations of the right ventricle and

the much finer trabeculations seen in the apical part of the left ventricle (Fig. 2.49).

MORPHOLOGICALLY LEFT VENTRICLE

As with the right ventricle, the musculature of the left ventricle extends from the atrioventricular to the ventriculo-arterial junctions. It is again conveniently considered in terms of inlet, apical trabecular, and outlet components (Fig. 2.50). In the left ventricle, however, the inlet and outlet components overlap considerably. The inlet component surrounds, and is limited by, the mitral valve and its tension apparatus. Its two leaflets, supported by two prominent papillary muscles and their tendinous cords, have widely differing appearances (Fig. 2.51). The anterosuperior leaflet is short, squat and relatively square. This leaflet, in fibrous continuity with the aortic valve, is better termed the aortic leaflet. The other leaflet is narrower, and its junctional attachment more extensive, being supported by the parietal part of the left atrioventricular junction. Positioned posteroinferiorly, it is accurately termed the mural leaflet. Because the aortic leaflet

of the mitral valve forms part of the outlet of the left ventricle, the distinction of inlet and outlet is somewhat blurred. The papillary muscles of the valve, although basically located in anteroinferior and posterosuperior positions, are close to each other at their origin (Fig. 2.52). Unlike the tricuspid valve, the leaflets of the mitral valve have no direct septal attachments, since the deep posteroinferior diverticulum of the subaortic outflow tract displaces the aortic leaflet of the valve away from the muscular ventricular septum (Fig. 2.53). The trabecular component of the left ventricle extends to the ventricular apex and has characteristically fine

trabeculations (Fig. 2.49). As in the right ventricle, the myocardium is surprisingly thin at the apex. This feature is important to the cardiac surgeon, who has reason to place catheters and electrodes in the right ventricle, or drainage tubes in the left side. Immediate perforation, or delayed rupture, may occur. This may be a particular problem should catheters stiffened by hypothermia be pushed against the apical endocardium as the heart is manipulated during surgery on the coronary arteries[19]. The outlet component of the left ventricle supports the aortic valve. Unlike its right ventricular counterpart, it is not a

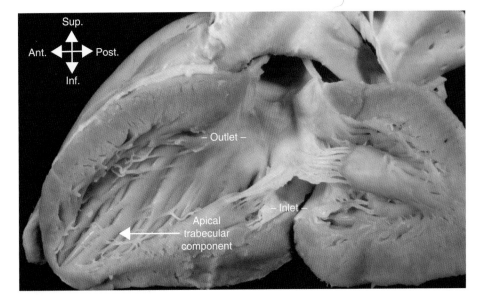

Fig. 2.50 In this specimen, viewed from the front in anatomic orientation, the morphologically left ventricle is opened in clam fashion to show its three components.

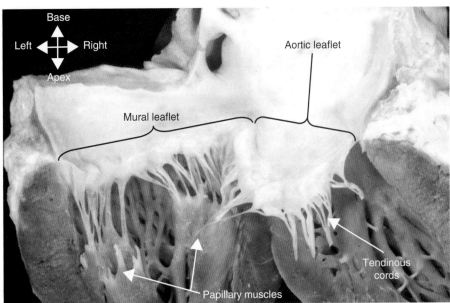

Fig. 2.51 This specimen, viewed from behind, and opened through a cut in the left atrioventricular junction adjacent to the septum, demonstrates the marked differences in the arrangement of the aortic and mural leaflets of the mitral valve.

complete muscular structure. The septal wall is largely composed of muscle, but in this area is found the membranous septum, forming part of the central fibrous body in the subaortic outflow tract (Fig. 2.34). The posterolateral portion of the outflow tract is composed exclusively by fibrous tissue, namely the fibrous curtain joining the leaflets of the aortic valve to the aortic leaflet of the mitral valve. The left lateral quadrant, continuing around to the septum, is a muscular structure representing the lateral margin of the inner heart curvature, separating the cavity of the left ventricle from the transverse sinus.

The muscular septal surface of the outflow tract is characteristically smooth, with the fan-like left bundle branch cascading down from the septal crest. The landmark of its descent is the membranous septum immediately beneath the zone of apposition between right coronary and non-coronary leaflets of

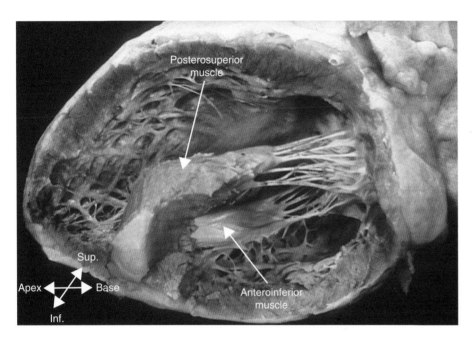

Fig. 2.52 This specimen, viewed from behind after the parietal wall of the left ventricle has been removed, is dissected to show the adjacency of the anteroinferior and posterosuperior papillary muscles of the mitral valve.

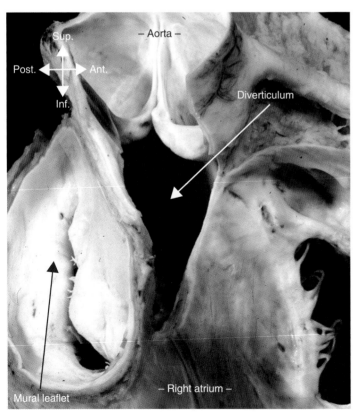

Fig. 2.53 This heart, seen from above and from the right in anatomical orientation, has been prepared by removing the atrial musculature and the non-coronary sinus of the aortic valve to illustrate the diverticulum separating the mitral valve from the septum.

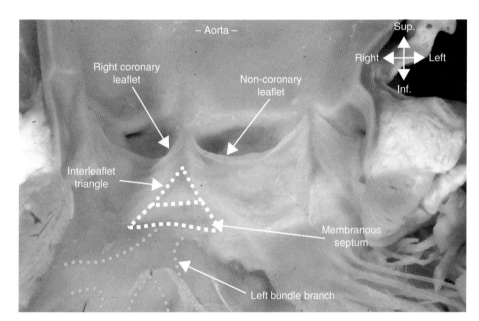

Fig. 2.54 This specimen, orientated in anatomical position, demonstrates the relationship of the left bundle branch to the zone of apposition between the right and non-coronary leaflets of the aortic valve. The dotted lines show the continuity between the membranous septum and the interleaflet triangle between the right coronary and non-coronary leaflets of the aortic valve. The green dotted lines show the location of the left bundle branch.

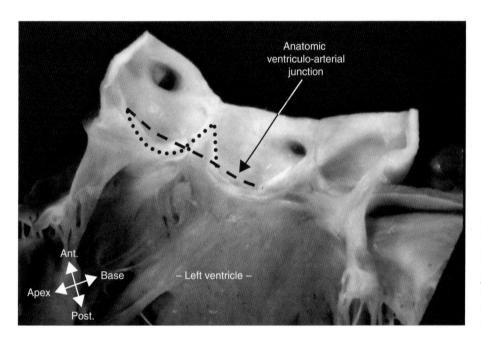

Fig. 2.55 This dissection demonstrates that, as in the pulmonary valve (see Fig. 2.42) the attachments of the leaflets of the aortic valve cross the anatomic ventriculo-arterial junction (dashed line) incorporating crescents of ventricular tissue into the arterial valvar sinuses, and triangles of arterial tissue into the ventricular base.

the aortic valve (Fig. 2.54). The bundle descends, initially, as a relatively narrow solitary fascicle, but soon divides into three interconnected fascicles that radiate into anterior, septal, and posterior divisions. The interconnecting radiations do not fan out to any degree until the bundle itself has descended to between one-third and one-half the length of the septum.

As with the pulmonary valve, the leaflets of the aortic valve are not attached in circular fashion to a supporting ring fibrocollagenous tissue. Instead, the leaflets are attached in semilunar fashion, with the hinge lines crossing the anatomic ventriculoaortic junction (Fig. 2.55). This arrangement again means that crescents of ventricular muscle are incorporated into the bases of two of the aortic sinuses, while three triangles of fibrous tissue are created beneath the sinutubular junction[20]. This arrangement is comparable to the semilunar attachment of the pulmonary valvar leaflets demonstrated in Figure 2.42. As an entity, the aortic valve itself forms the keystone of the heart, and is related to each of the other cardiac

chambers and valves. Its morphology is described in detail in Chapter 3.

THE AORTA

The ascending aorta begins at the distal extremity of the three aortic sinuses, the sinutubular junction, which lies at the line of opening of the free edge of the leaflets of the aortic valve (Fig. 2.56). The ascending aortic trunk then runs its short course, passing superiorly, and obliquely to the right, and slightly forward, toward the sternum. It is contained within the

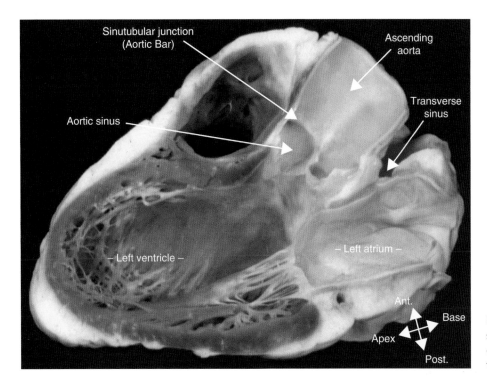

Fig. 2.56 This long axis section shows the sinutubular junction just at the line of opening of the free edge of the leaflets of the aortic valve.

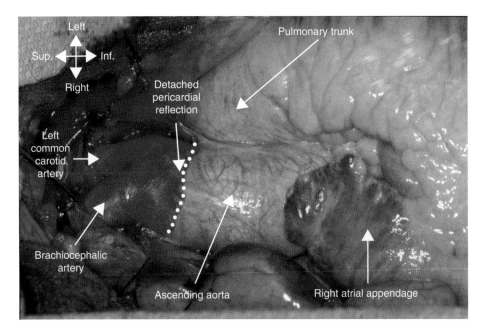

Fig. 2.57 This operative view through a median sternotomy shows the vascular pedicle leading to the beginning of the aortic arch, which gives rise to the brachiocephalic and left common carotid arteries just distal to the detached pericardial reflection (white dotted line). The origin of the left subclavian artery is not seen.

fibrous pericardial sac, so its surface is covered with serous pericardium. Its anterior surface abuts directly on the pulmonary trunk, which is also covered with serous pericardium. The two vessels together make up the so-called vascular pedicle of the heart (Fig. 2.57). The ascending aorta is related anteromedially to the right atrial appendage, and posterolaterally to the right ventricular outflow tract and the pulmonary trunk. Extrapericardially, the thymus gland lies between it and the sternum. The medial wall of the right atrium, the superior caval vein, and the right pleura relate to its right side. On the left, its principal relationship is with the pulmonary trunk. Posterior to the ascending aorta lies the transverse sinus of the pericardium (Fig. 2.56), which separates it from the roof of the left atrium and the right pulmonary artery.

The arch of the aorta begins at the superior attachment of the pericardial reflection just proximal to the origin of the brachiocephalic artery. It continues superiorly for a short distance, before coursing posteriorly and to the left,

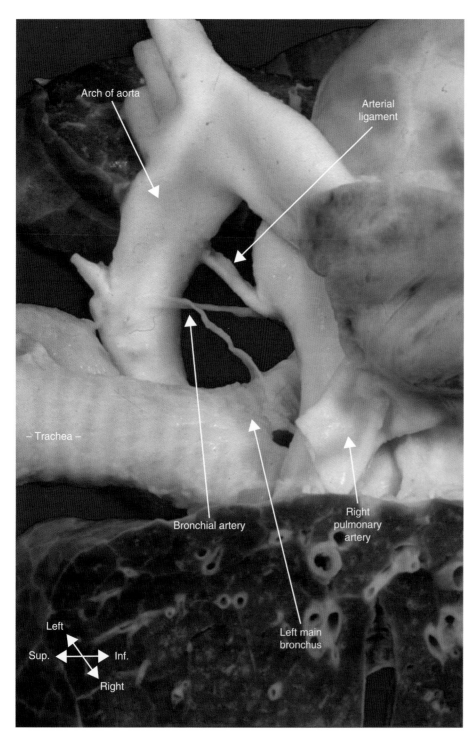

Fig. 2.58 This dissection, viewed from the right side in surgical orientation, shows a bronchial artery arising from the aorta in the midline and dividing to supply both bronchuses.

crossing the lateral aspect of the distal trachea, and finally terminating on the lateral aspect of the vertebral column. Here, it is tethered by the parietal pleura and the arterial ligament. During its course, it gives off the brachiocephalic, the left common carotid, and the left subclavian arteries. Bronchial arteries arise from the underside of the arch (Fig. 2.58). They can be particularly troublesome if

not carefully identified in the presence of aortic coarctation. The left phrenic and vagus nerves run over the anterolateral aspect of the arch just beneath the mediastinal pleura. The left recurrent laryngeal nerve takes origin from the vagus. It curls superiorly around the arterial ligament before passing on to the posteromedial side of the arch. Here, the arch relates to the tracheal bifurcation and

oesophagus on its medial border, but also to the left main bronchus and the left pulmonary artery inferiorly (Fig. 2.58).

The descending, or thoracic, aorta continues from the arch, running an initial course lateral to the vertebral bodies, and reaching an anterior position at its termination. It gives off many branches to the organs of the thorax throughout its course, as well as the prominent lower

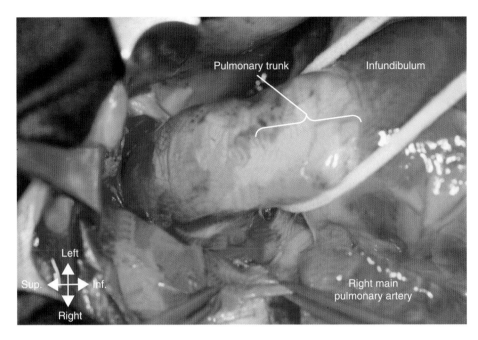

Pulmonary trunk   Infundibulum

Left
Sup.   Inf.
Right

Right main
pulmonary artery

Fig. 2.59 This operative view, taken through a median sternotomy, shows the short course of the pulmonary trunk to its bifurcation.

nine pairs of intercostal arteries. These latter vessels are of critical concern for the cardiac surgeon (see Chapter 9). In coarctation of the aorta, they serve as primary collateral vessels to bypass the obstructed aorta, accounting for the rib notching seen in older children with this lesion. These vessels, and their branches to the chest wall, can be a source of troublesome bleeding if not properly secured when operating on such patients. The surgeon must also remember that the dorsal branches of the intercostal vessels contribute a spinal branch that is important in supplying blood to the spinal cord. Because it is difficult to predict exactly the site of origin of these vital branches, the surgeon must make every attempt to protect their origin from permanent occlusion. The important bronchial arteries (Fig. 2.58) also arise from the descending segment of the thoracic aorta. These vessels can become dilated in the presence of pulmonary atresia, when they serve as a source of pulmonary vascular supply.

THE PULMONARY ARTERIES

The pulmonary trunk is a short vessel, usually less than five centimetres in length in the adult (Fig. 2.59). It is completely contained within the pericardium and, similar to its running mate, the ascending aorta, is covered with a layer of serous

pericardium except where the two vessels abut each other in the vascular pedicle. It takes origin from the most anterior aspect of the heart, lying just behind the lateral edge of the sternum and the second left intercostal space. Initially, the pulmonary trunk overlies the aorta and left coronary artery, but it soon moves to a side-by-side relationship with the ascending aorta. The left coronary artery turns abruptly anteriorly to lie between the left atrial appendage and the pulmonary trunk. The arterial ligament extends from the aorta to the very end of the pulmonary trunk as the latter divides into left and right pulmonary arteries. The left pulmonary artery then courses laterally in front of the descending aorta and the left main stem bronchus before it sends branches to the hilum of the lung. Posteroinferiorly, the left pulmonary artery is connected to the left superior pulmonary vein by a fold of serous pericardium that contains a ligamentous remnant of the left superior caval vein, the ligament of Marshall. The right pulmonary artery is somewhat longer than the left, having to traverse the mediastinum beneath the aortic arch, and then behind the superior caval vein, to reach the hilum of the lung. It lies in a posteroinferior position relative to the azygos vein, and is anterior to the left main bronchus. The right pulmonary artery often branches before reaching the lateral wall of the superior caval

vein posterior to the transverse sinus of the pericardium. In this situation, a large upper lobar branch may be mistaken for the right pulmonary artery itself.

References

1. Anderson KR, Ho SY, Anderson RH. The location and vascular supply of the sinus node in the human heart. *Br Heart J* 1979; **41**: 28–32.

2. James TN. *Anatomy of the Coronary Arteries.* Hoeber, New York. 1961; pp 103–106.

3. McAlpine WA. *Heart and Coronary Arteries. An Anatomical Atlas for Clinical Diagnosis, Radiological Investigation and Surgical Treatment.* Springer-Verlag, New York. 1975; p 152.

4. Busquet J, Fontan F, Anderson RH, Ho SY, Davies MJ. The surgical significance of the atrial branches of the coronary arteries. *Int J Cardiol* 1984; **6**: 223–234.

5. Barra Rossi M, Ho SY, Anderson RH, Rossi Filho RI, Lincoln C. Coronary arteries in complete transposition: the significance of the sinus node artery. *Ann Thorac Surg* 1986; **42**: 573–577.

6. Sweeney LJ, Rosenquist GC. The normal anatomy of the atrial septum in the human heart. *Am Heart J* 1979; **98**: 194–199.

7. Anderson RH, Webb S, Brown NA. Clinical anatomy of the atrial septum with reference to its developmental components. *Clin Anat* 1999; **12**: 362–374.

8. Anderson RH, Brown NA. The anatomy of the heart revisited. *Anat Rec* 1996; **246**: 1–7.

9. Ho SY, Anderson RH. How constant is the tendon of Todaro as a marker for the triangle of Koch? *J Cardiovasc Electrophysiol* 2000; **1**: 83–89.

10. Anderson RH, Ho SY, Becker AE. Anatomy of the human atrioventricular junctions revisited. *Anat Rec* 2000; **260**: 81–91.

11. James TN. The connecting pathways between the sinus node and the A-V node and between the right and the left atrium in the human heart. *Am Heart J* 1963; **66**: 498–508.

12. James TN, Sherf L. Specialized tissues and preferential conduction in the atria of the heart. *Am J Cardiol* 1971; **28**: 414–427.

13. Isaacson R, Titus JL, Merideth J, Feldt RH, McGoon DC. Apparent interruption of atrial conduction pathways after surgical repair of transposition of the great arteries. *Am J Cardiol* 1972; **30**: 533–535.

14. Anderson RH, Ho SY. Anatomic criteria for identifying the components of the axis responsible for atrioventricular conduction. *J Cardiovasc Electrophysiol* 2001; **12**: 1265–1268.

15. Janse MJ, Anderson RH. Internodal atrial specialised pathways – fact or fiction? *Eur J Cardiol* 1974; **2**: 117–137.

16. Anderson RH, Ho SY, Smith A, Becker AE. The internodal atrial myocardium. *Anat Rec* 1981; **201**: 75–82.

17. Goor DA, Lillehei CW. In: *Congenital Malformations of the Heart*. Grune and Stratton, New York. 1975; pp 1–37.

18. McFadden PM, Culpepper WS, Ochsner JL. Iatrogenic right ventricular failure in tetralogy of Fallot repairs: reappraisal of a distressing problem. *Ann Thor Surg* 1982; **33**: 400–402.

19. Breyer RH, Lavender S, Cordell AR. Delayed left ventricular rupture secondary to transatrial left ventricular vent. *Ann Thorac Surg* 1982; **3**: 189–191.

20. Sutton JPIII, Ho SY, Anderson RH. The forgotten interleaflet triangles: A review of the surgical anatomy of the aortic valve. *Ann Thorac Surg* 1995; **59**: 419–427.

3

Surgical anatomy of the valves of the heart

It is axiomatic that a thorough knowledge of valvar anatomy is a prerequisite for successful surgery, be it valvar replacement or reconstruction. The surgeon will also require a firm understanding of the arrangement of other aspects of cardiac anatomy to ensure safe access to a diseased valve or valves. These anatomical features were described in the previous chapter. Knowledge of the surgical anatomy of the valves themselves, however, must be founded on appreciation of their relationship to each other. This requires understanding of, first, the basic orientation of the cardiac valves, emphasising the intrinsic features that make each valve distinct from the others. This information must then be supplemented by emphasising the relationships of the valves to other structures that the surgeon must avoid, specifically, the conduction tissues and the major channels of the coronary circulation. Throughout our narrative, we will presume the presence of a normally structured heart, lying in its usual position without any congenital cardiac malformations.

POSITION OF THE VALVES WITHIN THE HEART

Fundamental to understanding valvar anatomy is a clear grasp of the relationship of the valves themselves. The close proximity of the valves to each other is best understood by examining the short axis cylindrical section of the heart through the atrioventricular and ventriculo-arterial junctions (Fig. 3.1). All four valves are contained in this cylinder. Indeed, the leaflets of three of them are in fibrous continuity with one another. Only the leaflets of the pulmonary valve are exclusively supported by muscle, that of the free-standing right infundibulum (Fig. 3.2). When considered in their position relative to the body, the pulmonary valve is the most anterior and superior valve, the tricuspid valve is the most inferior, while the mitral valve is the most posterior of the four. The central position of the aortic valve is readily evident from study of this cylinder, and its relationships are seen to the other valves. It used to be thought that there was an extensive fibrous skeleton within the cylinder that supported the leaflets of all four valves. This concept, appealing as it may be, is far from reality. As already emphasised, the leaflets of the pulmonary valve are supported by the free-standing sleeve of right ventricular muscular infundibulum. A fibrous skeleton does not uniformly support even the leaflets of the two atrioventricular valves.

Instead, the fibrous structures supporting the valvar leaflets are concentrated on the central position of the aortic valve. Thus, two of the leaflets of the aortic valve share fibrous continuity with one of the leaflets of the mitral valve (Fig. 3.2). The two ends of this area of fibrous continuity then anchor the aortic-mitral valvar unit across the short axis of the left ventricle (Fig. 3.3). At these points of attachment to the ventricular musculature, the fibrous tissue is thickened to form the right and left fibrous trigones. The right fibrous trigone is itself then continuous with the membranous septum, the conjunction of these two fibrous components forming the strongest part of the fibrous skeleton, named the central fibrous body (Fig. 3.4).

The base of the membranous septum itself then fills the gap between the bases of two of the semilunar hinges of the leaflets of the aortic valve, specifically the space between the non-coronary and right coronary leaflets (Figs. 3.4, 3.5). The fibrous tissue filling the gap between the leaflets, however, forming a septal structure at its point of attachment to the muscular ventricular septum, continues superiorly to the level of the aortic sinutubular junction (Fig. 3.5). This most apical part of the triangle of tissue interposed between the hinges of the

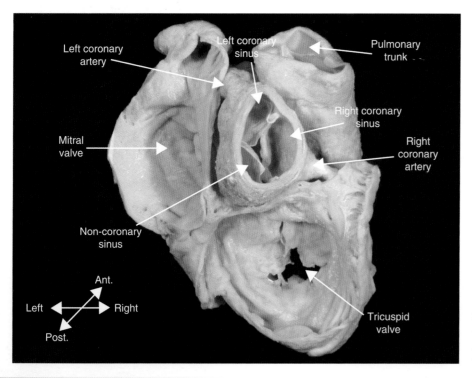

Fig. 3.1 This superior view of a cylindrical section of the heart through the atrioventricular and ventriculo-arterial junctions shows the relationship of the cardiac valves.

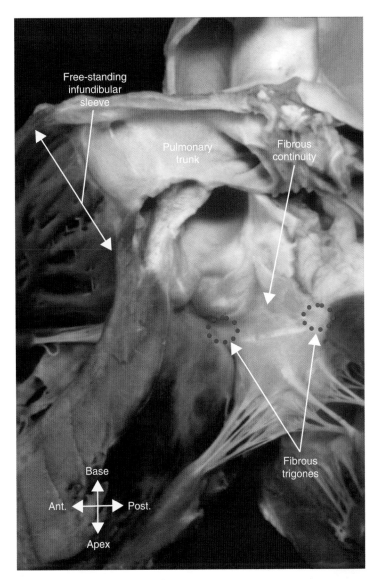

Free-standing
infundibular
sleeve

Pulmonary
trunk

Fibrous
continuity

Fibrous
trigones

Base

Ant. ← → Post.

Apex

Fig. 3.2 To produce this picture, the heart has been sectioned in the equivalent of the parasternal long axis echocardiographic plane. The arterial roots have been cleaned to show the free-standing sleeve of subpulmonary infundibular musculature that lifts the leaflets of the pulmonary valve away from the base of the ventricular mass. Note the area of fibrous continuity between the leaflets of the aortic and mitral valves forming the roof of the left ventricle. The ends are thickened to form the fibrous trigones (red dotted circles).

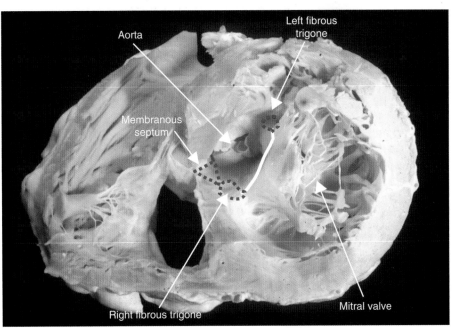

Aorta

Left fibrous
trigone

Membranous
septum

Right fibrous trigone

Mitral valve

Fig. 3.3 This view of the cardiac short axis, seen from beneath in anatomic orientation, shows the area of fibrous continuity (white line) between the leaflets of the aortic and mitral valves, which is thickened at both ends (red dotted circles) to form the fibrous trigones. The right fibrous trigone is continuous with the membranous septum (blue dotted triangle), the combined mass of fibrous tissue being described as the central fibrous body.

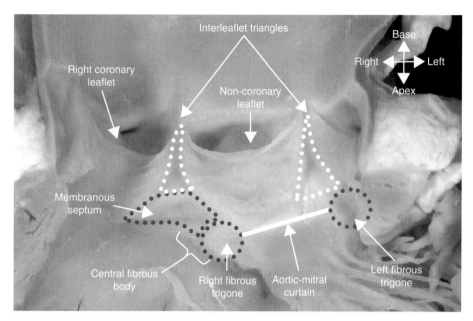

Fig. 3.4 This dissection shows the area of the central fibrous body as seen from the left ventricle in anatomic orientation. The white dotted triangles delimit the interleaflet fibrous triangles between the semilunar attachments of the leaflets of the aortic valve. Note that the triangle between the right and non-coronary leaflets is continuous inferiorly with the membranous septum (blue dotted line), itself continuous with the right fibrous trigone (red dotted circle) to form the central fibrous body. The interleaflet triangle between the non- and left coronary leaflets is continuous with the area of fibrous continuity between the aortic and mitral valves (white line) and the left fibrous trigone (red dotted circle).

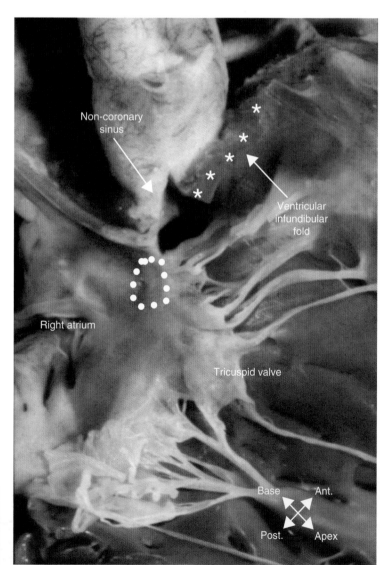

Fig. 3.5 This heart has been prepared by removing the interleaflet triangle between the right and non-coronary aortic leaflets, and is photographed from the right side. The base of the triangle is formed by the interventricular component of the membranous septum, itself continuous with the atrioventricular component (dotted white area). The asterisks show the cut edge of the ventriculo-infundibular fold, forming the supraventricular crest.

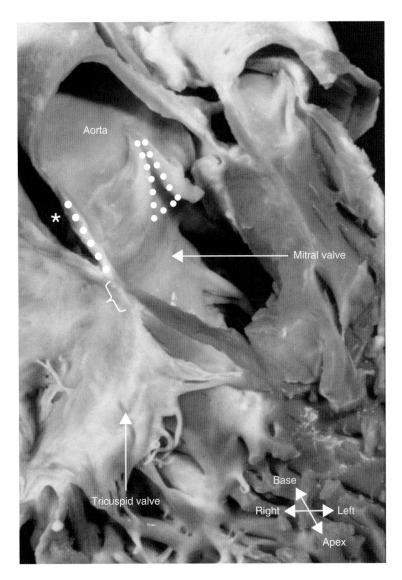

Aorta

*

Mitral valve

Tricuspid valve

Base

Right   Left

Apex

Fig. 3.6 This heart has been sectioned through the interleaflet triangle between the non-coronary and right coronary aortic leaflets. The bracket shows the membranous septum which forms the base of the interleaflet triangle, but the apex of the triangle (dotted white line) interposes between the left ventricular outflow tract and the transverse sinus (asterisk). The interleaflet triangle between the non-coronary and left coronary aortic leaflets is marked by the white dotted triangle.

valvar leaflets then separates the most distal part of the left ventricular cavity from the right side of the transverse sinus, in other words forms part of the parietal wall of the heart (Fig. 3.6).

A similar triangle of fibrous tissue, again confluent with the area of fibrous continuity between the aortic and mitral valves, fills the space between the hinges of the non-coronary and left coronary leaflets of the aortic valve. This fibrous tissue separates the left ventricular outflow tract from the middle part of the transverse sinus (Figs. 3.7, 3.8). Extensions of the fibrous tissue forming the crown-like aortic root are also to be found running from the fibrous trigones into the left atrioventricular junction, where they partly support the hinge of the mural leaflet of the mitral valve (Figs. 3.9, 3.10).

Their extent varies markedly from heart to heart[1]. It is rare to find a complete ring of fibrous tissue encircling the mitral valvar orifice. In many place, the hinge of the leaflet is supported by the fibrofatty tissue of the left atrioventricular groove, which also serves to insulate the atrial from the ventricular myocardium. This arrangement is the rule around the orifice of the tricuspid valve, where it is very rare to find the valvar leaflets supported by a fibrous annulus. Paradoxically, the persisting area of atrioventricular muscular continuity, the penetrating bundle of His, pierces the strongest part of the fibrous skeleton, specifically through the atrioventricular component of the membranous septum. This point is then marked by the attachment of another part of the skeleton, the tendon of Todaro,

to the right–sided aspect of the membranous septum, this forming an integral part of the so-called central fibrous body (Fig. 3.11).

It follows from the above discussion that it is incorrect to speak of either an aortic or a pulmonary valvar ring. Rather than being hinged in circular fashion from a ring, or an "annulus", the leaflets of the arterial valves have semilunar attachments (Figs. 3.12, 3.13). There is at least one annular area within the structure of each arterial valve, namely the anatomic junction between the arterial trunks and their supporting muscular ventricular structures. This ring is best seen in the pulmonary valve (Fig. 3.12). The semilunar attachments of the leaflets cross this ring. The upper extremity of each leaflet is then attached to a much more

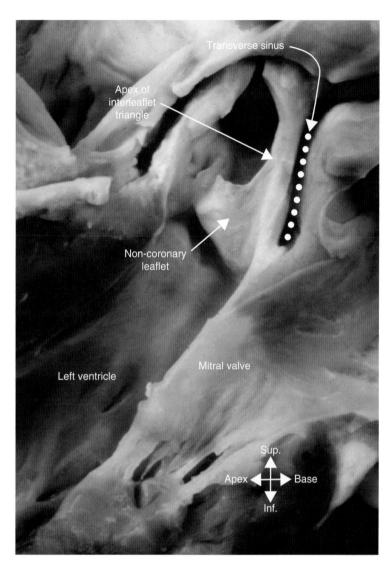

Fig. 3.7 In this heart, the left ventricular outflow tract is sectioned through the interleaflet triangle between the non-coronary and left coronary leaflets of the aortic valve. The fibrous wall separates the cavity of the left ventricle from the transverse sinus of the pericardium (dotted line).

obvious anatomic ring, namely the arterial wall forming the sinutubular junction at the peripheral points of attachment of the valvar leaflets. This is at an appreciably higher level than the deepest attachment of the leaflets within the ventricles[2,3]. This arrangement is of considerable surgical significance, since the triangular areas of outflow tract subjacent to the apex of the attachments of the three zones of apposition of the leaflets at the sinutubular junction (see Fig. 3.40) separate the ventricular cavity from the outside of the heart (see Figs. 3.5 & 3.8).

Although composed of arterial wall, the triangles are, in haemodynamic terms, part of the ventricles. In the case of the aortic valve, the two intercommissural triangles adjacent to the non-coronary leaflet are in relation to the transverse

sinus of the pericardium (Figs. 3.6, 3.7). The anterosuperior, or facing, triangle relates to a potential space between the aortic root and the right ventricular infundibulum (Figs. 3.14, 3.15). The perforating branches of the anterior interventricular coronary artery enter the muscular septum through the space. The leaflets of the aortic valve, therefore, are attached in part to the muscular component of the left ventricular outflow tract, and in part to the area of fibrous continuity with the mitral valve (Figs. 3.2, 3.13). In the case of the pulmonary valve, the attachments are exclusively to the musculature of the right ventricular outflow tract (Figs. 3.2, 3.12).

In contrast to the arterial valves, the leaflets of the two atrioventricular valves are attached to the atrioventricular

junction in truly annular, or ring-like, fashion. Even in this respect, nonetheless, there is a marked difference between the mitral and tricuspid valves in the extent to which this annulus is part of the fibrous skeleton. As described above, the strongest parts of the skeleton are the two ends of the area of fibrous continuity between the leaflets of the aortic and mitral valves, the right and left fibrous trigones (Figs. 3.2–3.4). The area of fibrous continuity itself is called the aortic–mitral curtain (Fig. 3.4). The fibrous skeleton forming the ring of the mitral valve extends septally and parietally from the two trigones, usually as a complete collagenous structure, albeit one that is not always cord-like[1]. It may have a linear structure rather than being a cord, and its structure varies markedly at different

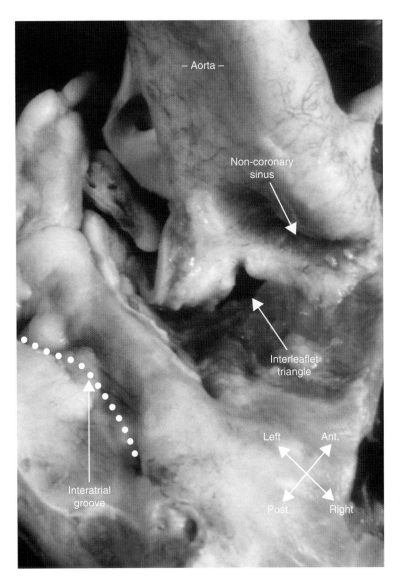

Aorta

Non-coronary
sinus

Interleaflet
triangle

Left   Ant.

Interatrial
groove

Post.   Right

Fig. 3.8 In this heart, the tip of the fibrous triangle between the left coronary and non-coronary aortic valvar leaflets has been removed. The heart is photographed from the transverse sinus, showing the location of the triangle. The white dotted line shows the interatrial groove.

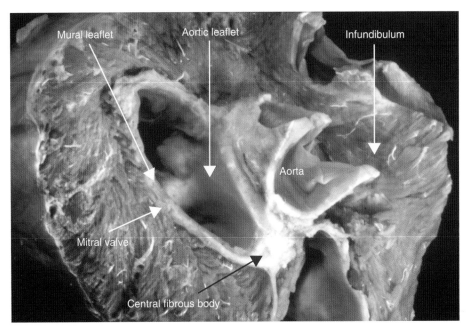

Mural leaflet   Aortic leaflet   Infundibulum

Aorta

Mitral valve

Central fibrous body

Fig. 3.9 This heart has been dissected by removing the entirety of the atrial myocardium, and is photographed from behind. The aorta has been removed at the level of the semilunar hingepoints of the valvar leaflets, showing the crown-like arrangement of the root. Fibrous extensions are seen running from the fibrous tissue of the aortic root into the orifices of the mitral and tricuspid valves.

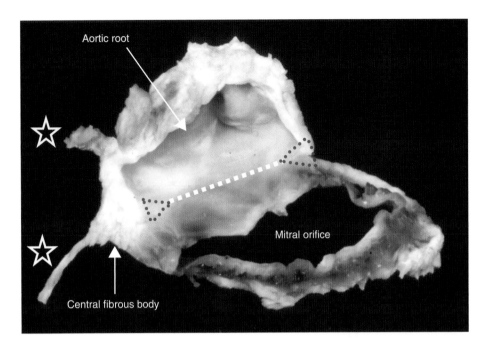

Fig. 3.10 The fibrous skeleton supporting the aortic-mitral unit has been removed from the heart shown in Fig. 3.9, and is photographed from beneath. The fibrous tissue extends only minimally into the tricuspid valvar orifice (stars). The white dotted line and the red dotted triangles show the continuity between the leaflets of the valves. The skeleton is also deficient at various points around the so-called "annulus" of the mitral valve.

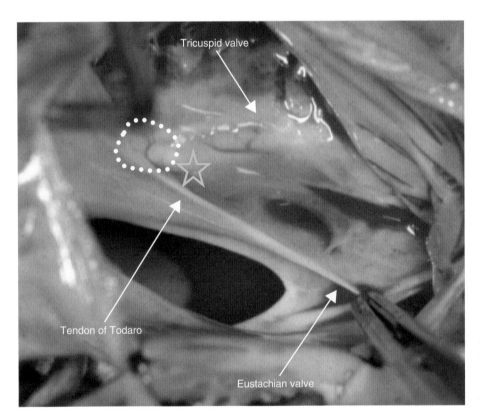

Fig. 3.11 This picture, taken in the operating room, shows the continuation of the Eustachian valve, the tendon of Todaro, which inserts into the membranous septum (white dotted circle). The star marks the site of the atrioventricular node at the apex of the triangle of Koch.

points around the junction. It usually tends to fade out or become attenuated around the mural leaflet of the valve. The right fibrous trigone brings both the mitral and aortic valves into fibrous continuity with the tricuspid valve. This part of the fibrous skeleton includes the membranous septum, which separates the left ventricular outflow tract from the right heart chambers (Fig. 3.16). Usually, the attachment of the septal leaflet of the tricuspid valve extends obliquely across the membranous septum, dividing it into atrioventricular and interventricular components. It is the right fibrous trigone, together with the membranous septum, that make up the central fibrous body (Fig. 3.4). The remainder of the attachment of the tricuspid valve around the right atrioventricular junction is the most weakly constructed part of the cardiac skeleton, particularly in its parietal part. Thus, it is rarely possible to dissect a complete collagenous ring

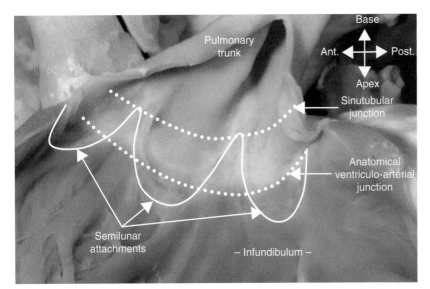

Fig. 3.12 In this specimen shown in anatomic orientation, the leaflets of the pulmonary valve have been removed to demonstrate their semilunar attachments, which have been emphasised by the bold lines. The dotted lines show the sinutubular and anatomic ventriculo-arterial junctions, respectively. Note that the semilunar attachments cross the anatomic junction.

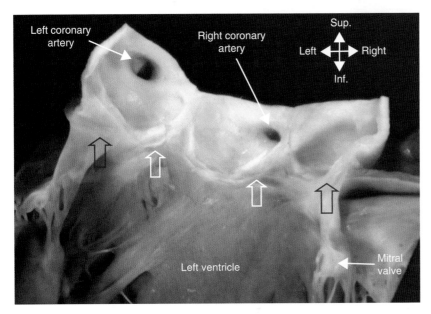

Fig. 3.13 This dissection is comparable to that shown in Fig. 3.12, but has removed the leaflets of the aortic rather than the pulmonary valve. The left ventricular outflow tract has been opened between the left coronary and the non-coronary aortic leaflets. Note that the two aortic sinuses giving rise to the coronary arteries are supported at their base by septal musculature (white arrows), with part of the left coronary leaflet, along with the non-coronary leaflet, in fibrous continuity with the aortic leaflet of the mitral valve (blue arrows).

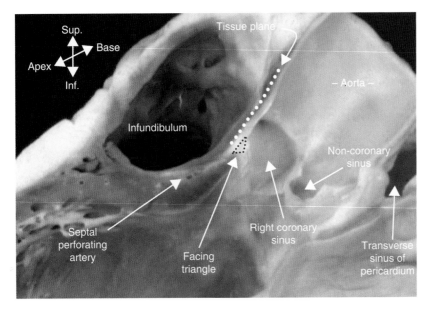

Fig. 3.14 This heart has been sectioned in parasternal long axis echocardiographic equivalent plane. Note how the apex of the interleaflet fibrous triangle between the two coronary aortic leaflets (blue dotted triangle) points into the tissue plane between the aortic sinuses and the subpulmonary infundibulum (dotted line).

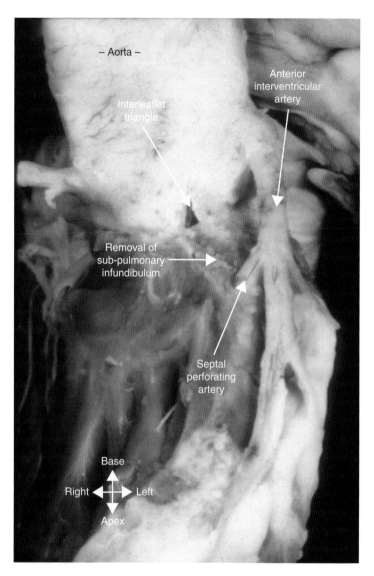

Aorta

Anterior interventricular artery

Interleaflet triangle

Removal of sub-pulmonary infundibulum

Septal perforating artery

Base

Right — Left

Apex

Fig. 3.15 This dissection shows the location of the interleaflet fibrous triangle between the two sinuses of the aortic valve that give rise to the coronary arteries. The triangle itself has been removed, as has the free-standing sleeve of sub-pulmonary infundibulum, and the heart is photographed from the right ventricular aspect. Note the position of the septal perforating artery.

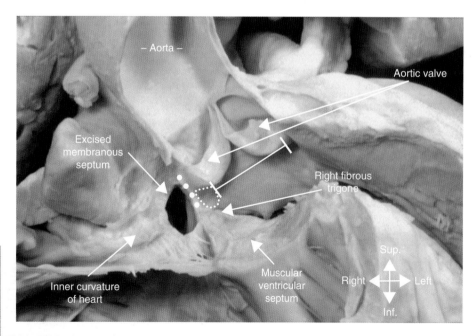

Aorta

Aortic valve

Excised membranous septum

Right fibrous trigone

Inner curvature of heart

Muscular ventricular septum

Sup.

Right — Left

Inf.

Fig. 3.16 This dissection is through the membranous septum (dotted line), showing how this structure produces fibrous continuity between the leaflets of the tricuspid and aortic valve, the aortic valve itself being in fibrous continuity with the mitral valve. The right end of the area of continuity with the mitral valve (white line) is thickened to form the right fibrous trigone (dotted area).

supporting the leaflets of the tricuspid valve (Fig. 3.10).

BASIC MORPHOLOGY OF THE ATRIOVENTRICULAR VALVES

The mitral and tricuspid valves have several important features in common, which collectively make up the valvar complex (Fig. 3.17). The first feature has already been described, namely the attachments of the valvar leaflets to the atrioventricular junctions. As emphasised above, in the case of the atrioventricular valves, this is appropriately termed the annulus. Another common feature is the arrangement of the leaflets. Histologically, these structures have a spongy atrial and a fibrous ventricular layer (Fig. 3.18). The atrial myocardium inserts for varying distances between the endocardium and the spongy layer. On rare occasions, rudimentary fibres of ventricular musculature may extend into the fibrous layer. In normal valves, blood vessels are found only within the segment of leaflet containing muscular fibres. The leaflets

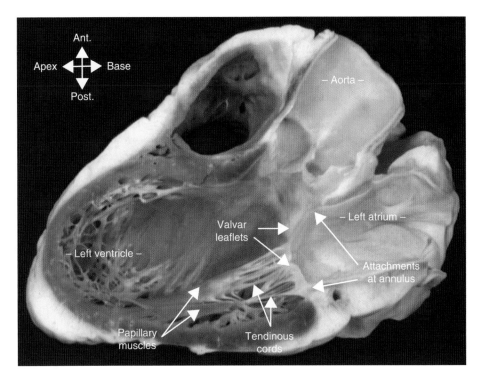

Fig. 3.17 This section in long axis parasternal echocardiographic equivalent shows the components of the atrioventricular valvar complex. All parts need to work in harmony to ensure normal valvar function.

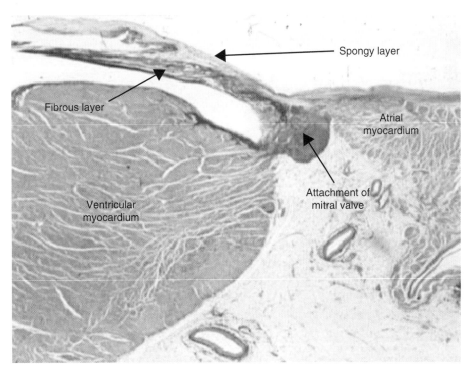

Fig. 3.18 This histological section is through the mural leaflet of the mitral valve, showing its spongy and fibrous layers. At this site, there is also a cord-like annulus anchoring the leaflet at the atrioventricular junction.

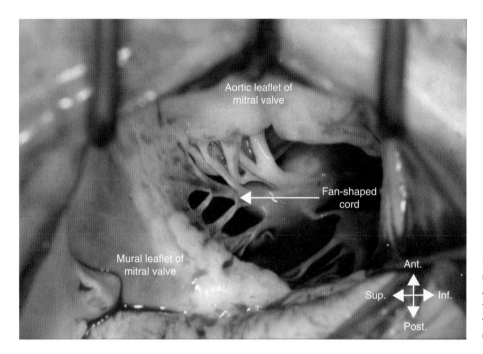

Aortic leaflet of
mitral valve

Fan-shaped
cord

Mural leaflet of
mitral valve

Ant.

Sup.   Inf.

Post.

Fig. 3.19 This surgical view of a rheumatic mitral valve, taken through a left atriotomy, shows a fan-shaped cord arising from the tip of its papillary muscle. This is the type of cord traditionally considered to represent a "commissural" cord.

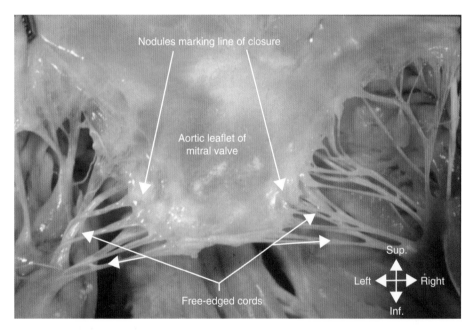

Nodules marking line of closure

Aortic leaflet of
mitral valve

Sup.

Left   Right

Inf.

Free-edged cords

Fig. 3.20 This anatomical specimen, viewed from the inlet aspect, shows the aortic leaflet of the mitral valve, with tendinous cords supporting the entirety of the free-edge of the valve. Note the nodules marking the area of overlap with the mural leaflet.

are supported by the tendinous cords, which themselves insert into the papillary muscles, or else directly into the ventricular myocardium. These cordal attachments are the third feature common to both tricuspid and mitral valves, although there are fundamental differences in the way each of the cordal units is arranged. This is also the case with the fourth feature, namely the papillary muscles. The differences in these

various features readily permit the morphological differentiation of the valves. Before describing these differences, it is important to emphasise again those features of the leaflets and their tension apparatus that are common to both valves.

Considered as a whole, the leaflets form a continuous skirt that hangs from the atrioventricular junction. The skirt itself is divided into discrete components, these individual sections of the skirt

representing the individual leaflets. There is no consensus as to how many leaflets there are in each valve, nor as to what constitutes the point of separation of one leaflet from the other. Traditionally, the tricuspid valve, as indicated by its name, has been considered to have three leaflets. More recently, some have argued that the valve has only two leaflets[4], albeit that our studies lend no support to this concept[5]. The alternative name for the mitral valve

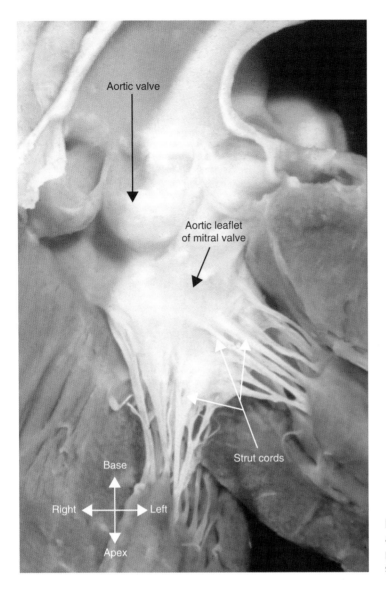

Fig. 3.21 Some cords to the rough zone of the ventricular aspect of the aortic leaflet of the mitral valve are particularly prominent, as shown in this illustration, and are defined as strut cords.

is the bicuspid valve. Yet it has been suggested that this valve is best considered as having four[6], or even six leaflets[7]. These ongoing arguments illustrate the difficulties which exist in defining individual leaflets. Some have sought to achieve this by identifying the so-called commissures between them. This then necessitates defining a commissure. Conventionally, a commissure is considered to represent the peripheral attachment of a breach in the skirt of valvar tissue, specifically one supported by a fan-shaped commissural cord[8], such a cord then inserting into a major papillary muscle or papillary muscle group (Fig. 3.19). This concept, therefore, depends on defining one variable structure in terms of another which is

itself variable. In terms of philosophy, this has been shown to be a poor principle[9]. Apart from anything else, so as to define commissures in this fashion, the valve is assessed when it is open. Yet, as all surgeons know, in order to function properly, the leaflets of the valve must fit together snugly when closed. Because of this, we prefer to define the extent of the leaflets according to the position of the zones of apposition between them.

The leaflets themselves are supported by tendinous cords. The ends of the zones of apposition between the adjacent leaflets are usually supported by fan-shaped cords as already considered (Fig. 3.19). In addition to the fan-shaped cord, nonetheless, the entire free edges of the leaflets are normally uniformly

supported by cords (Fig. 3.20). As was indicated by Frater[10] when discussing the exquisitely complex categorization of cords proposed by the group from Toronto[8], if any of these cords supporting the free-edge are cut, the valve may become regurgitant. We agree with Frater[10] that, for the purposes of categorisation, it is sufficient simply to distinguish those cords supporting the free-edge from those supporting the rough zone (Fig. 3.21). The detailed classification proposed by the Toronto group[8] has little, if any, surgical utility.

The cords from the rough zone are prominent structures that extend from the papillary muscles to the ventricular aspect of the leaflets. Some of the cords to the rough zone are particularly prominent

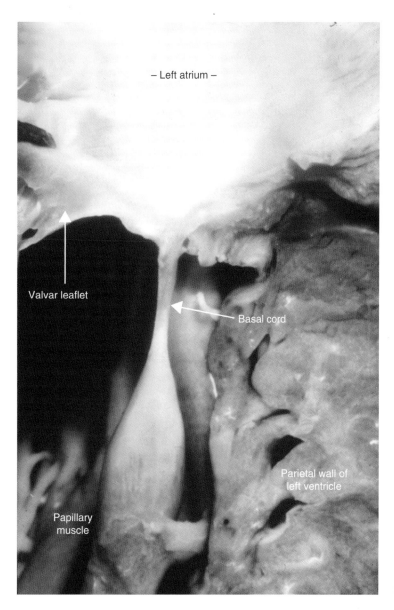

– Left atrium –

Valvar leaflet

Basal cord

Parietal wall of
left ventricle

Papillary
muscle

Fig. 3.22 This dissection has taken away most of the mural leaflet of the mitral valve, revealing a typically short cord with its own muscular belly. This is a basal cord.

in the mitral valve, and are called strut cords (Fig. 3.21). There is then a third type of cord that extends from the ventricular wall close to the atrioventricular junction, and again inserts into the ventricular aspect of the leaflet. These are the basal cords (Fig. 3.22). There is little point in further characterizing the pattern of branching and the generations of these cords, as long as it is appreciated that, normally, all parts of the leaflets receive good cordal support. Lack of uniform cordal support is very likely a mechanism leading to prolapse of a leaflet[11,12].

As has been emphasized in the setting of the mitral valve[13], the different components of the atrioventricular valve

making up the overall valve complex (Fig. 3.17) must function in concert so as to produce a competent valvar mechanism. The reason that the atrioventricular valves have such a complex tension apparatus is that, while in their closed position, they must withstand the full brunt of systolic ventricular pressure. A lesion of any of the valvar components can result in regurgitation. Thus, it is essential that the atrioventricular junction be of normal size and not overly dilated. The leaflets must coapt snugly. This demands an area of overlap (Fig. 3.23). Often, particularly in aged valves, this point of closure is marked by a series of nodules (Fig. 3.20). The point of closure away from the free edge gives a margin of safety for dilation of the

valvar orifice. Equally significant to competent closure, however, is the support of the leaflet by cords attached to the free edge. As discussed above, this feature is highly significant to the mechanism of prolapse of the valve leaflets. It has been suggested[14] that prolapse of the leaflets of the mitral valve is one of the most common congenital lesions. There is, as yet, no consensus as to the etiology of such prolapse. Morphologic observations[11,12] certainly suggest that lack of cordal support to the free edge of the leaflets can contribute to prolapse. And uniform support of the free edges of the leaflets is an integral part of a normal valve. Also important in the

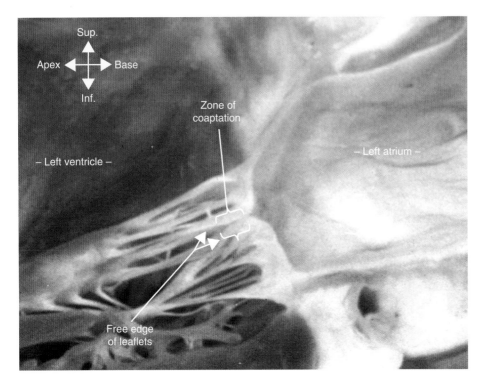

Fig. 3.23 This close-up of the section shown in Fig. 3.17 illustrates the overlapping zones of the mural and aortic leaflets of the mitral valve that produce the zone of coaptation (brackets).

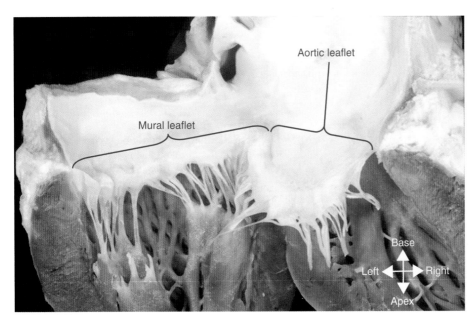

Fig. 3.24 Opening the mitral valve through the end of the zone of apposition between the leaflets closest to the septum, and spreading the valve, illustrates the widely dissimilar lengths of the two leaflets at their hingepoints from the atrioventricular junction.

maintenance of competence is the correct action of the papillary muscles and the ventricular myocardium. Not only must the papillary muscles be viable, but they must also be in their appropriate position of mechanical advantage relative to the axis of the valve. Taken together, all parts of the valvar unit are significant in the normal function of the valve[13].

THE MITRAL VALVE

The mitral valve has two major leaflets supported by paired papillary muscles. The two leaflets have widely dissimilar circumferential lengths (Fig. 3.24). The ends of the solitary zone of apposition between them, traditionally labelled the commissures, together with the papillary muscles, are positioned in inferoanterior position adjacent to the septum, and

superoposteriorly arising from the posterior ventricular wall, so that there is an angle between the axis of opening of the valve and the plane of the inlet septum (Fig. 3.25). The posterior extension of the subaortic outflow tract is wedged into this angle, this arrangement being important in terms of the disposition of the axis of atrioventricular conduction tissue (see Chapter 5). The two leaflets are frequently described as being "anterior" and

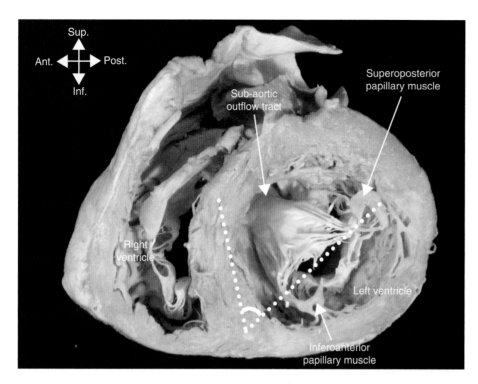

Fig. 3.25 This short axis of the ventricular mass, photographed from beneath, shows the angle between the line of the zone of apposition between the leaflets of the mitral valve and the plane of the inferior part of the ventricular septum (dotted lines). Note that, contrary to the usual descriptions, the papillary muscles are positioned inferoanteriorly and superoposteriorly when considered in attitudinally correct orientation (see compass).

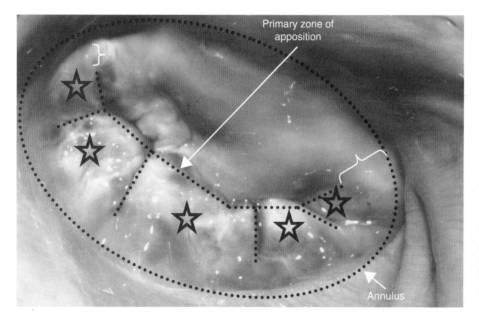

Fig. 3.26 The mitral valve is viewed from above in closed position, as it might be seen by the surgeon. There is a solitary zone of apposition between its two major leaflets, with slits in the mural leaflet producing a number of potential subcomponents in the mural leaflet (stars). Note that the ends of the zone of apposition do not extend to the atrioventricular junction (brackets). The original photograph of the mitral valve was kindly sent to us by Dr Van S. Galstyan, from Armenia, and we thank him for permitting us to use it in our book.

"posterior". Strictly speaking, they are anterosuperior and posteroinferior, the axis of opening of the valve being oblique relative to the anatomical axes of the body. Because of this, we prefer to describe the leaflets as being aortic and mural, this accounting well for both their morphology and position.

The aortic leaflet is attached to only one-third of the annular circumference. It is trapezoidal, or more semicircular, in shape than the mural leaflet (Fig. 3.24). The mural leaflet, attached to two-thirds of the annulus, is a long, rectangular, structure, although its middle component can also be somewhat semicircular. It is the segments of the mural leaflet closest to the ends of the zone of apposition with the aortic leaflet that show the most variation in morphology. Often these segments are almost completely separate from the central component, producing the so-called scallops of the mural leaflet (Fig. 3.26). Carpentier[15] has coded these scallops in alphanumeric fashion, along with the facing segments of the aortic leaflet, and this convention has widespread surgical use (Fig. 3.27). Yacoub[6] has gone so far as to nominate the scallops as separate leaflets of a quadrifoliate valve. Others, such as Kumar and colleagues[7], point out that the parts of the leaflet adjacent to the ends of

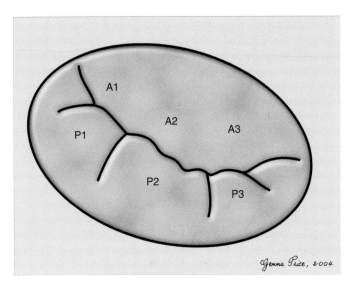

Fig. 3.27 The classification of Carpentier[15] recognises three major scallops in the mural leaflet (P1 through P3), and also names the facing segments of the aortic leaflet in alphanumeric fashion (A1 through A3). This classification, however, ignores the potential subcomponents of the leaflet at the ends of the solitary zone of apposition (see Fig. 3.28).

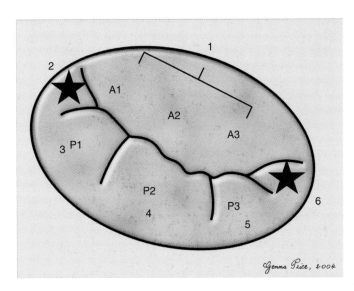

Fig. 3.28 Kumar and colleagues[7], in their suggested classification, also took into account the components of the mural leaflet adjacent to the ends of the solitary zone of apposition between the two major leaflets (stars), giving six rather than four potential subcomponents for the entire valvar skirt (compare with Fig. 3.27).

the zone of apposition can also take a "scallop-like" appearance (Fig. 3.28). In our opinion, all these categorisations are artificial. Because of the marked variability that occurs normally in the valve, sometimes the mural leaflet is comprised of four, five, or even more components. It is better to recognise that there are a variable number of slits in the mural leaflet, and that these slits act as pleats so that the normal valve can close snugly[16]. In the setting of prolapse, nonetheless, individual components of the divided mural leaflet may be deformed in isolation, and must then be recognised as such.

The cords supporting the leaflets attach them either to the papillary muscles, in the form of the cords to the free-edge and rough-zone, or else directly to the wall of the ventricle, as seen with the basal cords. The cords at the ends of the zone of apposition attach adjacent sides of both the leaflets to the apex of each of the papillary muscles (Fig. 3.29). Supplementary heads of both papillary muscles then support other cords to the free-edge, which usually attach uniformly along the leading edge of the leaflets, although, as we have discussed, the degree of support can be quite variable[11,12]. The cords supporting the divisions between the scallops of the mural leaflet also often have a fan-shaped appearance. When attached to a

prominent supplementary head of a papillary muscle, they can be markedly similar to the cords supporting the two ends of the zone of apposition between the leaflets. The cords to the rough-zone run from the papillary muscles to the ventricular aspect of the leaflets. Two or more of these cords, running from each papillary muscle to the undersurface of the aortic leaflet, are particularly prominent, and are called strut cords (Fig. 3.21). The basal cords attach only to the ventricular aspect of the mural leaflet, running directly from miniature muscle heads on the parietal wall of the ventricle (Fig. 3.22).

Almost always, the papillary muscles of the mitral valve are prominent paired

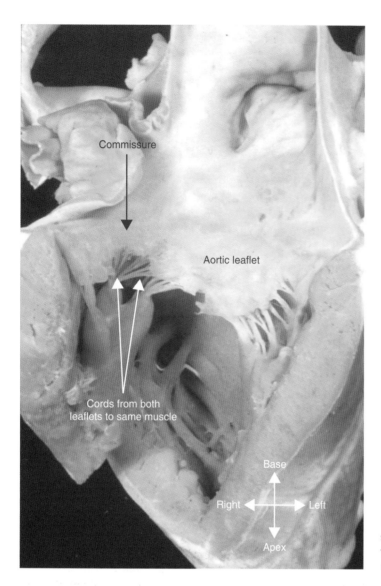

Commissure

Aortic leaflet

Cords from both
leaflets to same muscle

Base

Right ← → Left

Apex

Fig. 3.29 This anatomic specimen, seen from behind,
shows the opened mitral valve, with the cords supporting
the free-edge of both leaflets attached to the same papillary
muscles.

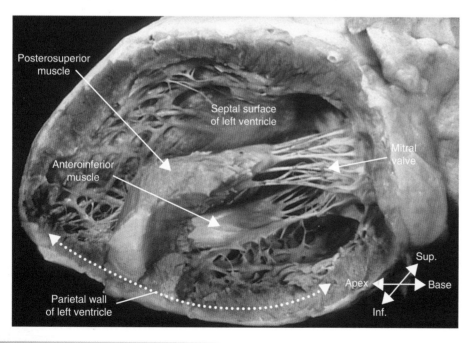

Posterosuperior
muscle

Septal surface
of left ventricle

Mitral
valve

Anteroinferior
muscle

Sup.

Apex ← → Base

Parietal wall
of left ventricle

Inf.

Fig. 3.30 The parietal wall of the left
ventricle has been removed (dotted line),
and the heart photographed from behind
and beneath. Note that the origins of the
papillary muscles are adjacent.

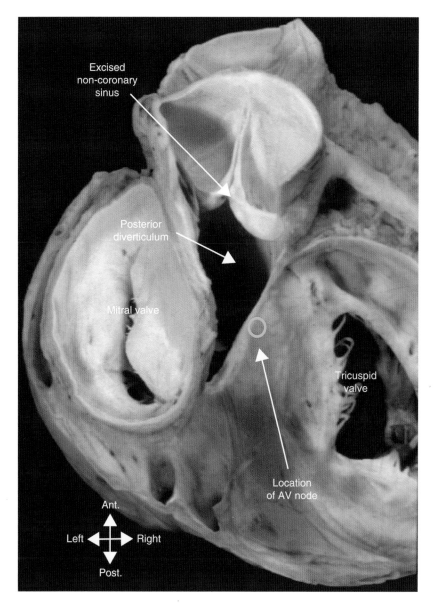

Excised
non-coronary
sinus

Posterior
diverticulum

Mitral valve

Tricuspid
valve

Location
of AV node

Ant.

Left ←→ Right

Post.

Fig. 3.31 In this heart, the atrial chambers have been removed, along with the non-coronary sinus and leaflet of the aortic valve, revealing the deep posteroinferiordiverticulum of the left ventricular outflow tract. Note the position of the atrioventricular node (green circle) relative to the mitral valve.

structures located on inferoanterior and superoposterior aspects of the parietal ventricular wall (Fig. 3.30). Although detailed study reveals considerable variation in the precise morphology of each muscle[11], neither arises from the septum, in contradistinction to the attachments of the tricuspid valve within the right ventricle. When the valve is dissected in its natural position within the left ventricle, the muscles can be seen to be adjacent to each other at the junction of the apical and middle third of the parietal ventricular wall (Fig. 3.30).

In terms of its relationships, the area of the valvar orifice related to the right fibrous trigone and central fibrous body is most vulnerable in terms of conduction

tissue, because here lays the atrioventricular node and penetrating bundle (Fig. 3.31). The area of the orifice between the two trigones, more or less the midportion of the aortic leaflet, is directly related to the commissure between the non-coronary and left coronary leaflets of the aortic valve. At this point, the aortic root is tented up, and an incision apparently through the atrial wall will extend into the subaortic outflow tract. If the incision is continued superiorly, it will pass into the transverse sinus of the pericardial cavity, which overlies the aortic-mitral curtain (Fig. 3.7). The deep inner curvature of the heart overlies and runs to either side of the curtain, and is lined by

the transverse sinus. Encircling the mural leaflet of the valve are the circumflex coronary artery from below and to the left (Fig. 3.32), and the coronary sinus from below and to the right (Fig. 3.33). The atrioventricular nodal artery also runs in close proximity to the right side of the mitral orifice, particularly when arising from a dominant circumflex artery. Indeed, the margin directly related to the circumflex artery is markedly variable. When the left coronary artery is dominant, the entire attachment of the mural leaflet is intimately related to the coronary artery and its branch to the atrioventricular node (compare Figs. 3.32 & 3.34).

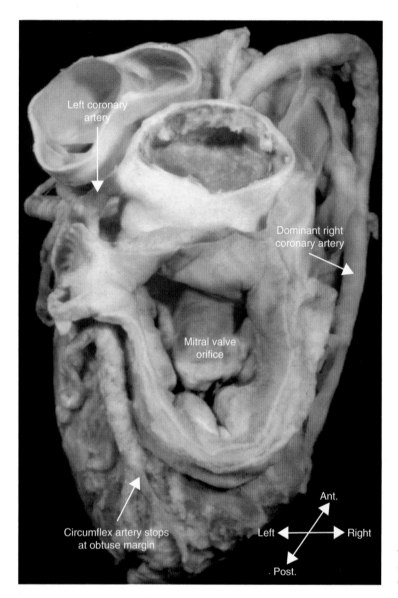

Left coronary artery

Dominant right coronary artery

Mitral valve orifice

Circumflex artery stops at obtuse margin

Ant.

Left ◄──► Right

Post.

Fig. 3.32 This dissection, taken from above and behind with the heart positioned anatomically, shows the relationship of the circumflex artery to the mitral valve when the right coronary artery is dominant.

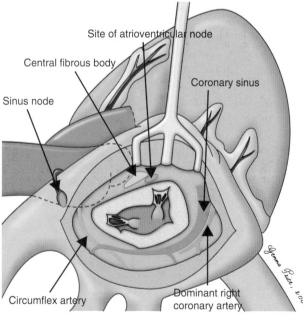

Site of atrioventricular node

Central fibrous body

Coronary sinus

Sinus node

Circumflex artery

Dominant right coronary artery

Fig. 3.33 In this cartoon, the components of the mitral valve are shown relative to structures of surgical significance.

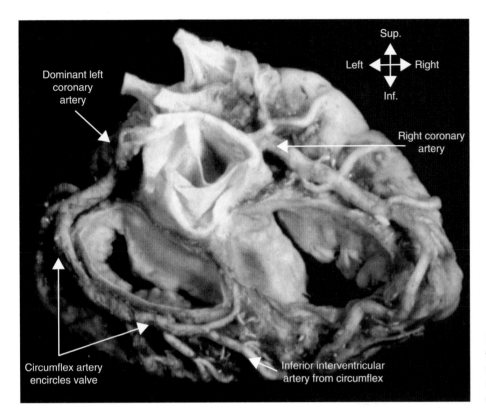

Dominant left coronary artery

Right coronary artery

Sup.

Left ↔ Right

Inf.

Circumflex artery encircles valve

Inferior interventricular artery from circumflex

Fig. 3.34 This dissection, photographed from above and behind, shows the relationship of the circumflex artery to the mitral valve when the left coronary artery is dominant.

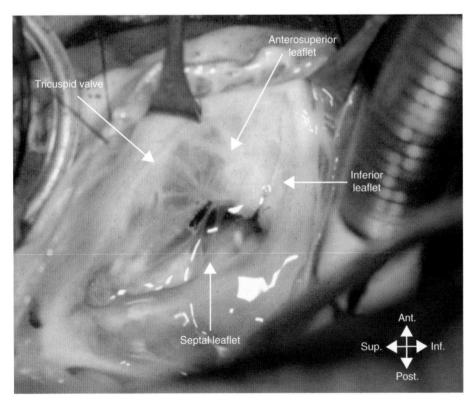

Anterosuperior leaflet

Tricuspid valve

Inferior leaflet

Septal leaflet

Ant.

Sup. ↔ Inf.

Post.

Fig. 3.35 This picture, taken in the operating room, shows the three leaflets of the tricuspid valve.

THE TRICUSPID VALVE

As judged on the basis of its pattern of closure[5], the tricuspid valve has three major leaflets (Figs. 3.35, 3.36), which are supported by papillary muscles of grossly disproportionate size. The septal leaflet extends from the somewhat indistinct and inconstant inferior papillary muscle to the much more constant medial papillary muscle, also known as the muscle of Lancisi, or the papillary muscle of the

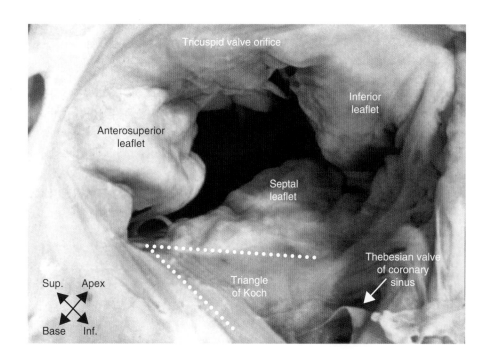

Fig. 3.36 This anatomic specimen is photographed in surgical orientation, demonstrating the leaflets of the tricuspid valve and the location of the triangle of Koch.

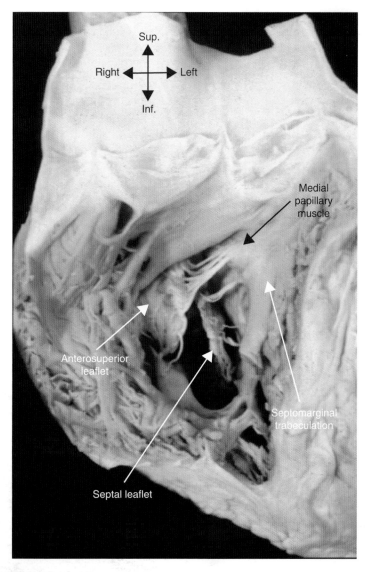

Fig. 3.37 The right ventricle is photographed from the infundibular aspect in anatomical orientation, showing the medial papillary muscle, also known as the muscle of Lancisi, supporting the superior end of the anterosuperior leaflet.

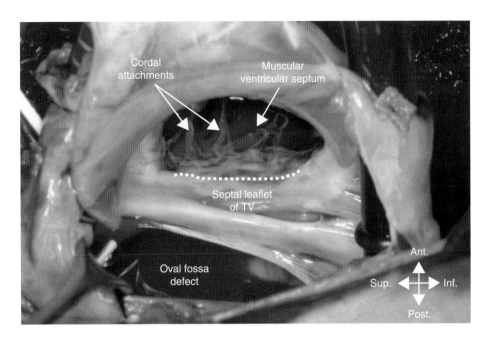

Fig. 3.38 This operative view through a right atriotomy shows the cordal attachments to the septum of the septal leaflet of the tricuspid valve. The patient also has a defect in the oval fossa.

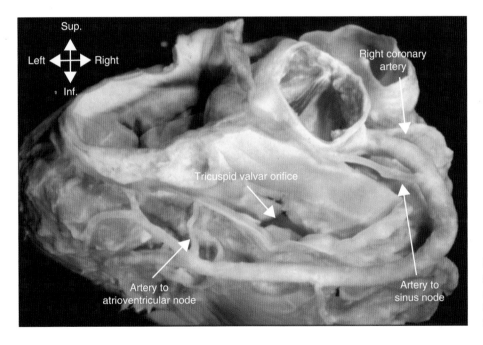

Fig. 3.39 This dissection of an anatomic specimen, photographed in anatomic orientation from above and behind, shows the relationship of the right coronary artery to the orifice of the tricuspid valve.

conus, which arises from the posterior limb of the septomarginal trabeculation (Fig. 3.37). The attachment of the septal leaflet crosses the membranous septum, dividing it into atrioventricular and interventricular components. The distal extent of the leaflet is attached by several cords running from the free edge directly to the septum (Fig. 3.38). As previously emphasised, it is this feature which serves to distinguish the valve from the leaflets of the mitral valve, which lacks any attachment to the septum. In the area where the septal leaflet extends across the membranous septum, the leaflet may be divided, resulting in a discrete cleft extending towards the central fibrous body.

The anterosuperior leaflet descends from the underside of the ventriculo-infundibular fold. It hangs like an extensive curtain between the inlet and outlet parts of the ventricle, its medial end being attached to the medial papillary muscle (Fig. 3.37). There is more variability in the arrangement of its lateral component. Usually, the end of the zone of apposition between it and the inferior leaflet is supported by the prominent anterior papillary muscle, which takes origin from the apical portion of the septomarginal trabeculation. The leaflet is then supported by cords to the free-edge, along with rough-zone and strut cords, in a fashion comparable with that seen in the aortic leaflet of the mitral valve. Less often, the anterior papillary muscle attaches directly to the midpoint of the anterosuperior leaflet. The muscle supporting the end of the zone of apposition with the inferior leaflet is then relatively indistinct. Frequently, there are extensions of muscle from either the papillary muscles or the ventriculo-infundibular fold into this leaflet.

The third leaflet of the tricuspid valve is the inferior, or mural, leaflet. It is much less constant than the other two, since the inferior papillary muscle is often indistinct and variable. The leaflet is attached to the parietal part of the atrioventricular junction, being supported distally by several cords to the free-edge attached either to small heads of muscle or directly into the ventricular wall. In terms of relationships, the entire parietal attachment of the tricuspid valve is usually encircled by the right coronary artery running in the atrioventricular groove (Fig. 3.39). As discussed, it is rare to find a well-formed collagenous tricuspid 'annulus'. Instead, the atrioventricular groove more or less folds itself directly into the leaflets of the tricuspid valve. The atrial and ventricular myocardial masses are then separated almost exclusively by the adipose tissue within the groove.

BASIC ARRANGEMENT OF THE ARTERIAL VALVES

The arterial valves are much simpler structures than the atrioventricular valves, since they do not need an intricate arrangement of tension apparatus to ensure their competence. Instead, their design is simplicity itself. There are three semilunar leaflets (Fig. 3.40). These leaflets open into the arterial sinuses during ventricular systole, and collapse together during diastole, being held in their closed position by the hydrostatic pressure of the column of blood they then support. In terms of histological structure, the leaflets have a fibrous core with an endothelial lining (Fig. 3.41). The fibrous core is thickened at the free edge, particularly at the central portion short of the free edge where, with age, a distinct fibrous nodule is seen, called the nodule of Arantius. The leaflets of the valve do not close at their free edge. Rather the closure line is some distance from the free edge, towards the semilunar attachment. Not infrequently, the leaflets may be perforated beyond the line of closure in this outer component. Such perforations

are a normal finding, and do not affect valvar function. The attached margin of the valve is of half-moon shape (Figs. 3.12 & 3.13). When the valve is removed from the heart, the seat of the leaflets is seen to be arranged in the form of a coronet (Fig. 3.42). The attachments of the leaflets at the apex of their zones of apposition are then significantly higher than the attachments at their midportion. As already discussed, the site and nature of these attachments vary from aortic to pulmonary valve, being partly fibrous in the aorta and exclusively muscular in the pulmonary trunk[2,3]. In either case, it is incorrect to describe the arterial valves as having an "annulus" or "ring"[17]. There is a true ring within the extent of the arterial root, but this ring marks the area over which the fibrous walls of the arterial trunks are attached to the supporting ventricular structures. This is the anatomic ventriculo-arterial junction. But there is then a marked discrepancy between this ring-like anatomic junction and the haemodynamic junction, the latter being marked by the semilunar attachment of the leaflets (Figs. 3.12 & 3.13). By virtue of this arrangement, part of the arterial

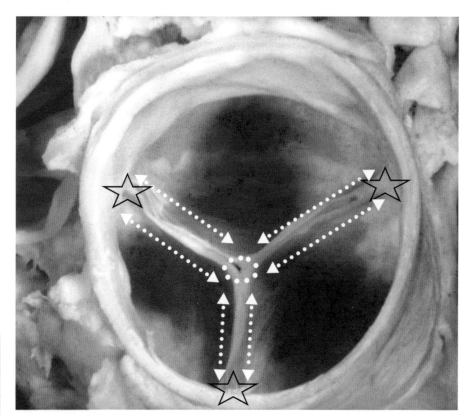

Fig. 3.40 This view of the aortic valve from above shows the valvar leaflets coapting snugly, held together by the diastolic pressure of the column of blood they support. The stars mark the peripheral attachments of the ones of apposition (white dotted lines) to the sinutubular junction, with the dotted circle showing the centroid of the valvar orifice.

wall is, haemodynamically, a ventricular structure. Part of the ventricle at the base of each sinus is, in contrast, within the arterial trunk. The zones of apposition in the arterial valves, traditionally termed the commissures, are directly comparable to those in the atrioventricular valves. They are simply the points of abutment of the semilunar leaflets, albeit that the peripheral attachments at the sinutubular junction mark a second well-formed ring at the top of the arterial root (Figs. 3.40, 3.42).

Also of significance in the normal functioning of the arterial valves are the sinuses located at the commencement of the arterial trunks. These dilations are arranged in clover-like fashion, permitting the valvar leaflets to close in the fashion of a Mercedes-Benz sign (Fig. 3.40). The valvar leaflets retract into the sinuses during ventricular systole so that there is unrestricted blood flow from ventricle to arterial trunk. Two of the aortic sinuses

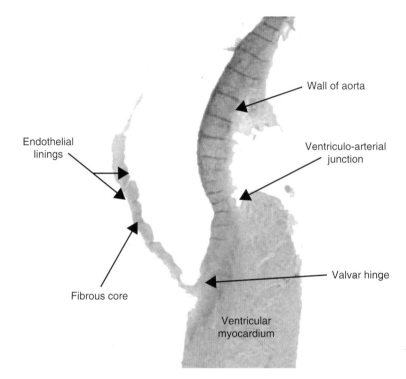

Wall of aorta

Endothelial linings

Ventriculo-arterial junction

Valvar hinge

Fibrous core

Ventricular myocardium

Fig. 3.41 The histological section shows the fibrous core of one leaflet of the aortic valves, with its endothelial linings on the arterial and ventricular aspects. Note that the valvar hinge is well below the anatomic ventriculo-arterial junction.

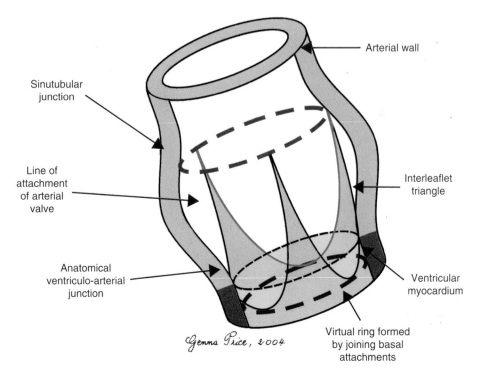

Sinutubular junction

Arterial wall

Line of attachment of arterial valve

Interleaflet triangle

Anatomical ventriculo-arterial junction

Ventricular myocardium

Virtual ring formed by joining basal attachments

Gemma Price, 2004

Fig. 3.42 The cartoon shows how the idealised arterial valve takes the form of a three-pronged crown when viewed in three dimensions. The base of the crown is a virtual ring, but the top of the crown is a true ring, the sinutubular junction, whilst the semilunar line of the attachments of the leaflets crosses an additional ring, the anatomic ventriculo-arterial junction.

are particularly significant, since they give rise to the major coronary arteries. The coronary arterial origin is usually within the sinus, beneath the sinutubular junction. There is, nonetheless, quite some variability in origin of the coronary arteries (see Chapter 4). The account thus far has presumed the presence of three leaflets of the arterial valve. In some instances, valves are found with four leaflets in either aortic or pulmonary position[18,19]. The variation that is of more significance is a valve with two leaflets, either in aortic[20] or pulmonary[3] position. These are congenital lesions of note. The bifoliate aortic valve is probably the most common congenital cardiac malformation[14].

THE AORTIC VALVE

As has already been described, the semilunar leaflets of the aortic valve are attached in part to the fibrous skeleton, and in part to the muscular outlet portion of the left ventricle (Fig. 3.43). When naming the aortic leaflets, advantage can be taken of the fact that, almost without exception, the major coronary arteries take origin from two of the aortic sinuses, but not the third. Thus, the aortic leaflets can accurately be described as being right coronary, left coronary, and non-coronary in position. It is the right and left coronary leaflets that have a predominantly muscular origin from the left ventricular

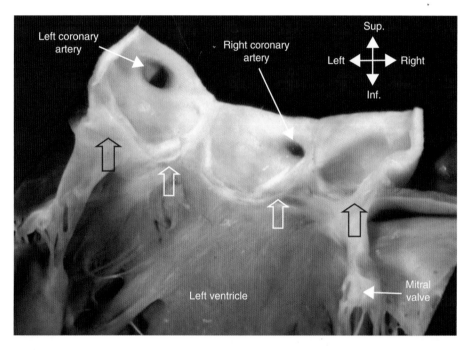

Fig. 3.43 The aortic root has been displayed by removing the leaflets of the aortic valve, having opened the outflow tract between the left coronary and the non-coronary aortic leaflets. The two sinuses giving rise to the coronary arteries have septal musculature at their base (white arrows), while part of the left coronary sinus, along with the non-coronary sinus, are supported by fibrous continuity with the aortic leaflet of the mitral valve (blue arrows).

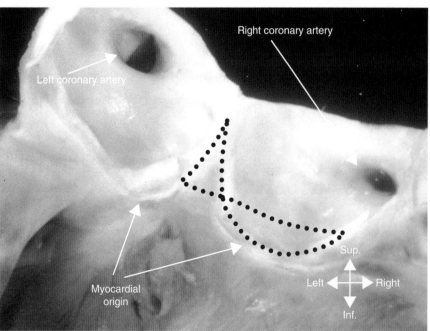

Fig. 3.44 The close-up of the right coronary sinus from the dissection shown in Fig. 3.43 shows the fibrous triangle rising to the sinutubular junction, and the crescent of musculature at the base of the sinus (dotted lines).

wall, the base of the myocardium being incorporated within the supporting aortic sinus (Fig. 3.44). These leaflets face the pulmonary trunk. Their more distal adjacent parts take origin from the free aortic wall. They face the potential space between it and the pulmonary infundibulum and trunk.

As the attachment of the right coronary leaflet is traced from its zone of apposition with the left coronary leaflet, it drops towards the crest of the muscular part of the septum in the area of the membranous septum. It then rises again to the apex of the zone of apposition with the non-coronary leaflet. The attachment of this posterior part of the right coronary leaflet is an integral part of the fibrous skeleton. All of the non-coronary leaflet has a fibrous origin, and is incorporated in the fibrous skeleton. Half of it, extending from the zone of apposition with the right coronary leaflet, is attached to the area of the membranous septum (Fig. 3.45). The

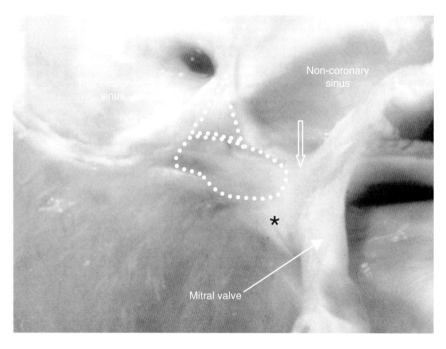

Fig. 3.45 This close-up of the triangle between the right coronary aortic leaflet and the non-coronary leaflet shows the interventricular part of the membranous septum (dotted white oval), the atrioventricular part (blue asterisk), and the apex of the triangle rising to the sinutubular junction (white dotted triangle). The white arrow shows the continuity with the aortic leaflet of the mitral valve. The view showing this area from the right side subsequent to its removal is shown in Fig. 3.5.

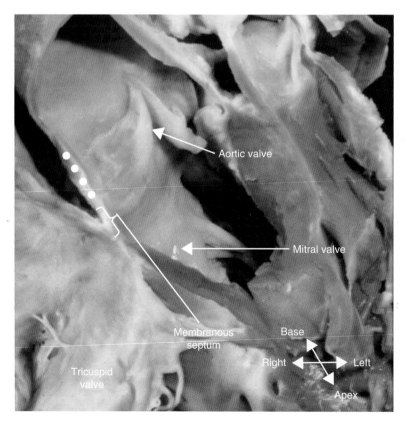

Fig. 3.46 This dissection shows the relationships between the fibrous triangle between the right and non-coronary leaflets of the aortic valve, which is in the plane of the section, to the right atrium and right ventricle. The dotted line shows the apex of the triangle, which separates the left ventricular outflow tract from the transverse sinus.

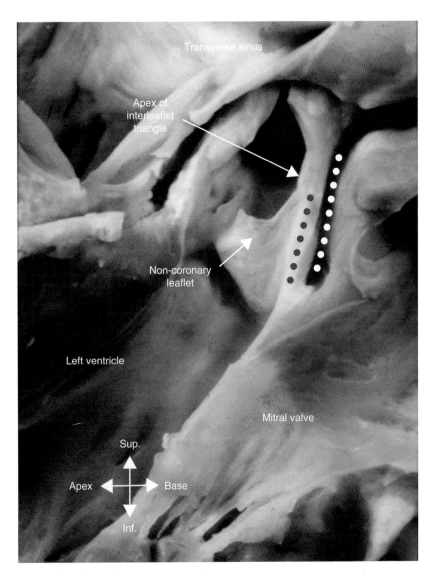

Transverse sinus

Apex of
interleaflet
triangle

Non-coronary
leaflet

Left ventricle

Mitral valve

Sup.

Apex ←→ Base

Inf.

Fig. 3.47 The left ventricular outflow tract in this heart is bisected through the fibrous triangle between the non- and left coronary aortic leaflets. The fibrous wall (red dotted line) separates the outflow tract from the transverse sinus (white dotted line).

triangle between these leaflets has important relationships to both right atrium and right ventricle (Fig. 3.46). The extensive posterior extension, or diverticulum, of the left ventricular outflow tract lies beneath the non-coronary leaflet, limited anterolaterally by the atrioventricular component of the membranous septum. Reaching its nadir at the attachment to the right fibrous trigone, the non-coronary leaflet then rises to the apex of its zone of apposition with the left coronary leaflet. The apex of the triangle between these leaflets is in close relationship with the transverse sinus (Fig. 3.47). The adjacent parts of both leaflets in this area are attached to the free aortic wall distally, and proximally are continuous with the

aortic leaflet of the mitral valve. In this way, they form the aortic–mitral curtain. As indicated, the curtain separates the left ventricular outflow tract not from the left atrium, but from the transverse sinus of the pericardium. Thus, cutting through the fibrous curtain takes the surgeon outside the heart and into the transverse sinus of the pericardial cavity (Fig. 3.47). Beyond this area, the left coronary leaflet then adjoins a short segment of parietal myocardium before extending anteriorly to reach the zone of apposition with the right coronary leaflet. The apex of this interleaflet triangle 'points' to the space between aorta and pulmonary trunk (Fig. 3.48). The trough of the attachment of the left coronary leaflet is related to the area of the left fibrous

trigone, and to the parietal wall of the left ventricle, while the anterior ascending component runs onto the free aortic wall posterior and superior to the ventricular septum. The precise attachments of the aortic leaflets vary from heart to heart, particularly with regard to that portion of the zone of apposition between the non-coronary and left coronary leaflets which is related to the aortic–mitral curtain. The length of the subaortic fibrous curtain also varies from heart to heart. In a small percentage of normal hearts, the aortic valve in this area is supported by a complete muscular infundibulum or sleeve[21]. These individual variations do not distort the basic anatomical relationships as described above.

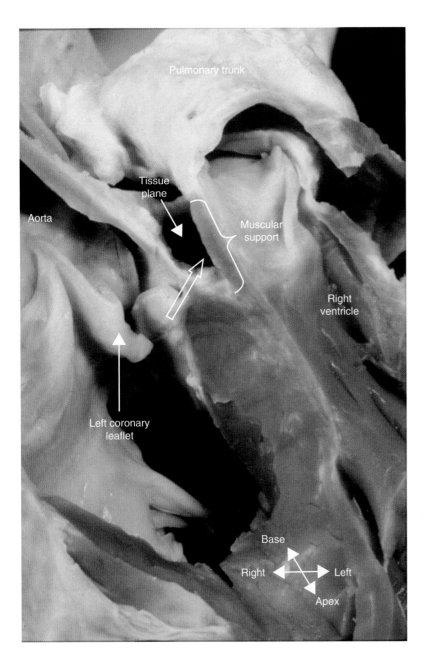

Labels on image: Pulmonary trunk, Tissue plane, Aorta, Muscular support, Right ventricle, Left coronary leaflet, Base, Right, Left, Apex

Fig. 3.48 In this heart, a window has been cut through the posterior wall of the free-standing subpulmonary infundibulum, extending into the left ventricular outflow tract. The superior border of the window passes through the fibrous triangle that separates the two coronary leaflets of the aortic valve. The tip of the fibrous triangle (white arrow) separates the cavity of the left ventricle from the tissue plane between the aortic sinuses and the free-standing subpulmonary infundibulum (white bracket).

The non-coronary leaflet is attached above the extensive posterior diverticulum of the outflow tract. This is the part of the valve directly related to the right atrial wall. From the inferior attachment of the non-coronary leaflet in relation to the right atrium, the valve tents up again to the zone of apposition between the non-coronary and right coronary leaflets. Consequently, the ascending part of the non-coronary leaflet is then positioned directly above the part of the atrial wall containing the atrioventricular node, while the zone of apposition itself is above the penetrating atrioventricular bundle and the membranous septum (Fig. 3.49). The zone of apposition between the right coronary and left coronary leaflets is usually positioned opposite the corresponding zone of apposition between the facing leaflets of the pulmonary valve. The adjacent parts of the two aortic coronary leaflets, therefore, are attached to the outlet part of the ventricular septum, and are thus directly related to the infundibulum of the right ventricle, albeit that a discrete extracardiac tissue plane interposes between them (Fig. 3.48). Incisions through the right ventricular outflow tract at this site, nonetheless, lead directly into the subaortic region (Fig. 3.50). This is the basis of the right ventricular approach for relief of subaortic obstruction. Beyond this point, the lateral part of the left coronary leaflet is the only part of the aortic valve not intimately related to another cardiac chamber. This is the part of the valve that takes origin from the lateral margin of the inner heart curvature. It is, consequently, in relationship externally with the free pericardial space.

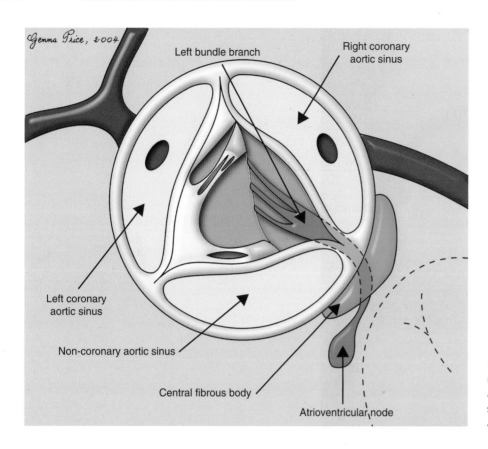

Fig. 3.49 This cartoon shows the relationships of the atrioventricular node and penetrating bundle as they would be seen by the surgeon working through the aortic valve.

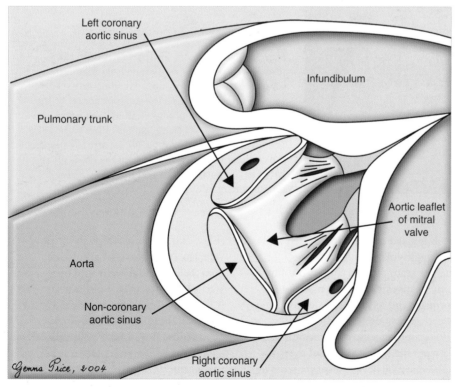

Fig. 3.50 This cartoon shows how an incision through the posterior wall of the subpulmonary infundibulum takes the surgeon into the subaortic outflow tract, the incision in the infundibular wall being carried into the muscular ventricular septum, and entering the left ventricular outflow tract between the two aortic sinuses giving origin to the coronary arteries.

THE PULMONARY VALVE

The pulmonary valve in the normal heart has exclusively muscular attachments to the infundibulum of the right ventricle (Fig. 3.51). Because of its oblique position, there is difficulty in naming the pulmonary leaflets according to the body co-ordinates. It is better to describe them according to their relationship to the aortic valve. As discussed above, the two leaflets of the aortic valve attached to the

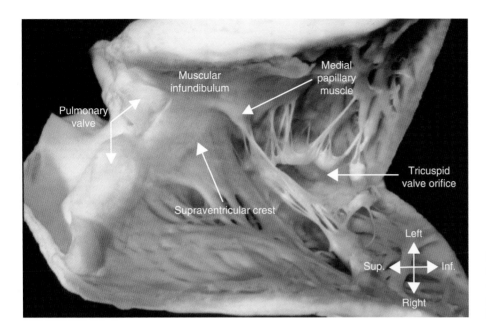

Fig. 3.51 This heart is opened along the parietal wall of the right ventricle, but orientated in surgical fashion. It shows how all leaflets of the pulmonary valve are supported by infundibular musculature, known as the supraventricular crest.

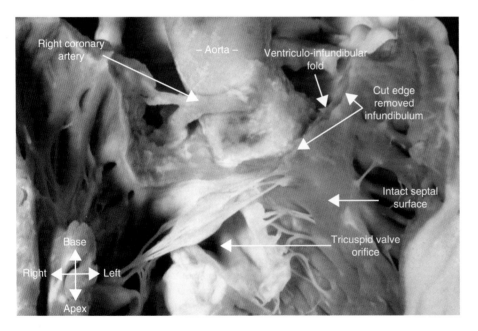

Fig. 3.52 The sleeve of subpulmonary infundibulum has been removed in this heart, positioned in anatomical orientation, showing the relationship to the aorta and the right coronary artery.

septum always face two leaflets of the pulmonary valve. These two leaflets of the pulmonary valve, therefore, can be called the right and left facing leaflets. The third leaflet is then described simply as the non-facing leaflet. The zone of apposition between the two facing leaflets has traditionally been considered to be attached to the muscular outlet septum immediately above the anterior limb of the septomarginal trabeculation. In reality, it is attached to a free-standing sleeve of infundibular musculature (Fig. 3.48). As the right facing leaflet drops down from

the apex of its facing zone of apposition with the other facing leaflet, it is supported by the inner curve of muscle that separates it from the tricuspid valve. This muscular mass is the supraventricular crest of the right ventricle (Fig. 3.51). That particular part between the atrioventricular and arterial valves is best termed the ventriculo-infundibular fold. The zone of apposition between the right and non-facing leaflets is then towards the parietal extent of this fold, and the non-facing leaflet is supported by the anterior parietal wall of

the infundibulum. The zone of apposition between the non-facing and left facing leaflets extends from the parietal attachment back towards the septum, so that the left facing leaflet runs from the parietal wall to the area of the septum. When considered as a whole, the valve can be liberated from the right ventricle together with its infundibular sleeve without damaging any vital structures (Figs. 3.52, 3.53). This is the feature which underscores the success of the Ross procedure[22].

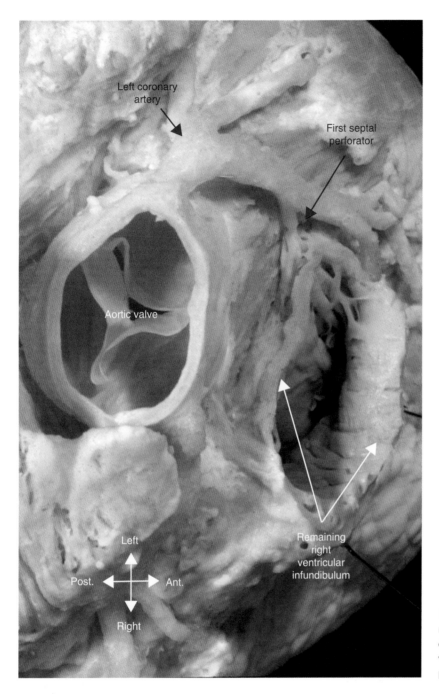

Left coronary artery

First septal perforator

Aortic valve

Left

Post. ◀▶ Ant.

Right

Remaining right ventricular infundibulum

Fig. 3.53 The subpulmonary infundibulum has been removed completely in this heart, showing how this can be achieved without transgressing on the left ventricle. Note the location of the first septal perforating artery.

RELATIONSHIPS OF THE VALVES TO OTHER VITAL CARDIAC STRUCTURES

As we have already discussed, positioned as they are mostly within the atrioventricular junctions, the tricuspid, mitral, and aortic valves are intimately related to two vital cardiac subsystems, namely the atrioventricular conduction system and the coronary circulation. It is mandatory to avoid damage to these structures during surgery, so it is important to know their precise locations. This must be learned relative to landmarks within the valves themselves, since the conduction tissues are largely invisible, and the course of the coronary vessels is likely to be hidden as the surgeon approaches the valves. Although we have mentioned these landmarks when discussing the individual valves, their importance is such that they justify a collective review.

THE SPECIALISED MUSCULAR AXIS FOR ATRIOVENTRICULAR CONDUCTION

In the normal heart, the penetrating atrioventricular bundle is the only muscular communication between the atrial and ventricular muscle masses. Since the bundle penetrates through the membranous septal component of the central fibrous body, it is, of necessity, intimately related to the leaflets of the mitral, tricuspid, and

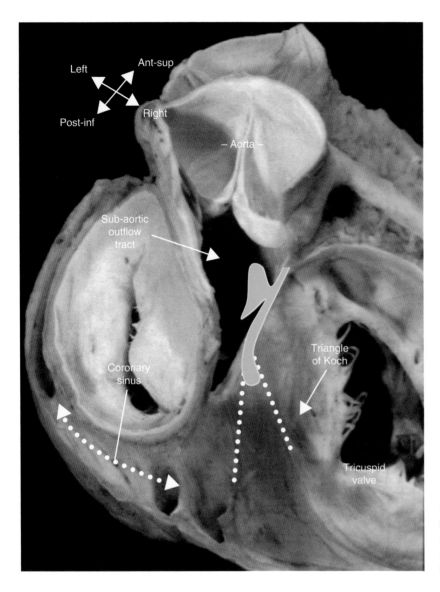

Fig. 3.54 The location of the conduction axis (green with yellow border) is superimposed on this dissection made by removing the non-coronary sinus and leaflet of the aortic valve. Note the location of the coronary sinus in the left atrioventricular groove.

aortic valves. The conduction axis takes its origin from the atrioventricular node and its atrial zones of transitional cells. The danger area for these atrial components of the conduction axis is contained exclusively within the triangle of Koch (see Chapter 5). The inferior extent of the triangle is the junctional attachment of the septal leaflet of the tricuspid valve. As the axis penetrates the septum, it immediately enters the subaortic region of the left ventricle (Fig. 3.54). The point of penetration is related to the anteroinferior end of the zone of apposition between the leaflets of the mitral valve. In this area, the atrioventricular node lies within 5 to 10 millimetres of the atrial attachment of the medial scallop

of the mural leaflet. Having reached the left ventricular outflow tract, the conduction axis begins to branch, either on the crest of the muscular ventricular septum, sandwiched between it and the interventricular membranous septum, or on the left ventricular aspect of the septum. This area is immediately beneath the zone of apposition between the non-coronary and right coronary leaflets of the aortic valve, but the height of the interleaflet fibrous triangle separates the valvar attachments from the conduction axis. When seen from the left ventricle, the left bundle branch fans out as a continuous sheet on the smooth left septal surface beneath the zone of apposition, splitting into its three divisions as it

approaches the ventricular apex. The right bundle branch is the continuation of the axis beyond the branching bundle. This dips back across the septum as a thin, insulated cord that emerges on the right ventricular aspect in the area of the medial papillary muscle. It then runs, usually intramyocardially, within the structure of the septomarginal trabeculation to ramify at the ventricular apex. When considered from the right side, the site of the branching segment of the conduction axis can be imagined as a line joining the apex of the triangle of Koch to the medial papillary muscle. This is a relatively safe area for the surgeon, since the axis is carried on the left side of the septum. Nonetheless, the axis is within 5 millimetres of the right ventricular septal surface.

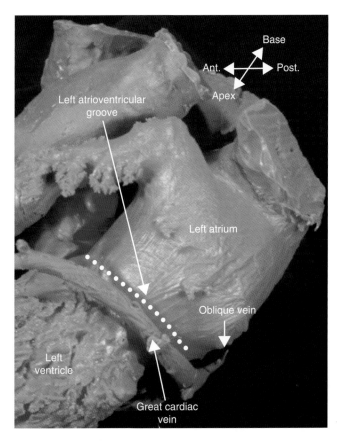

Fig. 3.55 This cast shows the location of the great cardiac vein in the left atrioventricular groove (white dotted line). The vein does not become the coronary sinus until it receives the oblique vein of the left atrium.

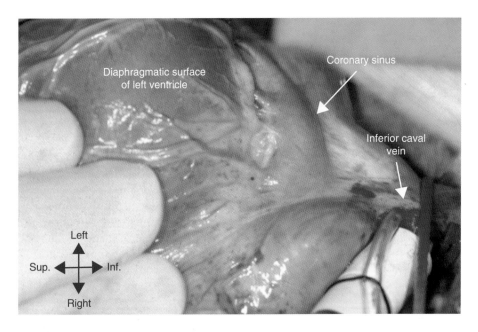

Fig. 3.56 This operative view, taken through a median sternotomy, with the surgeon having reflected the heart, shows the position of the coronary sinus in the inferior atrioventricular groove.

THE VULNERABLE CORONARY CIRCULATION

On the venous side of the circulation, the coronary sinus is the only noteworthy structure related to the valves. The great cardiac vein runs within the left atrioventricular groove, receiving the oblique vein as it turns into the inferior part of the groove (Fig. 3.55). This confluence marks the beginning of coronary sinus, which proceeds in the fatty tissue of the inferior atrioventricular groove to empty into the right atrium (Fig. 3.56). In its course in an adult, it may approach to within five to fifteen millimetres of the medial attachment of the mural leaflet of the mitral valve.

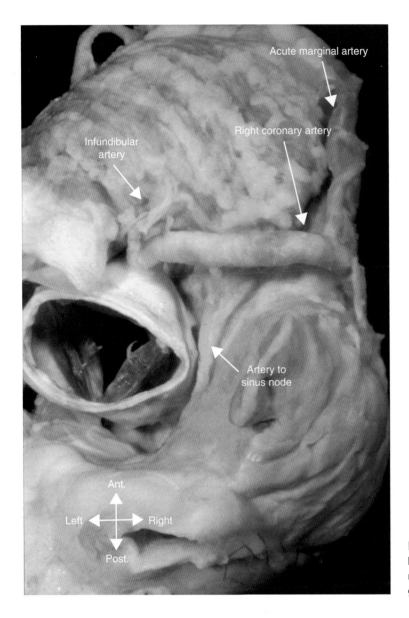

Acute marginal artery

Right coronary artery

Infundibular artery

Artery to sinus node

Ant.

Left ← → Right

Post.

Fig. 3.57 This heart is photographed from above and behind to show the right coronary artery emerging from the right coronary aortic sinus to enter the right atrioventricular groove immediately superior to the supraventricular crest.

Deeply placed sutures in this area during replacement of the mitral valve may lead to damage to the coronary sinus. This can cause extremely troublesome bleeding. Also, when removing a previously placed mitral valvar prosthesis, care must be taken not to enter the sinus with scalpel or suture. The normal anatomy may well have been distorted by the earlier operation.

The coronary arteries are intimately related to both the mitral and tricuspid valves, since much of their course is within the atrioventricular grooves. The main stem of the left coronary artery branches in the angle of the margin of the left-sided ventriculo–infundibular fold immediately above the left fibrous trigone. The anterior interventricular artery moves away from the valves, although its septal perforating branches extend into the septum immediately beneath the left facing leaflet of the pulmonary valve. This important artery could be damaged by extensive dissection in this area. It is the circumflex branch of the left coronary artery that is most intimately related to the mitral valve, particularly when the left coronary artery is dominant. When the right coronary artery is dominant, that is, gives rise to the inferior interventricular artery, as it does in about 90% of cases, the circumflex artery is related only to the area around the lateral scallop of the mural leaflet of the mitral valve (Fig. 3.32). When the circumflex branch becomes the inferior interventricular artery, its entire course is intimately related to the entirety of the mural leaflet (Fig. 3.34).

The right coronary artery always runs a circumferential course around the mural attachments of the tricuspid valve. The initial course of the artery is through the right atrioventricular groove (Fig. 3.57), where it lies on the epicardial aspect of the ventriculo-infundibular fold. It can be damaged by deeply placed sutures in this area[23]. The artery then encircles the attachment of the mural leaflet of the tricuspid valve before, in the majority of cases, turning to become the inferior interventricular artery. Just prior to its descent, the right coronary artery, when dominant, takes a prominent U-loop beneath

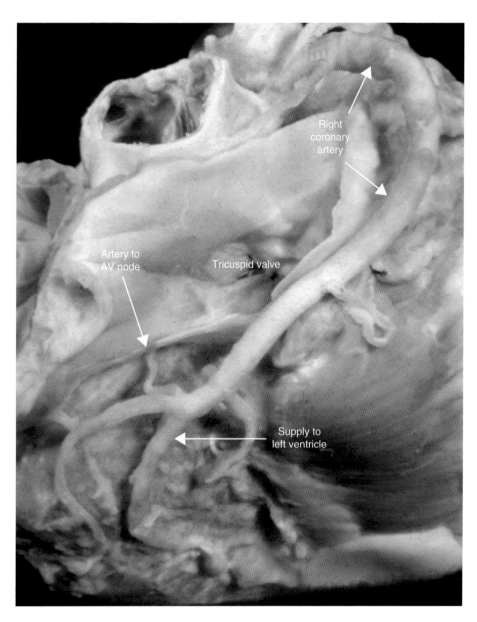

Fig. 3.58 This dissection, photographed from behind and beneath with the heart in anatomic position, shows the dominant right coronary artery giving rise to the artery to the atrioventricular node at the crux, before it continues into the left atrioventricular groove to give branches to the diaphragmatic surface of the left ventricle.

the floor of the coronary sinus, giving off the artery to the atrioventricular node at the apex of the loop (Fig. 3.58). In cases where the circumflex artery gives rise to the inferior interventricular artery, then the atrioventricular nodal artery originates from the circumflex artery (Fig. 3.34). Whether arising from a dominant left or right coronary artery, this small but important vessel is related to the inferior aspect of the annular attachment of the septal leaflet of the tricuspid valve.

References

1. Angelini A, Ho SY, Anderson RH, Davies MJ, Becker AE. A histological study of the atrioventricular junction in hearts with normal and prolapsed leaflets of the mitral valve. *Br Heart J* 1988; **59**: 712–716.

2. Sutton JPIII, Ho SY, Anderson RH. The forgotten interleaflet triangles: A review of the surgical anatomy of the aortic valve. *Ann Thorac Surg* 1995; **59**: 419–427.

3. Stamm C, Anderson RH, Ho SY. Clinical anatomy of the normal pulmonary root compared with that in isolated pulmonary valvular stenosis. *J Am Coll Cardiol* 1998; **31**: 1420–1425.

4. Victor S, Nayak VM. The tricuspid valve is bicuspid. *J Heart Valve Dis* 1994; **3**: 27–36.

5. Sutton JP111, Ho Sy, Vogel M, Anderson RH. Is the morphologically right atrioventricular valve tricuspid? *J Heart Valve Dis* 1995; **4**: 571–575.

6. Yacoub M. Anatomy of the mitral valve chordae and cusps. In: Kalmason D (ed). *The Mitral Valve. A Pluridisciplinary Approach*. London: Edward Arnold. 1976; pp 15–20.

7. Kumar N, Kumar M, Duran CM. A revised terminology for recording surgical findings of the mitral valve. *J Heart Valve Dis* 1995; **4**: 76–77.

8. Lam JHC, Ranganathan N, Wigle ED, Silver MD. Morphology of the human mitral valve. I. Chordae tendineae: a new classification. *Circulation* 1970; **41**: 449–458.

9. Van Praagh R, David I, Wright G B, Van Praagh S. Large RV plus small LV is not single RV. *Circulation* 1980; **61**: 1057–1058.

10. Frater R. Anatomy and physiology of the normal mitral valve. (Discussion) In: Kalmanson D (ed), *The Mitral Valve*. London: Edward Arnold. 1976; p 41.

11. Becker AE, de Wit APM. Mitral valve apparatus. A spectrum of normality relevant to mitral valve prolapse. *Br Heart J* 1979; **42**: 680–689.

12. Van der Bel-Kahn J, Duren DR, Becker AE. Isolated mitral valve prolapse: chordal architecture as an anatomic basis in older patients. *J Am Coll Cardiol* 1985; **5**: 1335–1340.

13. Perloff JK, Roberts WC. The mitral apparatus. Functional anatomy of mitral regurgitation. *Circulation* 1972; **46**: 227–239.

14. Roberts WC. The 2 most common congenital heart diseases. (Editorial) *Am J Cardiol* 1984; **53**: 1198.

15. Carpentier A, Branchini B, Cour JC, et al Congenital malformations of the mitral valve in children. Pathology and surgical treatment. *J Thorac Cardiovasc Surg* 1976; **72**: 854–866

16. Victor S, Nayak VM. Definition and function of commissures, slits and scallops of the mitral valve: analysis in 100 hearts. *AustralAs J Cardiac Thorac Surg* 1994; **3**: 8–16.

17. Anderson RH, Devine WA, Ho SY, Smith A, McKay R. The myth of the aortic annulus: the anatomy of the subaortic outflow tract. *Ann Thor Surg* 1991; **52**: 640–646.

18. Becker AE. Quadricuspid pulmonary valve. Anatomical observations in 20 hearts. *Acta Morphol Neerl Scand* 1972; **10**: 299–309.

19. Feldman BJ, Khandheria BK, Warnes CA, Seward JB, Taylor CL, Tajik AJ. Incidence, description and functional assessment of isolated quadricuspid aortic valves. *Am J Cardiol* 1990; **65**: 937–938.

20. Angelini A, Ho SY, Anderson RH, Devine WA, Zuberbuhler JR, Becker AE, Davies MJ. The morphology of the normal aortic valve as compared with the aortic valve having two leaflets. *J Thorac Cardiovasc Surg* 1989; **98**: 362–367.

21. Rosenquist GC, Clark EB, Sweeny LJ, McAllister HA. The normal spectrum of mitral and aortic valve discontinuity. *Circulation* 1976; **54**: 298–301.

22. Merrick AF, Yacoub MH, Ho SY, Anderson RH. Anatomy of the muscular subpulmonary infundibulum with regard to the Ross procedure. *Ann Thorac Surg* 2000; **69**: 556–561.

23. McFadden PM, Culpepper WS III, Ochsner JL. Iatrogenic right ventricular failure in tetralogy of Fallot repairs: reappraisal of a distressing problem. *Ann Thorac Surg* 1982; **33**: 400–402.

4

Surgical anatomy of the coronary circulation

The coronary circulation consists of the coronary arteries and veins, together with the lymphatics of the heart. Since the lymphatics, apart from the thoracic duct, are of very limited significance to operative anatomy, they will not be discussed further in this chapter. The veins, relatively speaking, are similarly of less interest, so this chapter is concentrated upon those anatomic aspects of arterial distribution that are pertinent to the surgeon.

THE CORONARY ARTERIES

The coronary arteries are the first branches of the ascending portion of the aorta, arising from the aortic root immediately above its attachment to the heart (Fig. 4.1). Normally, there are three sinuses at the aortic root, but only two coronary arteries. The sinuses can be named, therefore, according to whether or not they give rise to an artery, the normal arrangement being a right coronary, left coronary, and non-coronary aortic sinus (Fig. 4.2). In this respect, the terms 'right' and 'left' refer to the coronary sinuses giving rise to the right and left coronary arteries, rather than to the position of the sinuses relative to the right-left coordinates of the body. In the normal heart, the aortic root is obliquely situated, while, in malformed hearts, the root is frequently abnormally positioned. Whatever the position of the aortic root, however, almost always the two coronary arteries, when two are present, take origin from those aortic sinuses that are adjacent to the sinuses of the pulmonary trunk. Because of this, it is more convenient, and more accurate, to term these sinuses the left hand and right hand adjacent, or facing, sinuses, taking as the point of reference the observer standing within the non-adjacent sinus and looking towards the pulmonary trunk (Fig. 4.3). This convention, introduced by the group from Leiden[1], holds true irrespective of the relationships of the arterial trunks. It has now become convention to describe the right-handed sinus as "#1", and to distinguish the left hand sinus as "#2". The value of this convention will become evident when we discuss coronary arterial origins in malformed hearts (see Chapter 8). The coronary arteries usually arise from the aortic sinuses beneath the sinutubular junction, or aortic bar, the discrete transition between the aortic root and the tubular component of the ascending aorta (Fig. 4.4). The free edge of the leaflets of the aortic valve usually opens against this circular junction during ventricular systole. Deviations of origin of the coronary arteries relative to the junction are not uncommon[2]. When arising above the junction, they are considered abnormal only when they are more than one centimetre from the bar. According to Bader[3], this occurs in almost one-twentieth of normal hearts. The arterial opening can be deviated either toward the ventricle, so that the artery arises deep within the aortic sinus, or towards the aortic arch, so that the origin is outside the sinus (Fig. 4.5). Such displacement may lead to the artery taking an oblique course through the aortic wall, typically crossing the attachment of the zone of apposition between adjacent leaflets, a so-called intramural arrangement. This introduces the potential for luminal narrowing, and may provoke disturbances in myocardial perfusion[4].

The left coronary artery almost always takes origin from a single orifice within the left hand facing sinus. In contrast, in about half of all hearts, there are two orifices within the right hand facing sinus. In such instances, the orifices are unequal in size, the larger giving rise to the main trunk of the right coronary artery, while the considerably smaller second orifice usually gives rise to an infundibular artery, or rarely to the artery supplying the sinus node. In the series reported by Becker[5],

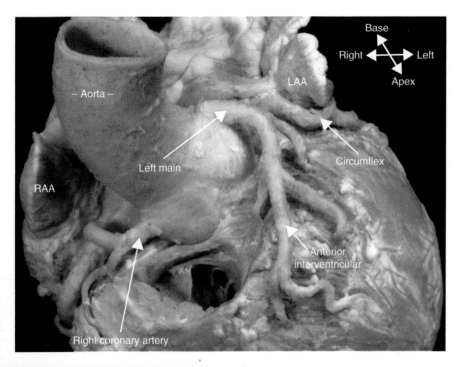

Base

Right ⟷ Left

Apex

LAA

– Aorta –

Left main

Circumflex

RAA

Anterior
interventricular

Right coronary artery

Fig. 4.1 The heart has been dissected by removing the subpulmonary infundibulum. It is photographed in anatomical orientation to show the origin of the coronary arteries from the aortic root. RAA, LAA = right and left atrial appendages.

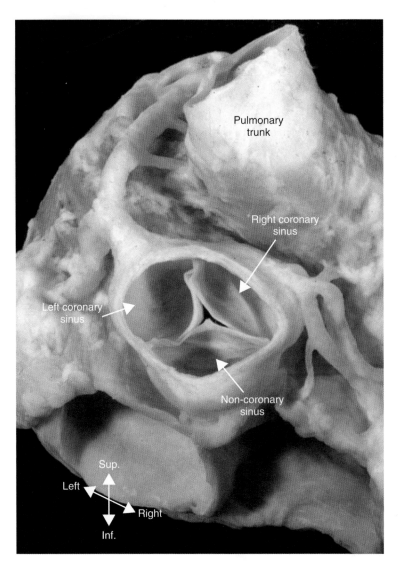

Fig. 4.2 The heart is photographed from above in anatomical orientation after removal of the atrial myocardium and the arterial trunks. It can be seen that two sinuses of the aortic valve give rise to coronary arteries, permitting them to be named as the right and left aortic coronary sinuses. The other sinus is the non-coronary sinus.

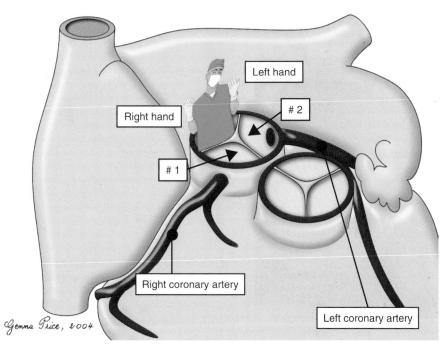

Fig. 4.3 This cartoon demonstrates the basis of the so-called Leiden convention. The surgeon stands, figuratively speaking, in the non-coronary sinus and looks towards the pulmonary trunk. Of the sinuses adjacent to the pulmonary trunk, one is then to the left hand. This is sinus #2. The other sinus, to the right hand, is sinus #1. Almost without exception, the coronary arteries take origin from one, or both, of these sinuses. In the usual arrangement, the right coronary artery arises from sinus #1, and the main stem of the left coronary artery from sinus #2.

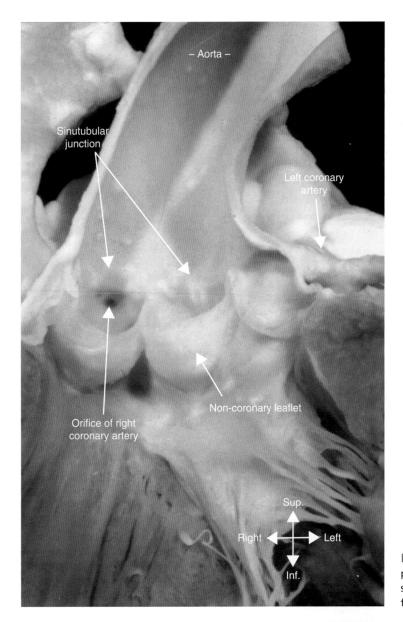

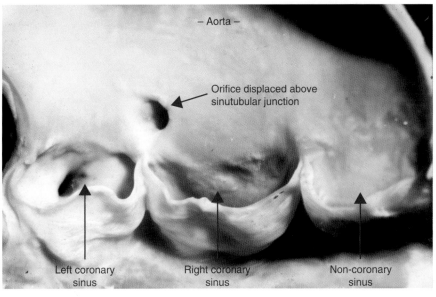

Fig. 4.4 The aortic root is opened from the front, and photographed in anatomic orientation, to show the sinutubular junction. Note the origin of the coronary arteries from the aortic sinuses immediately beneath the junction.

Fig. 4.5 In this heart, the aortic valve has been opened and the aortic root photographed from the front in anatomic orientation. The right coronary artery arises well above the sinutubular junction. Reproduced by kind permission of Professor Anton Becker, University of Amsterdam.

two orifices were found in the right hand facing sinus in 46 percent of cases, three orifices in 7 percent, and four orifices in 2 percent. These multiple orifices are of little surgical significance. In contrast, multiple orifices in the left hand facing sinus, although considerably more rare, being found in only eight of the 4250 patients reported by Engel and his colleagues[6], do have clinical significance. If unrecognised, they may create problems in the interpretation of coronary angiograms.

The coronary arteries can also arise, though very rarely, from a solitary orifice. This is usually within the right hand facing sinus. The artery supplied from the solitary orifice can take one of two patterns. It can divide immediately into right and left coronary arteries (Fig. 4.6). The left artery then passes either in front of or behind the pulmonary trunk, before dividing into anterior interventricular, or descending, and circumflex branches (Fig. 4.7). Alternatively, and less frequently, the single

artery initially follows the path of the normal right coronary artery. It then continues beyond the crux, encircling the mitral orifice through the territory usually supplied by the circumflex artery, before terminating as the anterior interventricular coronary artery (Fig. 4.8).

The epicardial course of the major coronary arteries follows the atrioventricular and interventricular grooves. The right coronary artery emerges from the right hand facing aortic

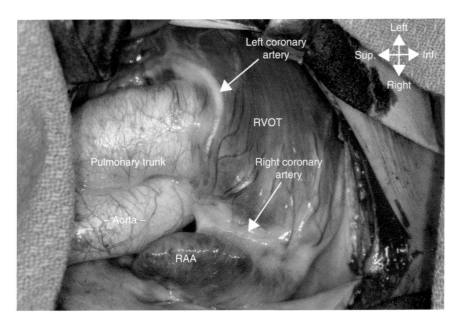

Fig. 4.6 This operative view, seen through a median sternotomy, shows a solitary coronary artery taking origin from the right hand aortic sinus (#1). It divides immediately into right and left branches, with the main stem of the left coronary artery crossing the subpulmonary infundibulum.

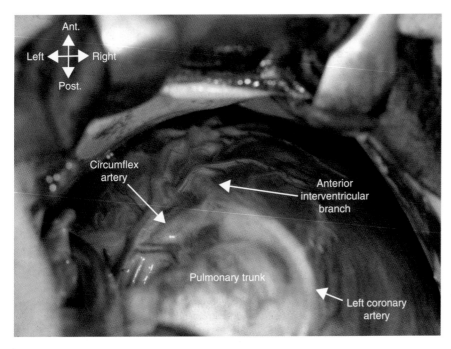

Fig. 4.7 A further view of the heart shown in Fig. 4.6 shows that the main stem of the left coronary artery, having crossed the subpulmonary infundibulum, divides into the anterior interventricular and the circumflex arteries.

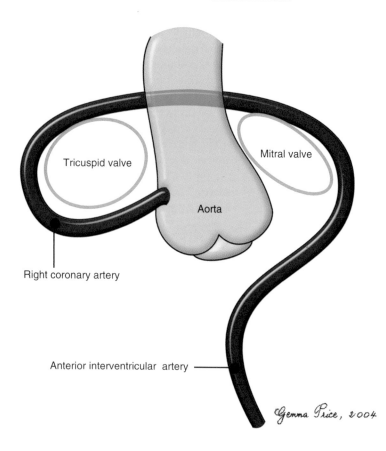

Tricuspid valve

Mitral valve

Aorta

Right coronary artery

Anterior interventricular artery

Gemma Price, 2004

Fig. 4.8 This cartoon, drawn in anatomic orientation, shows the arrangement in which a single coronary artery, having originated from the right coronary aortic sinus (#1), encircles both atrioventricular grooves. It encircles the tricuspid valve in the location of the right coronary artery, runs round the mitral valvar orifice in the course of the circumflex artery, and terminates as the anterior interventricular artery.

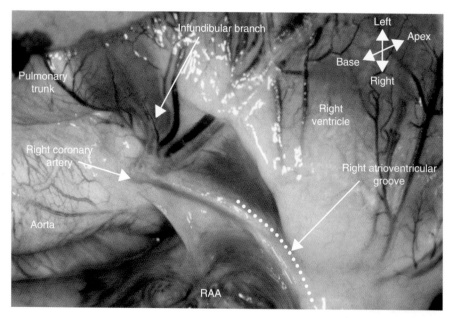

Fig. 4.9 In this operative view, seen through a median sternotomy, the right coronary artery emerges from its sinus into the right atrioventricular groove and immediately gives rise to an infundibular branch. RAA = right atrial appendage.

sinus and immediately enters the right atrioventricular groove (Fig. 4.9). It then encircles the tricuspid orifice within the fat pad of the groove (Fig. 4.10). In approximately nine-tenths of cases, the right coronary artery gives rise to an inferior interventricular artery at the crux, albeit that the artery is usually said to be posterior. In a good proportion of these cases, the artery then continues beyond the crux, where it supplies down going branches to the diaphragmatic surface of the left ventricle (Fig. 4.11). This is right coronary arterial dominance. As the artery encircles the tricuspid orifice, it is most closely related to the origin of the leaflets of the tricuspid valve near the take-off of its acute marginal branch. Other important branches also take origin from this encircling segment of the artery. Immediately after its origin, the artery is within the ventriculo–infundibular fold, where it gives rise to down going infundibular branches, which may also

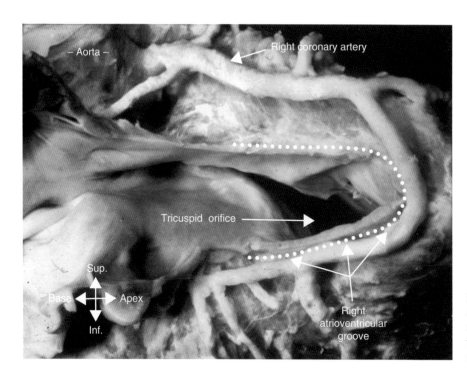

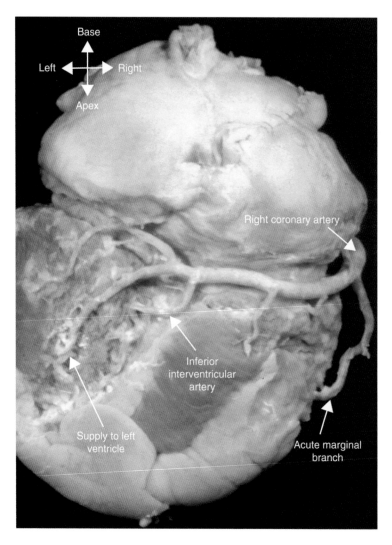

Fig. 4.10 This dissection, photographed in anatomic orientation from above and behind, shows the right coronary artery encircling the tricuspid orifice and running within the right atrioventricular groove (dotted line).

Fig. 4.11 This view of the diaphragmatic surface of the heart, shown in anatomical orientation, reveals the distribution of a dominant right coronary artery.

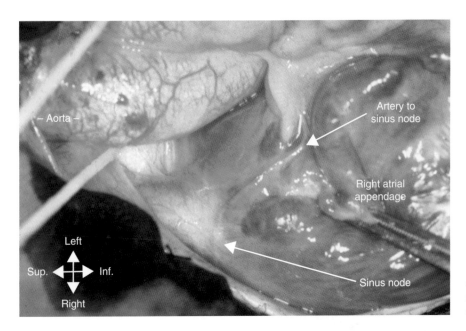

Fig. 4.12 This operative view, taken through a median sternotomy, shows the artery to the sinus node arising from the right coronary artery.

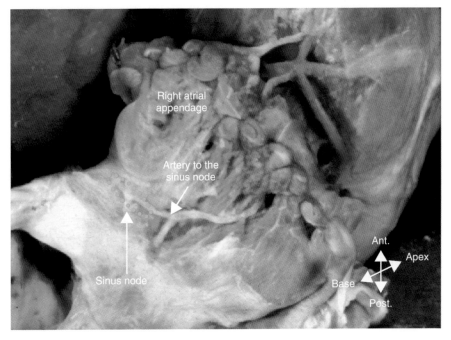

Fig. 4.13 In this specimen, photographed to replicate the view seen by the surgeon working through a median sternotomy, the artery to the sinus node takes a lateral origin from the right coronary artery. It then courses over the lateral margin of the right atrial appendage to reach the terminal groove. It has been divided by the standard atriotomy.

arise by separate orifices (see above). In just over half the cases, it gives rise to the artery supplying sinus node (Fig. 4.12). Very rarely, the nodal artery can arise more distally from the right coronary artery, coursing over the lateral margin of the appendage to reach the terminal groove. This is of major surgical significance (Fig. 4.13).

The left coronary artery has a short confluent stem, usually called the left main artery by the surgeon. It emerges from the left hand facing, or #2, sinus, and enters the left margin of the ventriculo-infundibular fold, being positioned behind the pulmonary trunk and beneath the left atrial appendage. It is a very short structure, rarely extending beyond one centimetre in length before bifurcating into its anterior interventricular and circumflex branches (Fig. 4.14). In some hearts, the left main artery trifurcates, with an intermediate branch present between the two major branches (Fig. 4.15). The intermediate branch supplies the pulmonary surface and obtuse margins of the left ventricle. The anterior interventricular, or descending, artery runs down within the anterosuperior interventricular groove, giving off diagonal branches to the pulmonary surface of the left ventricle, and the important perforating branches which pass inferiorly into the septum (Fig. 4.16). The first septal perforating branch (Fig. 4.17) is particularly important, since it is at major risk when the pulmonary valve is removed for use as a homograft. The interventricular artery then continues towards the apex, frequently curving under the apex onto the diaphragmatic surface of the ventricles.

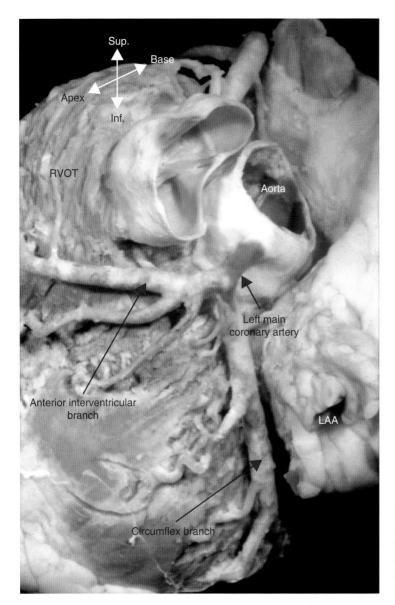

Sup.

Base

Apex

Inf.

RVOT

Aorta

Left main
coronary artery

Anterior interventricular
branch

LAA

Circumflex branch

Fig. 4.14 This dissection, photographed from the left side in anatomical orientation, shows the left coronary artery branching into its anterior interventricular and circumflex branches. The left atrial appendage has been reflected to show the bifurcation. LAA = left atrial appendage; RVOT = right ventricular outflow tract.

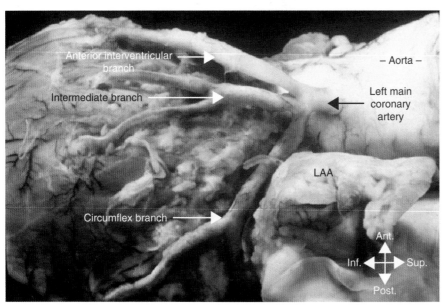

Anterior interventricular
branch

Intermediate branch

Circumflex branch

– Aorta –

Left main
coronary
artery

LAA

Ant.

Inf.   Sup.

Post.

Fig. 4.15 The left coronary artery in this specimen, photographed in anatomical orientation from the left side, gives rise to three, rather than two, branches. The intermediate branch supplies the obtuse margin of the left ventricle. LAA = left atrial appendage. Courtesy of Professor Anton Becker, University of Amsterdam.

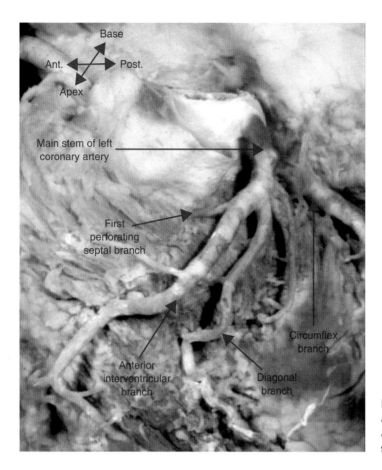

Fig. 4.16 This dissection, photographed from the front in anatomical orientation, shows the course and branches of the anterior interventricular artery. Note the location of the first septal perforating branch.

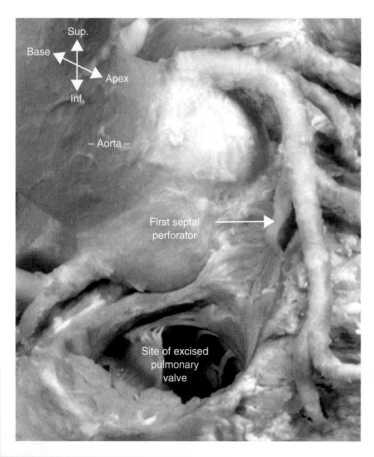

Fig. 4.17 This close-up view of a specimen, in anatomic orientation subsequent to excision of the pulmonary valve, shows the origin of the first septal perforating artery. Note its proximity to the subpulmonary infundibular area, putting it at risk when the pulmonary valve is removed for use as a autograft.

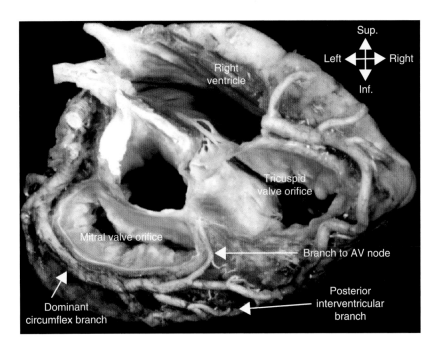

Right
ventricle

Sup.

Left ⟷ Right

Inf.

Tricuspid
valve orifice

Mitral valve orifice

Branch to AV node

Posterior
interventricular
branch

Dominant
circumflex branch

Fig. 4.18 This specimen, dissected and photographed to show the base of the heart in anatomical orientation, has a dominant circumflex branch passing behind the mitral orifice and giving rise to the posterior, in reality the inferior, interventricular branch at the crux.

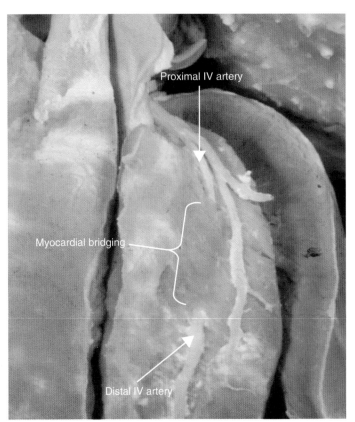

Proximal IV artery

Myocardial bridging

Distal IV artery

Fig. 4.19 In this specimen, photographed in anatomical orientation, there is extensive myocardial bridging across the anterior interventricular artery.

The circumflex branch of the left coronary artery passes backward to run in relationship with the mitral orifice. Its relationship to the orifice is most extensive when it gives rise to the inferior interventricular artery at the crux. In this circumstance, the left coronary artery is said to be dominant (Fig. 4.18).

A dominant left coronary artery, however, is found in only about one-tenth of cases. When the left coronary is not dominant, the circumflex artery usually terminates by supplying branches to the obtuse margin of the left ventricle. In almost half of normal individuals, the circumflex artery also

gives rise to the artery that supplies the sinus node.

Throughout much of their epicardial course, the arteries and their accompanying veins are encased in epicardial adipose tissue. In some hearts, the myocardium itself may form a bridge over segments of the artery (Fig. 4.19).

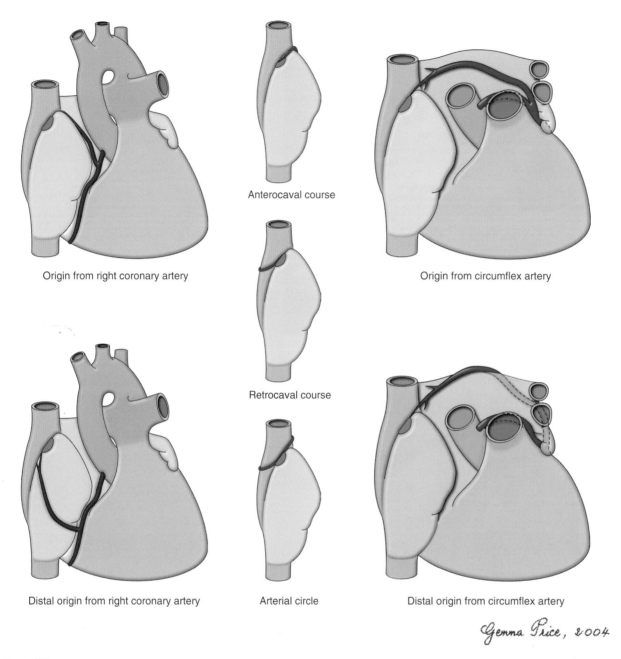

Anterocaval course

Origin from right coronary artery

Origin from circumflex artery

Retrocaval course

Distal origin from right coronary artery

Arterial circle

Distal origin from circumflex artery

Gemma Price, 2004

Fig. 4.20 The cartoon, drawn in anatomical orientation, shows the variations in the origin of the artery to the sinus node, and the variability relative to the cavoatrial junction. The left hand panels show the usual arrangement with origin from the right coronary artery, found in 55% of the population, with the rare variant of distal origin with coursing across the appendage (lower left hand panel). The right hand panels show proximal origin from the circumflex artery, found in around 45% of the population, with the rare variant of distal origin with coursing across the dome of the left atrium. The middle panels show the variation relative to the superior cavoatrial junction. The sinus node is shown in green.

The role of these myocardial bridges in the development of coronary arterial disease is not clear. They certainly can be an impediment to the surgeon in efforts to isolate the artery.

The origin of the important artery supplying the sinus node has already been discussed. This, the largest of the atrial arteries, originates from the right coronary artery in just over half of individuals, and from the circumflex artery in the remainder (Fig. 4.20). There are, however, rare variants that must also be recognised when present. The right lateral origin has already been discussed (Fig. 4.13). Equally rarely, the artery to the sinus node may take a lateral or terminal origin from the circumflex artery (Fig. 4.20). Although rare in normal individuals, our experience suggests that these variants are more frequent in congenitally malformed hearts[7]. The artery to the sinus node also takes a variable course relative to the cavoatrial junction. There are three possibilities (Fig. 4.20). Usually, the artery courses anterocavally across the crest of the appendage to reach the node. Alternatively, it runs deeply within Waterston's groove, and passes retrocavally. It is then intimately related to

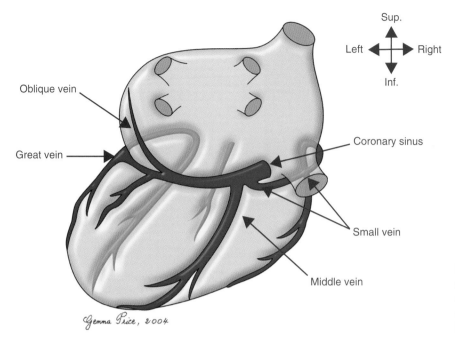

Sup.

Left ← → Right

Inf.

Oblique vein

Great vein

Coronary sinus

Small vein

Middle vein

Gemma Price, 2004

Fig. 4.21 The cartoon shows the diaphragmatic surface of the heart seen from behind in anatomic orientation. It illustrates the arrangement of the coronary veins that drain into the coronary sinus.

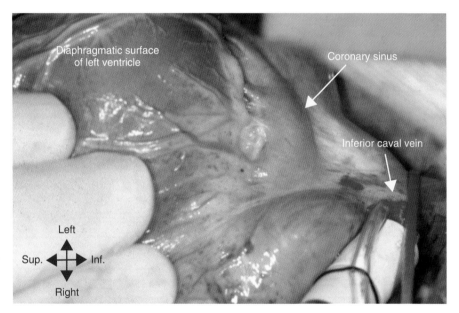

Diaphragmatic surface of left ventricle

Coronary sinus

Inferior caval vein

Left

Sup. ← → Inf.

Right

Fig. 4.22 This operative view, taken through a median sternotomy, with the apex of the heart being lifted, shows the coronary sinus running through the left atrioventricular groove.

the superior rim of the oval fossa. The third possibility is for the artery to branch, forming a circle around the cavoatrial junction (see Fig. 2.15).

The arterial supply to the ventricular conduction tissues is also of surgical significance. The atrioventricular nodal artery arises from the dominant coronary artery at the crux, usually from a U-turn of this artery beneath the floor of the coronary sinus. The nodal artery then passes toward the central fibrous body, running within the fibrofatty plane forming the "meat" in the atrioventricular muscular sandwich (Fig. 4.18). Having

traversed the node in some hearts, it then perforates the fibrous atrioventricular junction to supply a good part of the branching atrioventricular bundle. The septal perforating arteries from the anterior interventricular artery (Fig. 4.17) always supply the anterior parts of the ventricular bundle branches. Occasionally, they also supply the greater part of the inferior ventricular conduction tissues[8].

THE CORONARY VEINS

The coronary veins drain blood from the myocardium to the right atrium. The

smaller veins, known as the anterior and smallest cardiac veins, drain directly to the cavity of the atrium. They are not of surgical significance. The larger veins accompany the major arteries, and drain into the coronary sinus (Fig. 4.21). The great cardiac vein runs alongside the anterior interventricular artery. It becomes the coronary sinus as it encircles the mitral orifice to enter the inferior and leftward margin of the atrioventricular groove. The coronary sinus then runs within the groove (Fig. 4.22), lying between the left atrial wall and the ventricular myocardium, before draining into the right atrium between the

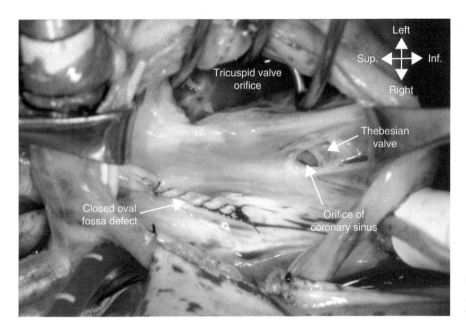

Tricuspid valve
orifice

Left

Sup. Inf.

Right

Thebesian
valve

Closed oval
fossa defect

Orifice of
coronary sinus

Fig. 4.23 This operative view, through a right atriotomy, shows the Thebesian valve guarding the orifice of the coronary sinus.

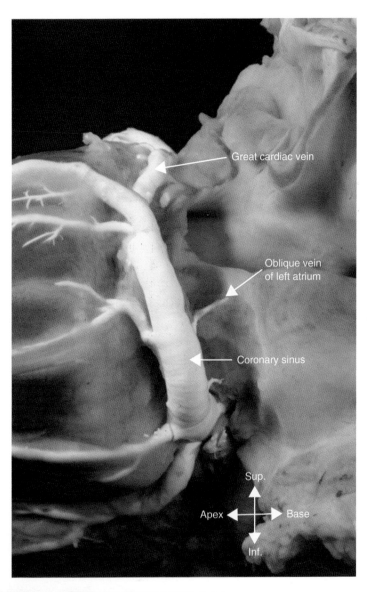

Great cardiac vein

Oblique vein
of left atrium

Coronary sinus

Sup.

Apex Base

Inf.

Fig. 4.24 This preparation was made by casting the coronary sinus with silastic, the heart then being photographed from behind in anatomic orientation. The great cardiac vein is seen entering the coronary sinus. The location of the site of drainage of the oblique vein marks the point at which the great vein becomes the coronary sinus.

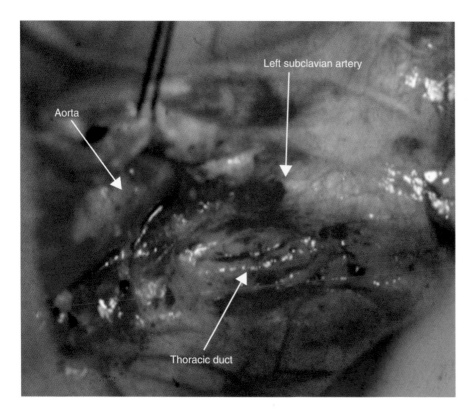

Aorta

Left subclavian artery

Thoracic duct

Fig. 4.25 This operative view, taken through a left thoracotomy, shows the location of the thoracic duct in the vicinity of the left subclavian artery and descending thoracic aorta.

sinus septum and the post-Eustachian sinus. At the crux, the sinus receives the middle cardiac vein, which has ascended with the inferior interventricular artery, and the small cardiac vein, which has encircled the tricuspid orifice in company with the right coronary artery. Occasionally, these latter two veins drain directly to the right atrium. The orifice of the coronary sinus is guarded by the Thebesian valve (Fig. 4.23), which, on very rare occasions, may be imperforate. A prominent valve is also found in the great cardiac vein where it turns round the obtuse margin of the left ventricle. This is called the valve of Vieussens[9]. Some consider that the valve marks the transition from the great cardiac vein to the coronary sinus. An alternative view is that the coronary sinus commences at the site of drainage of the oblique vein of the left atrium (Fig. 4.24).

THE CARDIAC LYMPHATICS

Little is known about the surgical implications of the lymphatic drainage of the heart itself, although lymphatic structures exist as superficial, myocardial, and subendocardial networks[10]. The most

important lymphatic channel within the thorax, nonetheless, is both well recognised and of particular importance. This is because, on occasion, the surgeon may need to ligate this vessel, the thoracic duct, in patients suffering with problems in lymphatic drainage subsequent to their conversion to the Fontan circulation. The thoracic duct originates within the abdomen in the confluence of lymphatic channels known as the cysterna chyli, this structure lying on the second lumbar vertebra. It enters the right paravertebral gutter of the thorax through the aortic opening of the diaphragm, and runs within the gutter to the level of the fourth thoracic vertebra. Within the lower part of the thorax, it lies on the vertebral column between the descending thoracic aorta and the azygos vein. Crossing obliquely the midline at the level of the fourth thoracic vertebra, it enters the left paravertebral gutter, running beneath the arch of the aorta (Fig. 4.25). It then continues superiorly and anteriorly, curving over the aortic arch between the left common carotid and subclavian arteries, to terminate in either the left subclavian or internal jugular vein as these structures join together to form the left

branchiocephalic vein. The duct has a fibromuscular coat, and contains several valves along its course, with a bifoliate valve characteristically present at its termination in the brachiocephalic vein[10].

References

1. Gittenberger-de Groot AC, Sauer U, Oppenheimer-Dekker A, Quaegebeur J. Coronary arterial anatomy in transposition of the great arteries: a morphologic study. *Pediatr Cardiol* 1983; **4 Suppl. I**: 15–24.

2. Neufeld HN, Schneeweiss A. *Coronary Artery Disease in Infants and Children*. Philadelphia: Lea & Febiger 1983; pp 73–75.

3. Bader G. Beitrag zur Systematic und Haufigkeit der Anomalien der Coronararterien des Menschen. *Virch Arch Path Anat* 1963; **337**: 88–96.

4. Gittenberger-de Groot AC, Sauer U, Quaegebeur J. Aortic intramural coronary artery in three hearts with transposition of the great arteries. *J Thorac Cardiovasc Surg* 1986; **91**: 566–571.

5. Becker AE. Variations of the main coronary arteries. In: Becker AE, Losekoot TG, Marcelletti C, Anderson RH. (Eds). *Paediatric Cardiology Volume 3*. Edinburgh: Churchill Livingstone. 1981: 263–277.

6. Engel HJ, Torres C, Page HL, Jr. Major variations in anatomical origin of the coronary arteries: angiographic observations in 4,250 patients without associated congenital heart disease. *Cathet Cardiovasc Diagn* 1975; **1**: 157–169.

7. Barra Rossi M, Ho SY, Anderson RH, Rossi Filho RI, Lincoln C. Coronary arteries in complete transposition: the significance of the sinus node artery. *Ann Thorac Surg* 1986; **42**: 573–577.

8. Anderson RH, Becker AE. *Cardiac Anatomy. An integrated text and colour atlas.* London: Gower Medical Publishing. 1980; pp 6.28–6.29.

9. Zawadzki M, Pietrasik A, Pietrasik K, Marchel M, Ciszek B. Endoscopic study of the morphology of Vieussen's valve. *Clin Anat*; **17**: 318–321.

10. Walmsley T. The Heart. In: Sharpey-Schafer E, Symington J, Bryce TH (eds). *Quain's Elements of Anatomy.* Eleventh Edition Vol IV, Part III. London: Longmans, Green and Co. 1929; p110.

5

Surgical anatomy of the conduction system

The disposition of the conduction system in the normal heart has already been discussed (see Chapter 2). In that earlier chapter, we emphasised the importance of avoiding the cardiac nodes and ventricular bundle branches, and scrupulously protecting the vascular supply to these structures. In this chapter, we will consider the anatomy of these tissues relative to the treatment of intractable problems of cardiac rhythm. Abnormal dispositions of conduction tissue secondary to congenital cardiac lesions, features now of much greater surgical significance, will be discussed in the sections devoted to those lesions in the chapters that follow.

LANDMARKS TO THE ATRIOVENTRICULAR CONDUCTION AXIS

In patients with intractable tachycardia, it may be necessary to ablate the atrioventricular bundle. Although this sometimes occurs inadvertently, it can be surprisingly difficult to divide this structure intentionally. The landmark to penetration of the atrioventricular conduction axis through the fibrous insulating plane is the apex of the triangle of Koch (Fig. 5.1). This is the point at which the tendon of Todaro inserts into the central fibrous body (Fig. 5.2). Just inferior to the apex of this triangle, the axis of atrioventricular conduction tissue

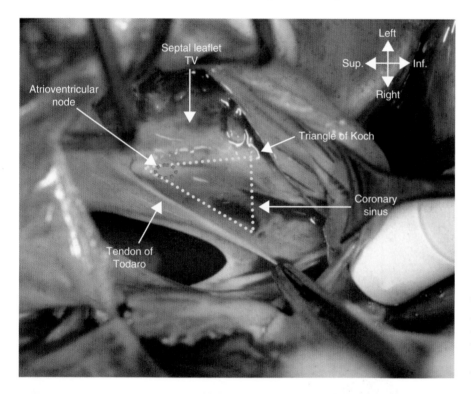

Fig. 5.1 This operative photograph, showing the surgeon's view through a right atriotomy in a patient with an atrial septal defect in the oval fossa, demonstrates the landmarks of the triangle of Koch (dotted line). Tension has been placed on the Eustachian valve to bring the tendon of Todaro into prominence.

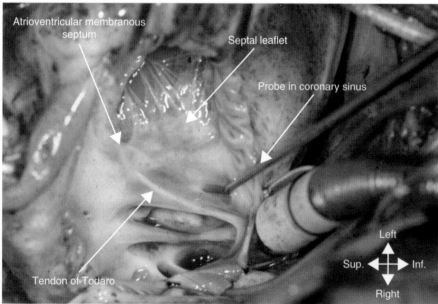

Fig. 5.2 Another operative view, in the same orientation as Fig. 5.1, shows the tendon of Todaro inserting into the atrioventricular part of the membranous septum.

gathers itself together, and enters the fibrous body (Fig. 5.3 & Fig. 5.4). It then penetrates to the left through the fibrous body. As the axis passes through the fibrous tissue, and divides into its branches, the fibrous tissue is crossed by the septal leaflet of the tricuspid valve. The latter structure divides the membranous septum into atrioventricular and interventricular components. Often the interventricular component is occupied by the axis of the conduction tissue. Further anteriorly, the axis is positioned on the crest of the muscular septum, immediately beneath the fibrous membranous septum (Fig. 5.5). When viewed from the left, the bundle is intimately related to the subaortic outflow tract, with the fibrous triangle separating the non-coronary and right coronary leaflets of the aortic valve marking the take-off of the left bundle branch (Fig. 5.6). Sometimes, the branching bundle lies below the septal crest, being carried on the left ventricular aspect of the septum[1]. From the left side, the right bundle branch then burrows intramyocardially to reach the right side of the septum, surfacing beneath the medial papillary muscle. Taken together, the site of the conduction axis is indicated by a line drawn from the apex of the triangle of Koch to the medial papillary muscle. The compact atrioventricular node, located within the triangle of Koch, is positioned some distance

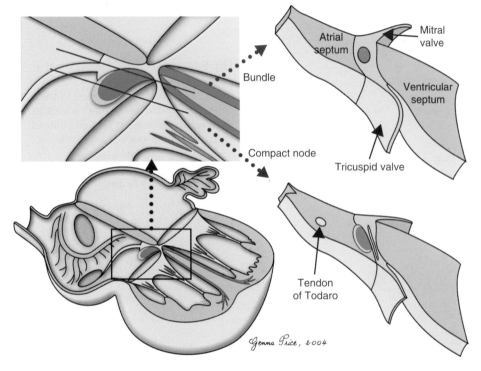

Fig. 5.3 This cartoon, drawn in anatomic orientation, shows the location of the conduction tissues within the triangle of Koch, and the mechanism of penetration of the axis of conduction tissue into the central fibrous body to form the bundle of His, the point of penetration serving to delimit the junction of the atrioventricular node with the penetrating bundle.

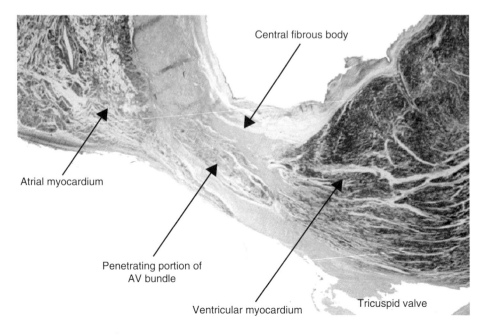

Fig. 5.4 Histological section showing the location of the penetrating atrioventricular bundle as an insulated structure within the central fibrous body. The section corresponds to the upper right hand panel of Fig. 5.3.

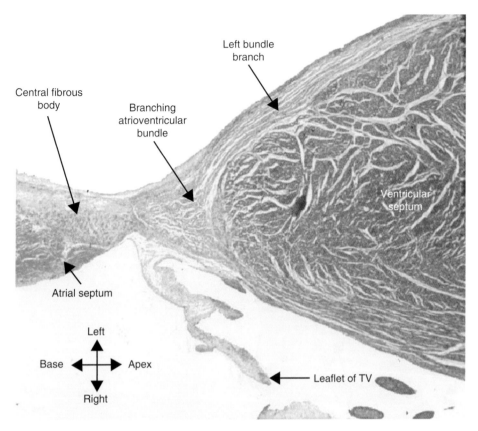

Central fibrous
body

Branching
atrioventricular
bundle

Left bundle
branch

Ventricular
septum

Atrial septum

Left

Base ←→ Apex

Right

Leaflet of TV

Fig. 5.5 This histological section, in the same anatomical orientation as Fig. 5.4, shows the branching component of the conduction axis. It lies astride the crest of the muscular ventricular septum sandwiched between septum and the central fibrous body, and is immediately adjacent to the septal leaflet of the tricuspid valve. Courtesy of Professor Anton Becker, University of Amsterdam.

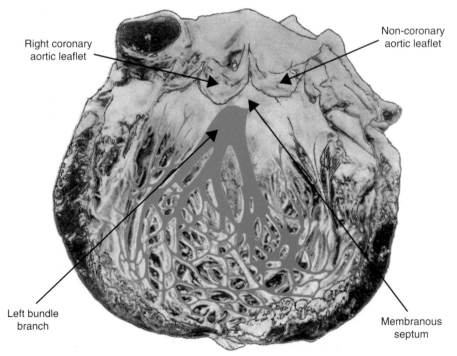

Right coronary
aortic leaflet

Non-coronary
aortic leaflet

Left bundle
branch

Membranous
septum

Fig. 5.6 This diagram is a reproduction of Tawara's original drawing. It shows the location of the left bundle branch (in green) relative to the aortic root. Tawara originally coloured the conduction tissue in red, but we have changed the colour to match our other illustrations.

posterior to the attachment of the septal leaflet of the tricuspid valve. It is located well superior to the orifice of the coronary sinus.

VENTRICULAR PRE-EXCITATION

Ventricular pre-excitation is a frequent problem of cardiac rhythm that

necessitates knowledge of the pertinent anatomy for its optimal treatment. Pre-excitation is the abnormal rhythm in which all, or part, of the ventricular

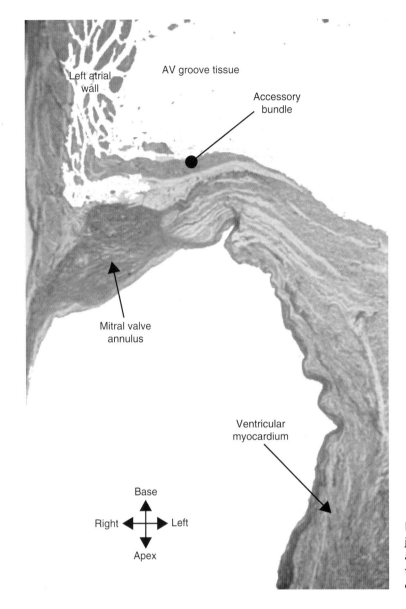

Fig. 5.7 This histological section across the atrioventricular junction shows the arrangement of the typical left-sided accessory muscular atrioventricular connection that produces the Wolff–Parkinson–White syndrome. Elastin stain. Courtesy of Professor Anton Becker, University of Amsterdam.

myocardium is excited earlier than would be expected had the impulse reached the ventricles by way of the normal atrioventricular conduction system[2]. There are various anatomical pathways, proven and hypothetical, that can produce this phenomenon. Essentially, they are pathways that short-circuit part, or all, of the normal delay induced by the atrioventricular conduction tissues. Most of this delay occurs within the atrioventricular node and its zones of transitional cells, but an increment of delay reflects the time taken for the impulse to traverse the ventricular bundle branches, since these structures are insulated from the septal myocardium. Accessory pathways can exist between the

atrium and the atrioventricular bundle, so-called atrio-Hisian tracts, and between the conduction axis and the crest of the ventricular septum, the latter first being described by Mahaim[3]. These are not amenable to surgical division. In contrast, the accessory atrioventricular pathways that produce the Wolff–Parkinson–White syndrome, probably the most common form of pre-excitation, are very much amenable to surgical division[4]. Nowadays, however, if division is necessary, the pathways will almost certainly be ablated in the catheter laboratory. The treatment of this arrhythmia, nonetheless, constituted an important step in the evolution of cardiac surgery. When treatment was first mooted, the bundles

were called, inappropriately, bundles of Kent[4]. The muscular strands which produce the abnormal rhythm join together the atrial and ventricular myocardial muscle masses outside the area of the specialised conduction tissues (Fig. 5.7). The best initial description of the bundles was given by Ohnell[5]. His illustration (Fig. 5.8) shows that the structures bear no resemblance to the node-like remnants described by Kent, and considered inappropriately by him to be part of the normal conduction system (Fig. 5.9). The abnormal accessory muscular bundles that produce the Wolff–Parkinson–White syndrome can be found anywhere around the atrioventricular junctions. They are best

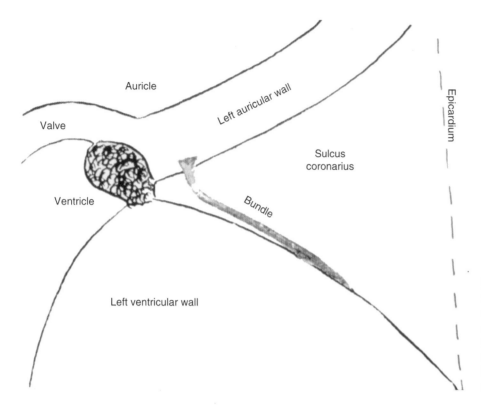

Fig. 5.8 Ohnell's drawing showing the arrangement of the typical left-sided accessory muscular atrioventricular connections that produce the Wolff–Parkinson–White syndrome. As can be seen by making comparison with Fig. 5.7, Ohnell was remarkably accurate with his drawing.

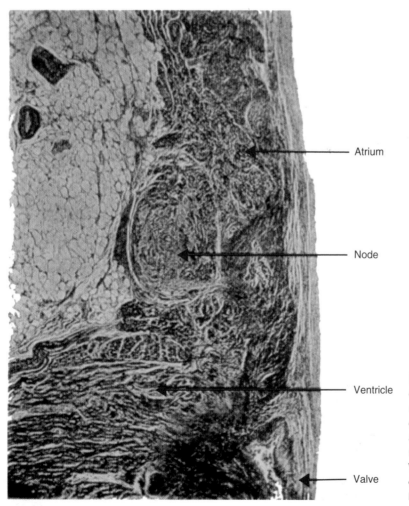

Fig. 5.9 This illustration, taken from one of Kent's demonstrations to the Society of Physiology, and re-labelled by us, shows the structure of remnants of conduction tissue found adjacent to the right atrioventricular junction. This structure bears no resemblance to the accessory connections that produce Wolff–Parkinson–White syndrome (see Figs. 5.7, 5.8), but can rarely give rise to an anomalous connection – see Fig. 5.15.

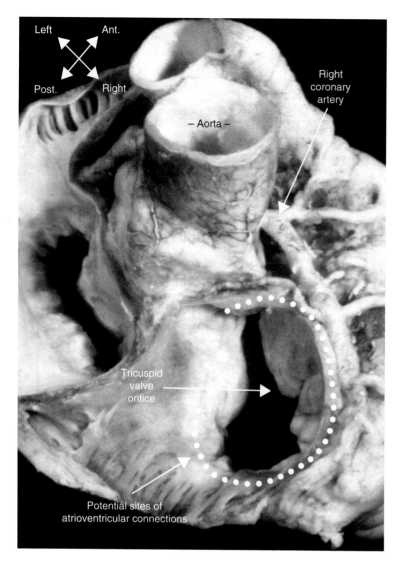

Left | Ant.
Post. | Right

Right coronary artery

– Aorta –

Tricuspid valve orifice

Potential sites of atrioventricular connections

Fig. 5.10 This dissection, photographed in anatomic orientation from above and behind, shows the potential sites of atrioventricular connections (dotted line) in the parietal aspect of the right atrioventricular junction.

described as left-sided, right-sided, and paraseptal pathways. The anatomy of each group shows significant differences.

Left-sided pathways are found at any point around the mural component of the mitral valvar orifice. They are exceedingly rare in the area of aortic-mitral valvar fibrous continuity. The pathways almost always run from atrial to ventricular muscle masses outside a well-formed fibrous annulus, the latter supporting the hinge of the mural leaflet of the mitral valve (Fig. 5.7). The atrial origin of the bundle is very close to the fibrous junction. The bundle itself usually skirts very close to the fibrous tissue, often branching into several roots which then insert into the ventricular myocardium. The bundles are rarely thicker than 1 to 2 millimetres in diameter, and are composed of ordinary myocardium. On occasions,

there may be more than one bundle in the same patient. If approached from within the atrium, incisions that divide the atrial myocardium, or ablative lesions placed above the origin of the leaflets of the mitral valve, are unlikely to divide the accessory muscle bundle itself. In order to ablate surgically the accessory connection, it was usually necessary to dissect within the fat pad on the epicardial aspect of the annulus, or to approach the pathway from the epicardium. If approached endocardially, it was necessary to reflect the coronary vessels to expose the accessory muscle bundles. When treated in the catheter laboratory, lesions are usually placed on the ventricular aspect of the hingepoint of the mitral valve.

Right-sided accessory pathways may also pass through the fat pad to connect the atrial and ventricular myocardial

masses. More frequently, bundles on the right side are found some distance away from the attachment of the leaflets of the tricuspid valve, which is rarely a firm and well-formed fibrous junction, as is usually the case on the mitral side. Right-sided connections can be multiple, and can coexist with left-sided pathways. They are frequently associated with Ebstein's malformation, and may need to be treated concomitantly with repair or replacement of the abnormal tricuspid valve. They can be found at any point within the parietal aspect of the tricuspid orifice, from the site of the membranous septum to the mouth of the coronary sinus (Fig. 5.10). The same rules for their ablation apply as discussed for left-sided connections.

It is connections in paraseptal position that constitute the greatest clinical challenge[6]. When viewed from the right

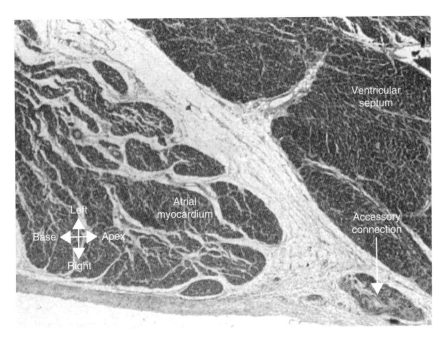

Fig. 5.11 This histological section, in anatomic orientation, shows a muscular accessory atrioventricular connection crossing the fibrofatty insulating plane of the right atrioventricular junction. The strand takes its origin from the distal insertion of the atrial myocardium into the area of attachment of the septal leaflet of the tricuspid valve, and crosses the groove to attach to the ventricular myocardium. Trichrome stain. Courtesy of Professor Anton Becker, University of Amsterdam.

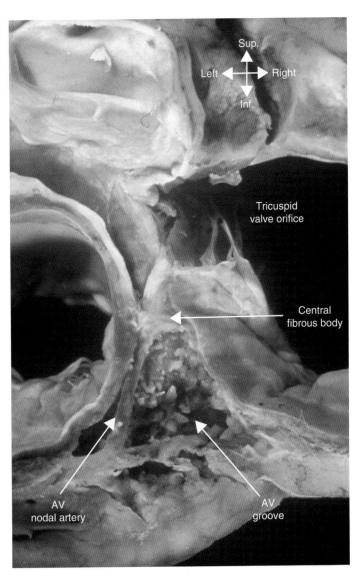

Fig. 5.12 This dissection, shown in anatomic orientation, shows the plane occupied by adipose tissue that runs superiorly and anteriorly beneath the mouth of the coronary sinus. It carries the artery to the atrioventricular node, in this case from a dominant left coronary artery.

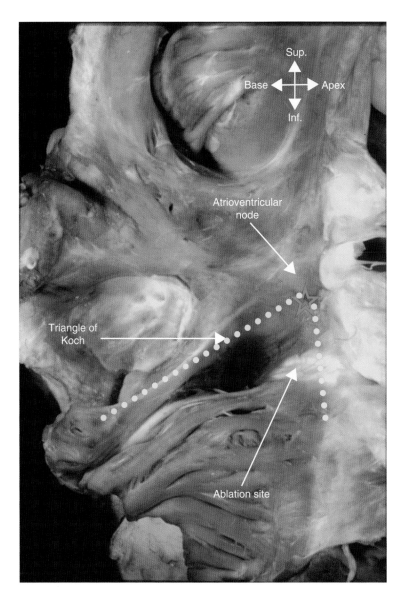

Sup.
Base ← → Apex
Inf.

Atrioventricular node

Triangle of Koch

Ablation site

Fig. 5.13 This photograph shows the site of ablation within the base of the triangle of Koch which cured a patient with atrioventricular nodal re-entry tachycardia. It is outside the area occupied by the specialised tissues of the atrioventricular node and its zones of transitional cells. Reproduced by kind permission of Dr Wyn Davies, St Mary's Hospital, London.

atrium, they can cross from the atrial to the ventricular myocardium at any point between the mouth of the coronary sinus and the supraventricular crest (Fig. 5.10). They present problems for ablation, firstly, because they may run deep within the atrioventricular area as viewed from the right atrium. The second problem is that the atrioventricular node and bundle are also found within this area. The anatomy of the area is best illustrated by a dissection of the floor of the coronary sinus. This shows that a continuation of the inferior atrioventricular groove extends superiorly as a layer of fibrofatty tissue between the atrial and ventricular muscle masses, extending to reach the

central fibrous body (Fig. 5.12). The artery to the atrioventricular node courses forwards within this tissue plane (Fig. 5.12). The atrioventricular node itself occupies the superior part of the atrial layer of this triangular sandwich. Accessory muscular connections may cross through the fibrofatty tissue at any point from the attachment of the mitral and tricuspid valves at either side of the septum. Indeed, the only connection that has been identified morphologically within this area[7] was located at the insertion of the tricuspid valve (Fig. 5.11). If necessary, the fibrofatty tissue plane can be entered surgically from the cavity of the right atrium, or can be reached by

dissection from the epicardial aspect. Incisions within the atrial component of this atrioventricular sandwich, interrupting the muscular approaches to the atrioventricular node, have also been shown to interrupt reciprocating atrioventricular nodal tachycardias[8]. Treatment of these arrhythmias is now also accomplished with efficiency and safety using catheter ablation (Fig. 5.13). When treating these arrhythmias, either surgically or by catheter ablation, it should be remembered that the triangle of Koch contains both the atrioventricular node and its nutrient artery. Unless performed with care, there is always the danger that intervention can produce complete atrioventricular dissociation.

Surgeons and catheter ablationists, attempting to treat arrhythmias, have often referred to this area containing the atrioventricular area as being "septal". They also describe an 'anterior' septum[9]. By this, they mean the area of the right atrioventricular junction that lies anterior and superior to the site of the membranous component of the septum. It is a mistake to describe this part of the right atrioventricular junction as 'septal', just as it is incorrect to consider the atrial aspect of the triangle of Koch as being part of a septal structure. In reality, the "anterior septum" is the medial margin of the ventriculo–infundibular fold. Muscular connections, if found in this area, will join the atrial wall to the supraventricular crest of the right ventricle (Fig. 5.14). Recent experience[10] has also shown that muscular connections running to the most lateral margin of the supraventricular crest at the acute margin of the right ventricle can produce the electrocardiographic pattern initially attributed to the so–called "Mahaim" fibres[3]. The muscular atrioventricular connections which have been removed surgically from the acute margin have been shown to resemble histologically the tissues of the atrioventricular node. We had previously identified[7] a similar pathway running across the right atrioventricular junction (Fig. 5.15). The atrial component of these

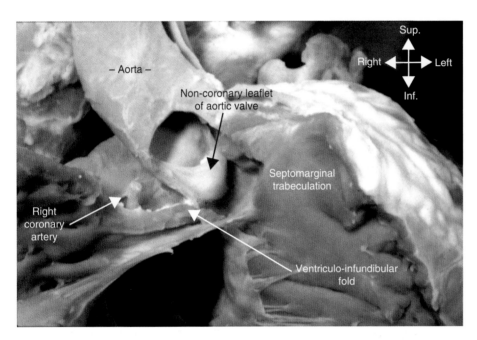

Fig. 5.14 This dissection, in anatomical orientation, illustrates how the area anterior to the membranous septum, which was previously considered to represent the 'anterior' septum, is part of the parietal wall of the right atrioventricular junction.

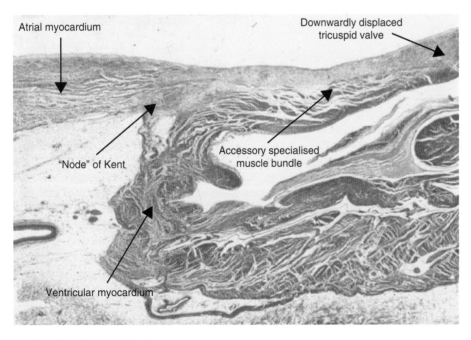

Fig. 5.15 This section is taken across the right atrioventricular junction, and comes from the heart of a patient who had ventricular pre-excitation. The tricuspid valve was deformed by Ebstein's malformation. An accessory muscular connection was identified taking origin from a nodal remnant as identified by Kent, and crossing the insulating plane to run within the muscularised leaflet of the tricuspid valve. Section reproduced by kind permission of Professor Anton Becker, University of Amsterdam.

connections is remarkably reminiscent of the illustrations provided by Kent (Fig. 5.9). As already discussed, Kent had argued, incorrectly, that the nodal remnants were pathways for normal atrioventricular conduction[11]. It does seem, nonetheless, that under abnormal circumstances[12] these 'nodes' can function as the atrial origin of specialised muscular accessory connections. It is these connections which are now known to produce ventricular pre-excitation of the so-called "Mahaim" type.

SUBSTRATES FOR OTHER SUPRAVENTRICULAR TACHYCARDIACS

Recent experience has also focussed the attention of both surgeons and interventionists on the substrates of so-called supraventricular tachycardias, particularly atrial flutter and fibrillation. Atrial flutter of the commonest type has shown itself to be especially amenable to interventional therapy. Thus, the "flutter circuit" is known to pass in counter-clockwise fashion (Fig. 5.16) down the terminal crest before ascending through the septal isthmus of the tricuspid valvar vestibule[13]. The most inferior part of the circuit passes through another muscular isthmus, this time limited by the orifice of the inferior caval vein and the hinge of the septal leaflet of the tricuspid valve (Fig. 5.17). The isthmus has three discrete areas (Fig. 5.18), containing various combinations of fibrous and muscular

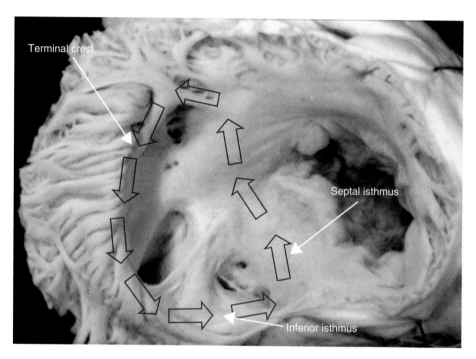

Fig. 5.16 The right atrium has been opened and photographed in anatomic orientation to show the circuit known to be responsible for the common variant of atrial flutter. The flutter wave descends the terminal crest, crosses through the inferior cavo-tricuspid isthmus, and then ascends through the septal isthmus to reach the superior aspect of the terminal crest before recommencing the circuit.

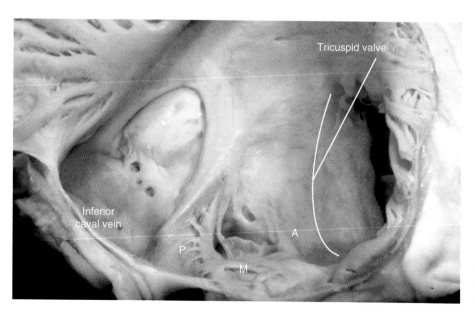

Fig. 5.17 The right atrium has been opened through the parietal wall, and photographed in anatomic orientation to show the structure of the inferior cavo-tricuspid isthmus. It has posterior (P), middle (M), and anterior (A) components.

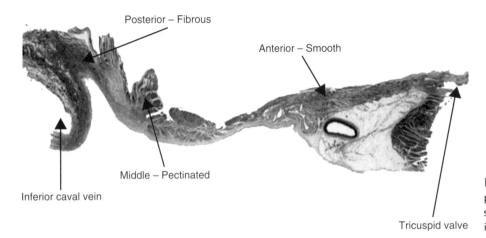

Posterior – Fibrous

Anterior – Smooth

Middle – Pectinated

Inferior caval vein

Tricuspid valve

Fig. 5.18 This histological section, prepared by Dr Siew Yen Ho, shows the structure of the three components of the inferior cavo-tricuspid isthmus.

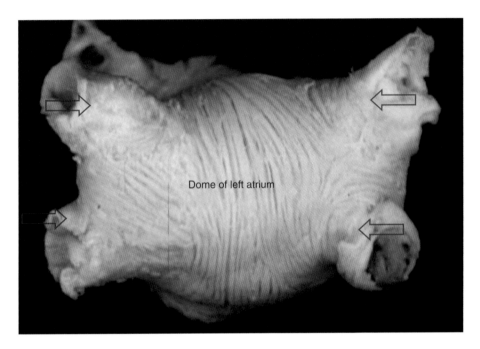

Dome of left atrium

Fig. 5.19 This dissection was made by Professor Damien Sanchez-Quintana. It shows the dome of the left atrium, having removed the epicardium to illustrate the organisation of the myocardial fibres. Sleeves of myocardium (red arrows) can be seen to extend onto the pulmonary veins for varying distances. These sleeves are now known to be the sources of focal activity in some variants of atrial fibrillation.

tissue[14], but interventionists are now able to construct lines of block with great facility so as to cure flutter. Such lines would obviously be made surgically with equal facility. Indeed, the group from Chicago[15] has now shown that, when contemplating atrial surgery for congenital cardiac malformations, it is advisable to design incisions so as not to leave potential isthmuses that could act as substrates for macro-re-entry. If it is impossible to avoid creating such bridges, then it is probably wise to divide them with a suitably constructed line, either created surgically or by cryoablation[15].

The other lesion now becoming increasingly amenable to interventional therapy is atrial fibrillation. It has long been known that surgical techniques that create mazes[16] or corridors[17] can certainly ameliorate, if not cure, this troublesome arrhythmia. But the operative procedures are complex and time-consuming, and the maze procedure, for example, has undergone many modifications[18] that are beyond the context of our description. More recently, nonetheless, interventionists have shown themselves capable of constructing lines within both the left and right atriums that can provide successful treatment for atrial fibrillation[19,20]. Even more recently, it has been shown that a proportion of cases of fibrillation can be cured by making focal lesions in the mouth of the pulmonary veins[21]. This is because the atrial myocardium extends for variable distances along the pulmonary veins from the venoatrial junctions (Fig. 5.19). These sleeves of myocardium contain bundles of fibres running in different directions, along with separating sheaths of fibrous tissue which set the scene for the focal triggering that produces the fibrillation[22,23]. Arguments continue as to whether these sleeves are "histologically specialised". Although a very recent study has shown that some of the cells have a characteristic ultrastructural appearance[24], the arrangements described bear no resemblance to the structure of the cardiac nodes and bundle branches.

References

1. Massing GK, James TN. Anatomical configuration of the His bundle and bundle branches in the human heart. *Circulation* 1976; **53**: 609–621.

2. Durrer D, Schuilenburg RM, Wellens HJJ. Pre-excitation revisited. *Am J Cardiol* 1970; **25**: 690–698.

3. Mahaim I. *Maladies Organiques du Faisceau de His-Tawara*. Paris; Masson et Cie. 1931.

4. Sealy WC, Gallagher JJ, Pritchett ELC. The surgical anatomy of Kent bundles based on electrophysiological mapping and surgical exploration. *J Thorac Cardiovasc Surg* 1978; **76**: 804–815.

5. Ohnell RF. Preexcitation, a cardiac abnormality. Pathophysiological, patho-anatomical and clinical studies of an excitatory spread phenomenon. *Acta Med Scand ?Year* **Suppl 152**: 1–167.

6. Sealy WC, Gallagher JJ. The surgical approach to the septal area of the heart based on experience with 45 patients with Kent bundles. *J Thorac Cardiovasc Surg* 1980; **79**: 542–551.

7. Becker AE, Anderson RH, Durrer D, Wellens HJJ. The anatomical substrates of Wolff-Parkinson-White syndrome. A clinicopathologic correlation in seven patients. *Circulation* 1978; **57**: 870–879.

8. Johnson DC, Ross DL, Uther JB. The surgical cure of atrioventricular junctional reentrant tachycardia. In: Zipes DP, Jalife J (eds). *Cardiac Electrophysiology from Cell to Bedside*. London; W.B. Saunders Company. 1990: 921–923.

9. Guiraudon GM, Klein GJ, Sharma AD, Yee R, Pineda EA, McLellan DG. Surgical approach to anterior septal accessory pathways in 20 patients with the Wolff-Parkinson-White syndrome. *Eur J Cardio-thorac Surg* 1988; **2**: 201–206.

10. Guiraudon CM, Guiraudon GM, Klein GJ. "Nodal ventricular" Mahaim pathway: histologic evidence for an accessory atrioventricular pathway with an AV node-like morphology. *Circulation* 1988; **78 Suppl. II**: 40–40.

11. Kent AFS. The structure of the cardiac tissues at the auriculo-ventricular junction. *J Physiol* 1913; **47**: 17–18.

12. Anderson RH, Ho SY, Gillette PC, Becker AE. Mahaim, Kent and abnormal atrioventricular conduction. *Cardiovasc Res* 1996; **31**: 480–491.

13. Cosio FG, Lopez-Gil M, Giocolea A, Arribas F, Barroso JL. Radiofrequency ablation of the inferior vena cava-tricuspid valve isthmus in common atrial flutter. *Am J Cardiol* 1993; **71**: 705–709.

14. Cabrera JA, Sanchez-Quintana D, Ho SY, Medina A, Anderson RH. The architecture of the atrial musculature between the orifice of the inferior caval vein and the tricuspid valve: the anatomy of the isthmus. *J Cardiovasc Electrophysiol* 1998; **9**: 1186–1195.

15. Mavroudis C, Backer CL, Deal BJ, Johnsrude C, Strasburger J. Total cavopulmonary conversion and maze procedure for patients with failure of the Fontan operation. *J Thorac Cardiovasc Surg* 2001; **122**: 863–871.

16. Cox JL, Boineau JP, Schuessler RB, Jaquiss RD, Lappas DG. Modification of the maze procedure for atrial flutter and atrial fibrillation. I. Rationale and surgical results. *J Thorac Cardiovasc Surg* 1995; **110(2)**: 473–484.

17. Defauw JJ, Guiraudon GM, van Hemel NM, Vermeulen FE, Kingma JH, de Bakker JM. Surgical therapy of paraoxysmal atrial fibrillation with the "corridor" operation. *Ann Thorac Surg* 1992; **53**: 564–570.

18. Cox JL, Ad N. New surgical and catheter-based modifications of the Maze procedure. *Semin Thorac Cardiovasc Surg* 2000; **12**: 68–73.

19. Goya M, Ouyang F, Ernst S, Volkmer M, Antz M, Kuck KH. Electroanatomic mapping and cather ablation of breakthroughs from the right atrium to the superior vena cava in patients with atrial fibrillation. *Circulation* 2002; **106**: 1317–1320.

20. Pappone C, Oreto G, Rosanio S, Vicedomini G, Tocchi M, Gugliotta F, Salvati A, Dicandia C, Calabro MP, Mazzone P, Ficcara E, di Gioia C, Guletta S, Nardi S, Santinella V, Benussi S, Alfieri O. Atrial electroanatomic remodelling after circumferential radiofrequency pulmonary vein ablation: Efficacy of an anatomic approach in a large cohort of patients with atrial fibrillation. *Circulation* 2001; **104**: 2539–2544.

21. Shah DC, Haissaguerre M, Jais P. Catheter ablation of pulmonary vein foci for atrial fibrillation. PV foci ablation for atrial fibrillation. *Thorac Cardiovasc Surgeon* 1999; **47 Suppl 3**: 352–356.

22. Ho SY, Cabrera JA, Tran VH, Farré J, Anderson RH, Sánchez-Quintana D. Architecture of the pulmonary veins: relevance to radiofrequency ablation. *Heart* 2001; **86**: 265–270.

23. Hocini M, Ho SY, Kawara T, Linnenbank AC, Potse M, Shah D, Jaïs P, Janse MJ, Haïssaguerre M, de Bakker JMT. Electrical conduction in canine pulmonary veins. Electrophysiological and anatomical correlation. *Circulation* 2002; **105**: 2442–2448.

24. Perez-Lugones A, McMahan JT, Ratliff NB, Saliba WI, Schweikert RA, Marrouche NF, Saad EB, Navia JL, McCarthy PM, Tchou P, Gillinov AM, Natale A. Evidence of specialized conduction cells in human pulmonary veins of patients with atrial fibrillation. *J Cardiovasc Electrophysiol* 2003; **14**: 803–809.

6

Analytic description of congenitally malformed hearts

Systems for describing congenital cardiac malformations have frequently been based upon embryological concepts and theories. As useful as these systems have been, they have often had the effect of confusing the clinician, rather than clarifying the basic anatomy of a given lesion. As far as the surgeon is concerned, the essence of a particular malformation lies not in its presumed morphogenesis, but in the underlying anatomy. An effective system for describing this anatomy must be based upon the morphology as it is observed. At the same time, it must be capable of accounting for all congenital cardiac conditions, even those that, as yet, might not have been encountered. To be useful clinically, the system must be not only broad and accurate, but also clear and consistent. The terminology used, therefore, should be unambiguous. It should be as simple as possible. The sequential segmental approach is such a system[1], particularly when the emphasis is placed on its surgical applications[2]. The basic philosophy of the system is initially to analyse, separately, the architectural make-up of the atrial chambers, the ventricular mass, and the arterial segment. Emphasis is then given to the nature of the junctional arrangements (Fig. 6.1). Still further attention is then devoted to the interrelationships of the cardiac structures within each of the individual segments. This provides the basic framework within which all other associated malformations can then be catalogued. As indicated, such an

approach is particularly useful to the surgeon[2], since it focuses on demonstrable anatomical derangements, rather than diverting attention to speculative embryological theory.

ATRIAL ARRANGEMENT

The first step in analysing any malformed heart is to determine the arrangement of the chambers within the atrial mass. Based on the anatomy of the appendages, which are the most constant components of the atriums, specifically on the extent of the pectinate muscles relative to the atrial vestibules[3], the atrial chambers can only be of morphologically right or morphologically left type. As described in Chapter 2, the morphologically right appendage has a broad triangular shape, whereas the morphologically left appendage is finger-like, and much narrower (Fig. 6.2), often with several constrictions along its length, and a constricted neck. The shape of the appendages permits their distinction in most instances. Only in ambiguous circumstances will it prove necessary to inspect the extent of the pectinate muscles, but this feature, of course, is readily visible to the surgeon once the heart has been opened.

When judged on the extent of the pectinate muscles, there are only four topological ways in which the appendages can be arranged within the atrial mass (Fig. 6.3). Almost always, the atrium possessing the appendage in which the

pectinate muscles extend to the crux is right-sided, while the one with a smooth posterior vestibule is left-sided. This usual arrangement is often called "situs solitus". Rarely, the appendages can be disposed in mirror-image fashion, so-called "situs inversus". More common than the mirror-imaged topologic arrangement, but still rare, is where the appendages of both chambers in the atrial mass have the same morphology. This can occur in two forms, with morphologically right (Fig. 6.4) or morphologically left (Fig. 6.5) appendages on both sides. These bilaterally symmetrical topologic patterns, or isomeric arrangements, have traditionally been named according to the arrangement of the abdominal organs, particularly the spleen. This is because they usually exist with jumbled up abdominal arrangement, or so-called "visceral heterotaxy"[4,5]. It is far more convenient, as well as more accurate, to designate them in terms of their own intrinsic morphology[6,7], particularly since this can readily be determined by the surgeon in the operating room. It should then be remembered, nonetheless, that isomerism of the right appendages is usually, but not always, found with absence of the spleen and right bronchial isomerism, while isomerism of the left appendages is typically found, but again not always, with multiple spleens and left bronchial isomerism.

The topologic arrangement of the atrial appendages can be predicted with a high degree of accuracy by studying the relationships of the abdominal great

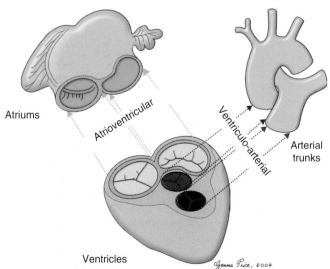

Atriums

Atrioventricular

Ventriculo-arterial

Ventricular-arterial

Arterial trunks

Ventricles

Gemma Price, 2004

Fig. 6.1 The cartoon shows the three segments of the heart. These are the atriums, the ventricular mass, and the arterial trunks. The segments are joined together at the atrioventricular and ventriculo-arterial junctions.

vessels as determined with cross-sectional ultrasonography[8]. When identified, knowledge of isomerism of the atrial appendages is of value in two additional ways. First, it alerts the surgeon to unusual dispositions of the sinus node. In right isomerism, the sinus node, being a morphologically right atrial structure, is duplicated. A node is found laterally in each of the terminal grooves[9]. In left isomerism, there are no terminal grooves (Fig. 6.5). In this situation, the sinus node is a poorly formed structure, without a constant site[10]. Usually the node is found in the anterior interatrial groove, close to the atrioventricular junction[10].

The second advantage of recognizing isomeric appendages is that the

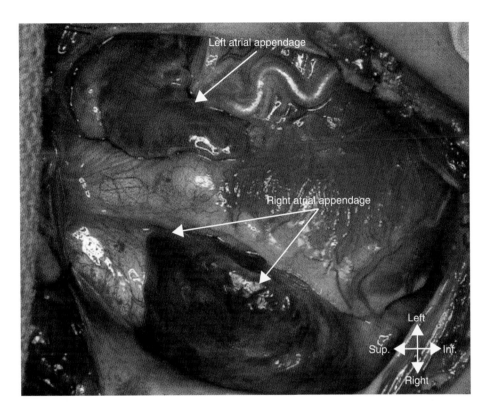

Fig. 6.2 This operative view, taken through a median sternotomy, shows the differences between the broad triangular morphologically right atrial appendage and the narrow finger-like morphologically left atrial appendage.

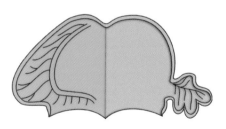

Usual

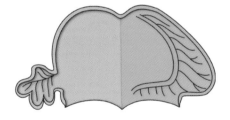

Mirror-imaged

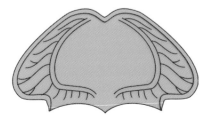

Isomeric right

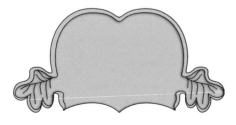

Isomeric left

Fig. 6.3 This diagram shows the four possible arrangements of the atrial appendages. The appendages cannot always be distinguished on the basis of their shape. The best means of distinguishing between them is to establish the extent of the pectinate muscles. They extend all the way to the crux in the morphologically right atrial appendage, but are confined around the mouth of the appendage in the morphologically left atrial appendage, leaving a smooth posterior vestibule. Using this criterion, all congenitally malformed hearts have appendages fitting within one of the four groups shown in the cartoon.

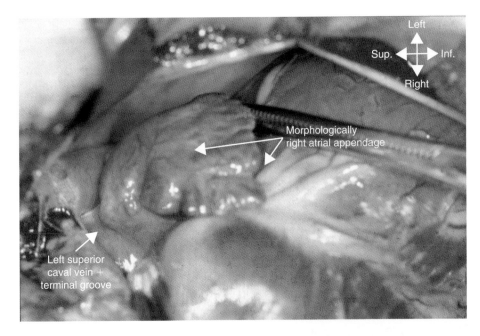

Fig. 6.4 This surgical view, through a median sternotomy, shows a left-sided atrial appendage of morphologically right pattern. The right-sided appendage is also of right morphology, so the patient has isomerism of the right atrial appendages. Note the crest of the appendage in relation to the left superior caval vein and the terminal groove. When examined internally, pectinate muscles encircled both atrioventricular junctions.

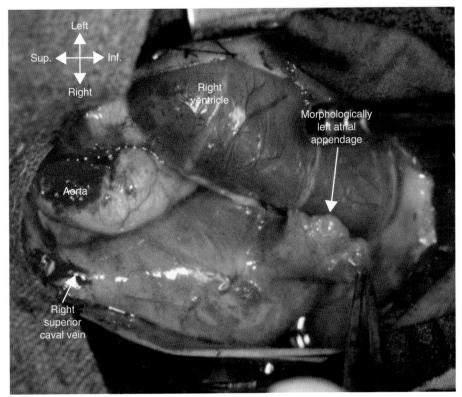

Fig. 6.5 This surgical view, through a median sternotomy, shows a right-sided atrial appendage of morphologically left pattern. The left-sided appendage is also of left morphology, so the patient has isomerism of the left atrial appendages. Note the absence of any terminal groove. Internal inspection confirmed the presence of smooth bilateral posterior vestibules.

arrangements are known to be harbingers of complex intracardiac lesions. Hearts with isomerism of either type tend to have bilateral superior caval veins, an effectively common atrial chamber, albeit with two isomeric appendages, and common atrioventricular valves[3]. Right isomerism is always associated with totally anomalous pulmonary venous connection, even if the pulmonary veins are joined to one or other atrium. It is also seen most frequently with pulmonary stenosis or atresia, and in association with a univentricular atrioventricular connection, typically double inlet ventricle through a common valve. Left isomerism, in the majority of cases, is associated with interruption of the inferior caval vein, with continuation of the venous drainage from the abdomen through the azygos system of veins.

THE ATRIOVENTRICULAR JUNCTIONS

Once the arrangement of the atrial appendages has been established, it is then necessary to analyse the atrioventricular junctions. For this, the surgeon needs to know how the atrial chambers are, or are not, connected to the ventricular mass, along with the morphology of the valves

Usual arrangement

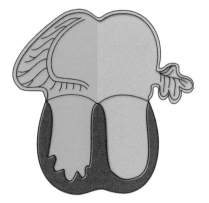

Concordant

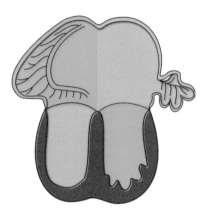

Discordant

Mirror-imaged pattern

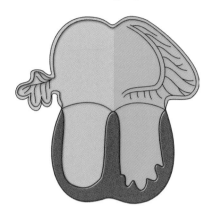

Concordant

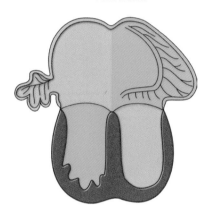

Discordant

Gemma Price, 2004

Fig. 6.6 This cartoon shows how the atrial chambers can be connected to the ventricles in concordant or discordant fashion, with each pattern existing in usual and mirror-imaged variants.

that guard the atrioventricular junctions. These are separate and independent features.

There are five distinct and discrete ways in which the atrial chambers may be connected to the ventricular mass, the final one having two subtypes along with an intriguing further variation. Most often, the atrial chambers are connected to their morphologically appropriate ventricles. This pattern is called concordant atrioventricular connections. When each atrium is connected in this way to its own ventricle, there is rarely any difficulty in distinguishing the morphology of the ventricles, even when the ventricles themselves are unusually related (see below). In the second pattern, which is discordant each atrium is connected with a morphologically inappropriate ventricle.

Concordant and discordant connections can exist with either the usual or mirror-imaged arrangement of the atrial appendages (Fig. 6.6), but not with isomeric appendages. When the appendages are isomeric, and each atrium is connected to its own ventricle, then of necessity one junction will be concordantly connected, but the other junction will be discordantly connected (Fig. 6.7). This will occur irrespective of the topologic pattern of the ventricular mass (see below). This is a third discrete pattern, namely biventricular and ambiguous atrioventricular connections.

In the three connections described thus far, each atrium is connected to its own ventricle. This means that the atrioventricular connections themselves are biventricular. The essential feature in the remaining two types of

atrioventricular connection is that the atrial chambers, with one exception, connect to only a single ventricle. In one of these patterns, both atrial chambers connect to the same ventricle. This is double inlet atrioventricular connection (Fig. 6.8). In the other variant, one of the atrial chambers is connected to a ventricle, but the other atrium has no connection with the ventricular mass. This is absence of one atrioventricular connection. The latter arrangement can be divided into two subtypes, with either the right-sided (Fig. 6.9) or the left-sided (Fig. 6.10) atrioventricular junction being absent. The intriguing variation seen with this latter pattern is when the atrioventricular connection, either right-sided or left-sided, is absent, but the solitary atrioventricular valve straddles the septum to be attached in both ventricles. This produces a uniatrial, but

Right isomerism

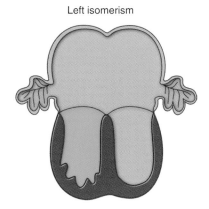

Right hand topology

Left isomerism

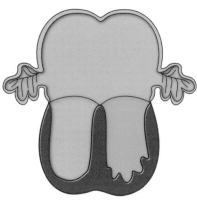

Right hand topology

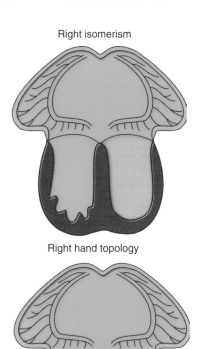

Left hand topology

Left hand topology

Gemma Price, 2004

Fig. 6.7 This cartoon demonstrates the atrioventricular connections when there are isomeric atrial appendages, and each atrium is connected to its own ventricle. In each pattern, half of the heart is concordantly connected, and the other half is discordant. It is essential in these settings, therefore, to describe both the type of isomerism, and the specific ventricular topology (see Fig. 6.22).

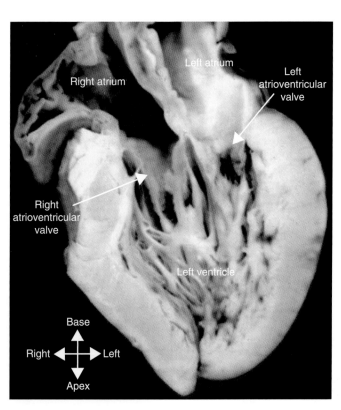

Fig. 6.8 When both atriums are connected to only one ventricle, the atrioventricular connection is univentricular. In this heart, showing a four-chamber section in anatomic orientation, there is double inlet to a dominant left ventricle.

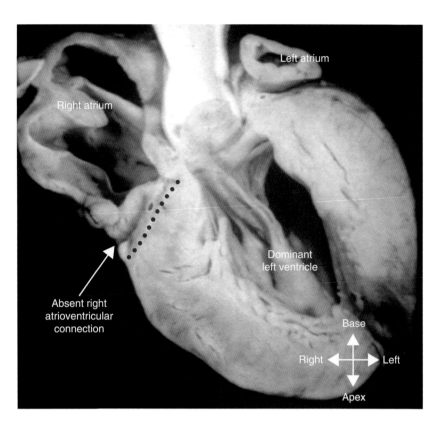

Left atrium

Right atrium

Dominant
left ventricle

Absent right
atrioventricular
connection

Base

Right ⟷ Left

Apex

Fig. 6.9 This anatomical specimen, seen in 'four chamber' orientation, shows absence of the right atrioventricular connection (dotted line), another form of univentricular atrioventricular connection. In this case, the morphology is that of classical tricuspid atresia, with the left atrium connected to a dominant left ventricle.

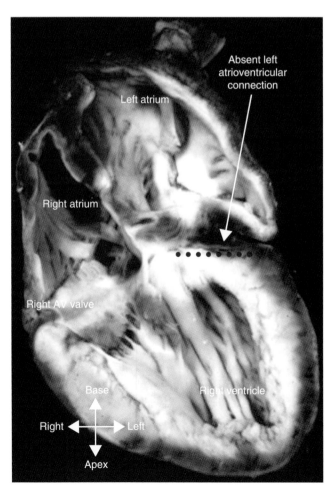

Absent left
atrioventricular
connection

Left atrium

Right atrium

Right AV valve

Base

Right ⟷ Left

Apex

Right ventricle

Fig. 6.10 This anatomical specimen, again seen in 'four chamber' orientation (compare with Figs. 6.8 and 6.9), shows absence of the left atrioventricular connection (dotted line), giving the third variant of univentricular atrioventricular connection. In this example, the right atrium is connected to a dominant right ventricle through a right-sided atrioventricular (AV) valve.

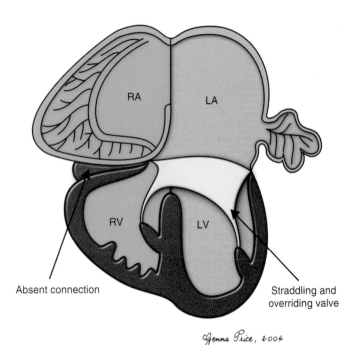

Absent connection

Straddling and overriding valve

Gemma Price, 2004

Fig. 6.11 This cartoon illustrates the arrangement when there is absence of the right atrioventricular connection, but with the solitary atrioventricular valve straddling the ventricular septum. This produces a uniatrial but biventricular atrioventricular connection, shown here in the setting of usual atrial arrangement with right hand ventricular topology. RA, LA, right and left atriums; RV, LV right and left ventricles.

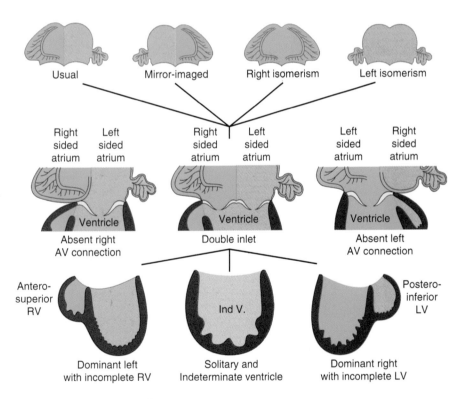

Fig. 6.12 This cartoon shows the multiple possibilities for univentricular atrioventricular connection that can be produced by combining the variations in atrial morphology, atrioventricular connection, and ventricular morphology. It takes no account of the further variations possible according to ventricular relationships, ventriculo-arterial connections, and so on. RV, LV, morphologically right and left ventricles.

biventricular, atrioventricular connection (Fig. 6.11).

The hearts in which the atrial chambers connect to only one ventricle, whether due to a double inlet or to absence of one connection, have been the source of much controversy. Previously, such hearts have been classified as single ventricle, common ventricle, or, more recently, as univentricular hearts. This is

despite the fact that, almost always, the ventricular mass contains more than one chamber. By focussing on the fact that the atrioventricular connection is, in reality, joined to only one ventricle, we are able to achieve a satisfactory solution for this dilemma. Thus, the hearts can logically and accurately be described in terms of their anatomic univentricular atrioventricular connection, which

produces a functionally univentricular arrangement. The ventricle supporting the atrioventricular junction or junctions may have one of three morphologies: right, left, or indeterminate (Fig. 6.12). Most frequently, the ventricle will be a morphologically left ventricle, as judged from the pattern of its apical trabecular component. Almost always, there will be a complementary right ventricle, perforce

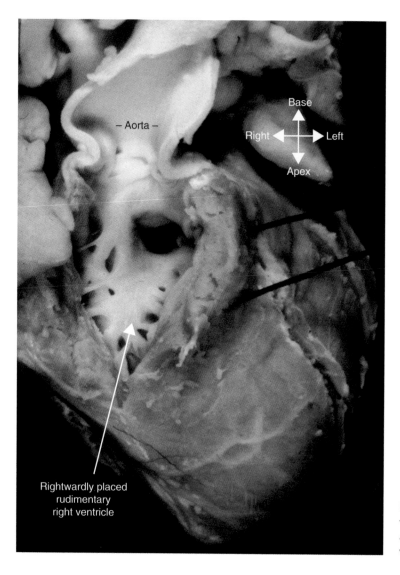

Aorta

Base

Right ← → Left

Apex

Rightwardly placed
rudimentary
right ventricle

Fig. 6.13 In this anatomical specimen with double inlet left ventricle, the rudimentary right ventricle is positioned anterosuperiorly and to the right of the dominant left ventricle.

rudimentary and incomplete because it lacks any atrioventricular connection, in other words, without its inlet portion. Such incomplete right ventricles are always found anterosuperiorly relative to the dominant left ventricle, irrespective of whether there is double inlet, absent right, or absent left atrioventricular connection. They can, however, be positioned either to the right (Fig. 6.13), or to the left (Fig. 6.14) of the dominant ventricle.

More rarely, the atrial chambers may be connected to a dominant right ventricle. This happens most frequently in the absence of the left atrioventricular connection (Fig. 6.15), but can be found with double inlet or, rarely, with absence of the right atrioventricular connection. When only the right ventricle is connected

to the atrial chambers, it is the left ventricle that is incomplete and rudimentary, lacking its atrioventricular connection and, hence, its inlet portion. The incomplete left ventricle will always be found in posteroinferior position. Usually it is left-sided, although rarely it can be right-sided.

The third morphological configuration found with double inlet or, rarely, with absence of either atrioventricular connection, is when the atrial chambers connect to a solitary ventricle that has indeterminate apical trabecular morphology (Fig. 6.16). Incomplete and rudimentary second ventricles are never found in this variant of univentricular atrioventricular connection, in which the only septal structure in the ventricle is found separating the outflow tracts.

VALVAR MORPHOLOGY

The atrioventricular valvar morphology is independent of the way in which the atrial chambers connect with the ventricles. Valvar morphology, therefore, constitutes a separate feature of the atrioventricular junctions. With concordant, discordant, ambiguous, or double inlet connections, both atrial chambers are connected to the ventricular mass. The two atrioventricular junctions can then be guarded by two separate atrioventricular valves (Fig. 6.17), or by a common valve (Fig. 6.18). When there are two valves, either can be imperforate. An imperforate valve must be distinguished from absence of an atrioventricular connection, since either can produce atrioventricular valvar 'atresia'. With an imperforate valve, the

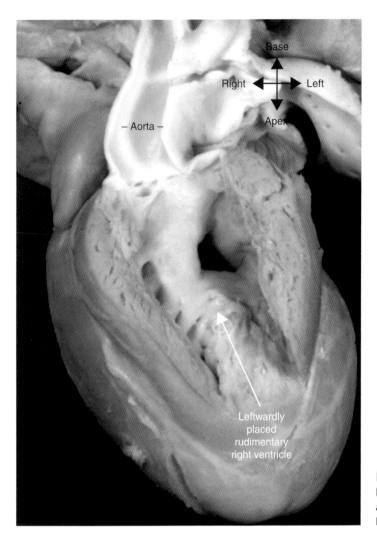

Base

Right ← → Left

Apex

— Aorta —

Leftwardly placed rudimentary right ventricle

Fig. 6.14 This anatomical specimen, again with double inlet left ventricle, has the rudimentary right ventricle in anterosuperior and leftward position relative to the dominant left ventricle.

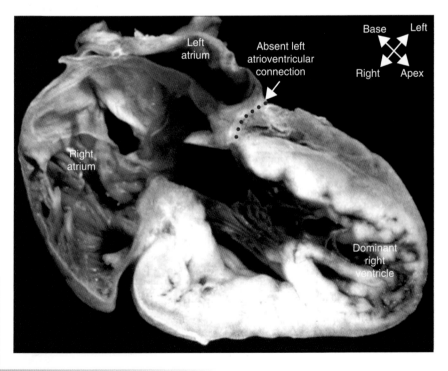

Base — Left

Left atrium

Absent left atrioventricular connection

Right — Apex

Right atrium

Dominant right ventricle

Fig. 6.15 This section through a specimen in 'four-chamber' orientation shows absence of the left atrioventricular connection (red dotted line) with the right atrium connected to a dominant right ventricle.

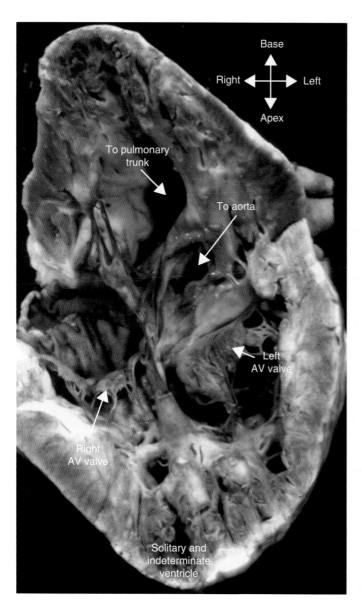

Fig. 6.16 This heart, opened in 'clam-like' fashion, has double inlet to, and double outlet from, a solitary and indeterminate ventricle, the ventricle itself having very coarse apical trabeculations.

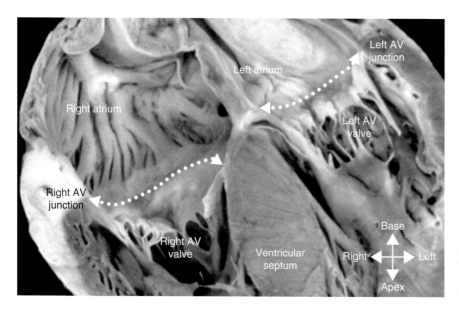

Fig. 6.17 This example of a normal heart, sectioned in 'four-chamber' orientation, shows the right and left atrioventricular junctions (dotted lines) guarded by separate atrioventricular valves.

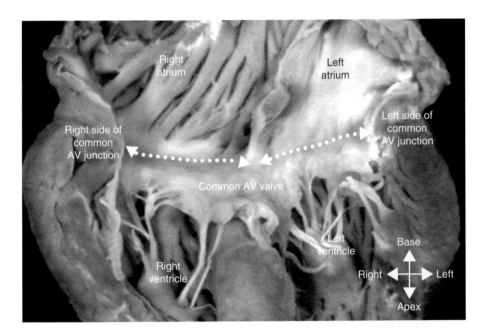

Fig. 6.18 This section, again in 'four-chamber' orientation (compare with Fig. 6.17), shows that the right and left atrioventricular junctions (dotted lines) are guarded by a common atrioventricular valve.

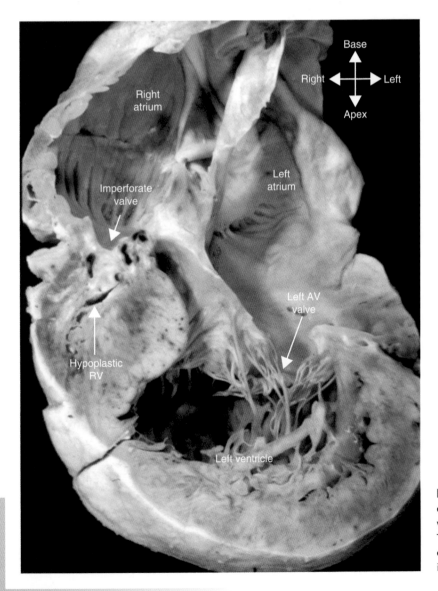

Fig. 6.19 This section of a heart in 'four-chamber' orientation shows an imperforate right atrioventricular valve connecting to a hypoplastic right ventricle (RV). The atrioventricular (AV) connections remain concordant, even though the right valve is imperforate.

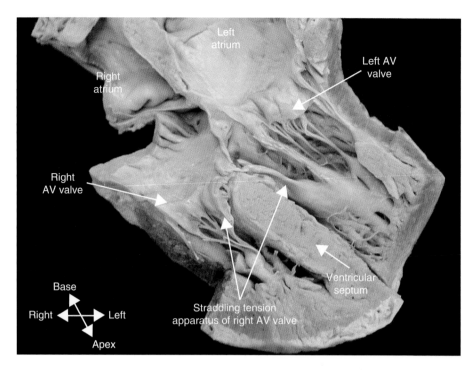

Fig. 6.20 This section of a heart, in 'four-chamber' orientation, shows how the tension apparatus of the straddling right atrioventricular (AV) valve is attached to both sides of the ventricular septum, while the orifice of the right atrioventricular junction is overriding.

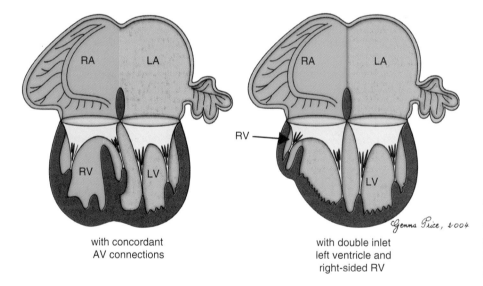

with concordant AV connections

with double inlet left ventricle and right-sided RV

Gemma Price, 2004

Fig. 6.21 In presence of an overriding junction, be it atrioventricular or ventriculo-arterial, the junction is considered to belong to the ventricle supporting its greater part. This is the so-called "50% rule", illustrated here for the atrioventricular junctions.

connection has formed but is blocked by a valvar membrane (Fig. 6.19). When the connection is absent, the floor of the atrium involved is completely separated from the ventricular mass by the fibrofatty tissue of the atrioventricular groove (see Fig. 6.8).

Either of two valves, or a common valve, can also straddle a septum within the ventricular mass. In this respect, we distinguish straddling of the tension apparatus of a valve from overriding of its annulus. Straddling is considered present when the tension apparatus is attached to each side of a septum (Fig. 6.20). Overriding is present when the junction is connected to both ventricles. The degree of override, which usually coexists with straddling, determines the precise atrioventricular connection present. So as to adjudicate the connection in the presence of overriding, the overriding valve is assigned to the ventricle connected to its greater part. This is called the "50% rule" (Fig. 6.21). The possible arrangements are much more limited when one atrioventricular connection is absent. In this case the solitary valve present can either be committed in its entirety to one ventricle, or else it can straddle and override. When the valve straddles and overrides in this setting, then the atrioventricular connection itself is uniatrial but biventricular (Fig. 6.11).

VENTRICULAR MORPHOLOGY AND TOPOLOGY

From the discussion above, it will be appreciated that the nature of an atrioventricular connection is inextricably linked with the architectural arrangement of the ventricular mass. Concordant or discordant atrioventricular connections cannot be defined until the morphology of the ventricles is known. Ambiguous, double inlet, and absent connections can all be identified without mention of ventricular morphology. It is always necessary, nonetheless, to give more information concerning the arrangement of the ventricular mass. For instance, in the case of an ambiguous connection, it is important to describe the pattern in which the morphologically right ventricle is structured relative to the morphologically left ventricle. This ventricular pattern can take only one of two topological arrangements. This is because, when there is an ambiguous connection, the right-sided atrium, with either a morphologically right or left appendage, can be connected to either a morphologically right or a morphologically left ventricle (see Fig. 6.7). When there is right isomerism, and the right-sided atrium is connected to a morphologically right ventricle, the ventricular mass is typically as seen in hearts with concordant atrioventricular connections and usual atrial arrangement. In contrast, when there is right isomerism, and the right-sided atrium is connected to a morphologically left ventricle, the ventricular mass is as usually found in the presence of

discordant atrioventricular connections and usual atrial arrangement.

These two basic patterns of ventricular topology can conveniently be described according to the way in which the hands can be placed, figuratively speaking, palm downwards upon the septal surface of the morphologically right ventricle. The other hand will then fit in the morphologically left ventricle in similar fashion, but it is the arrangement of the morphologically right ventricle that is chosen for the purposes of description. When the ventricles are found with the usual atrial arrangement and concordant atrioventricular connections, only the right hand can be placed so that the thumb is in the ventricular inlet and the fingers are in the outlet. When the usual atrial arrangement exists with discordant atrioventricular connections, it is the left hand that can be placed in this manner. These two patterns[11] are respectively termed 'right hand' and 'left hand' patterns of ventricular topology (Fig. 6.22). The significance of this feature in hearts with ambiguous and biventricular connections is that the ventricular topology determines the disposition of the atrioventricular conduction tissues[9]. This topic discussed further in Chapter 8.

When the atrial chambers connect to only one ventricle, the morphology of that

ventricle must always be described. This is because, as already stated, the dominant ventricle may be of left ventricular, right ventricular, or solitary and indeterminate pattern. It is also necessary to determine whether a rudimentary and incomplete ventricle is present and, if present, to describe its relationship to the dominant ventricle.

VENTRICULAR RELATIONSHIPS

Ventricular relationships, as opposed to ventricular topology, should generally be described as a separate feature of the heart. Where each atrium is connected to its own ventricle, the relationships are almost always in harmony with both the connection and topology present. When the atrial chambers are in their usual position with concordant atrioventricular connections, the relationships described in the setting of the heart within the chest are almost always for the morphologically right ventricle to be right-sided, anterior, and inferior to the morphologically left ventricle. In mirror-imaged atrial arrangement, with concordant atrioventricular connections, the morphologically right ventricle is almost invariably left-sided, anterior, and inferior to the morphologically left ventricle.

With the atrial chambers in their usual arrangement, and discordant

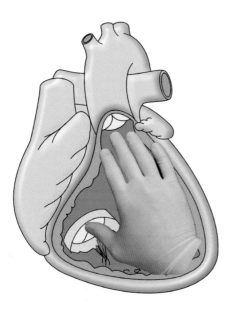

Right hand topology

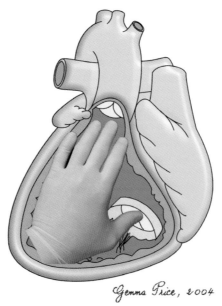

Left hand topology

Gemma Price, 2004

Fig. 6.22 The cartoon shows how the patterns of ventricular topology can be described, figuratively speaking, in terms of the way that the palmar surface of the hands can be placed on the septal surface of the morphologically right ventricle. The fingers point up the outlet, and the thumb lies in the inlet, giving right hand and left hand patterns. In the arrangements shown, the atrioventricular connections are concordant, but the ventriculo-arterial connections are discordant, with the aorta arising from the morphologically right ventricle ("transpostion").

atrioventricular connections, there is almost always left hand pattern of ventricular topology. The usual relationship is for the morphologically right ventricle to be left-sided, anterior, and inferior. When discordant atrioventricular connections accompany mirror-imaged atrial arrangement, there is usually right hand topology. The ventricular relationships are then similar to those seen in the normal heart. When the relationships are as anticipated, it is unnecessary to describe them. But, very occasionally, the relationships of the ventricles are not as anticipated for the connections present. This disharmony between connections and relationships underscores the anomaly known as the 'criss-cross heart'[12,13]. With these hearts, and also those with so-called 'superoinferior ventricles'[11], connections and relationships must be described separately, using as much detail as is necessary to achieve unambiguous categorization. The essence of the 'criss-cross heart', therefore, is that the ventricular relationships are not as expected for the atrioventricular connection present. Even more rarely, the ventricular topology may be disharmonious with the atrioventricular connection[14]. All features must then be described.

In hearts with univentricular atrioventricular connection, the relationship of the incomplete and rudimentary ventricle, if present, must be described. When the left ventricle is dominant, the incomplete right ventricle is always anterosuperior, but can be right- or left-sided. The sidedness of the ventricle does not affect the basic disposition of the atrioventricular conduction tissues in these hearts. With dominant right ventricle, the incomplete and rudimentary left ventricle, if present, is always posteroinferior, but again can be right- or left-sided. In this case, the sidedness of the rudimentary ventricle does affect the disposition of the atrioventricular conduction tissue (see below).

When considering the atrioventricular junctions, therefore, there are four different features to take into account. These are, first, the way the atrial myocardium is connected to the ventricular mass, second, the morphology of the atrioventricular valves guarding the junctions, third, the ventricular morphology and topology, and finally the ventricular relationships. All are of importance to the surgeon because they influence the disposition of the atrioventricular conduction axis.

VENTRICULO-ARTERIAL JUNCTIONS

Analysis of the ventriculo-arterial junctions proceeds as described for the atrioventricular junctions, with morphology of the connection, the valvar morphology, and the relationships of the arterial trunks being different facets requiring separate description in mutually exclusive terms. It is also necessary to take account of infundibular morphology.

Ventriculo-arterial connections

There are four discrete ways in which the arterial trunks can be connected to the ventricular mass, namely in concordant, discordant, double outlet, and single outlet fashion. Concordant ventriculo-arterial connections exist when the arterial trunks are connected to morphologically appropriate ventricles. Discordant connections account for the trunks being connected with morphologically inappropriate ventricles. Double outlet connections exist when both great arteries are connected to the same ventricle, which may be of right, left, or indeterminate morphology. A single outlet arrangement is seen when only one arterial trunk is connected to the heart. This may be a common trunk, supplying directly the systemic, pulmonary and coronary arteries, or it may be an aortic or pulmonary trunk when the complementary arterial trunk is atretic, and its connection to a known ventricle cannot be established (Fig. 6.23). Rarely, in the absence of intrapericardial pulmonary arteries, it may be more accurate to describe an arterial trunk as solitary rather than common (Fig. 6.23).

Arterial valvar morphology

The morphological arrangement of the arterial valves is limited because they have no tension apparatus. Furthermore, a common valve can exist only with a common trunk, and as an integral part of the connection. The different patterns, therefore, involve one of two arterial valves. Usually both valves are perforate, but either or both may override the ventricular septum. When a valvar orifice is overriding, the '50%' rule can

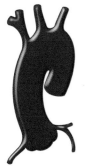

Aorta

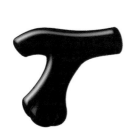

Pulmonary trunk

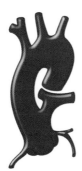

Common arterial trunk

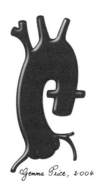

Solitary arterial trunk

Gemma Price, 2004

Fig. 6.23 This cartoon shows the patterns which identify the morphology of the arterial trunks. When there is absence of the intrapericardial pulmonary arteries, there is no way of knowing if, had there been an atretic pulmonary trunk, it would have originated from the base of the heart or from the aorta. This pattern, therefore, is best described as a solitary arterial trunk.

again be applied to assign the valve to the ventricle connected to its greater part, thus avoiding the need for intermediate categories. The other pattern of valvar morphology is when one of the arterial valves is imperforate. As with the atrioventricular junctions, an imperforate arterial valve must be distinguished from absence of one ventriculo-arterial connection, since both can produce arterial valvar 'atresia'.

Infundibular morphology

Describing the morphology at the ventriculo-arterial junctions also involves the arrangement of the musculature within the ventricular outflow tracts. This is infundibular morphology. Although the outlet regions are integral parts of the ventricular mass, it is traditional to consider them in concert with the great arteries. The two outflow tracts together make a complete cone of musculature. This cone has parietal components, a septal component, and a component adjacent to the atrioventricular junction (Fig. 6.24). The parietal components make up the anterior free wall of the outflow tracts. The septal component is the outlet, or infundibular, septum. This has a body, with septal and parietal insertions. The component adjacent to the atrioventricular junction always separates the leaflets of

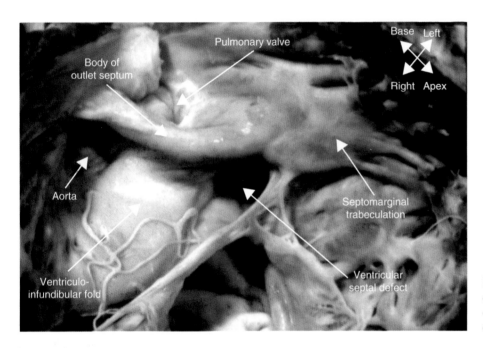

Fig. 6.24 This view of a heart with double outlet right ventricle, seen in anatomical orientation, shows the muscular components of the ventricular outflow tracts.

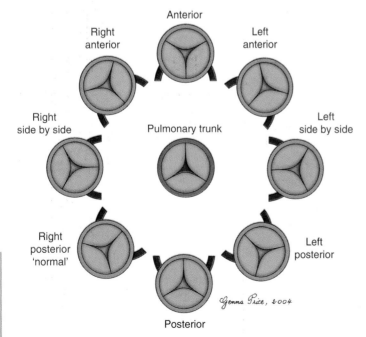

Fig. 6.25 This cartoon shows the combination of anterior to posterior, and right to left, co-ordinates that are used to describe the interrelationships of the aortic and pulmonary valves.

arterial from atrioventricular valves. It is termed the ventriculo-infundibular fold, although the fold may be attenuated to give arterial-atrioventricular valvar fibrous continuity (Fig. 6.24).

The infundibular structures never contain or overlie conduction tissue. It is vital, therefore, to distinguish them from another structure, namely the septomarginal trabeculation, or septal band. This latter structure is part of the ventricular septum, reinforcing its right ventricular aspect. It has a body that continues apically as the moderator band, and two limbs. The anterior limb, in the normal heart, extends to the pulmonary valve, overlying the outlet septum. The posterior limb runs beneath the interventricular membranous septum. This posterior limb usually overlies the branching part of the atrioventricular bundle, with the right bundle branch passing down to the apex of the right ventricle within the body of the trabeculation.

Although each outflow tract is potentially a complete muscular structure, in most hearts it is only the outflow tract of the right ventricle that is a complete muscular cone. This is because, within the left ventricle, part of the ventriculo-infundibular fold is usually attenuated to permit fibrous continuity between the leaflets of the arterial and atrioventricular valves. In the normal heart, therefore, there is a muscular subpulmonary infundibulum in the right ventricle, and fibrous valvar continuity in the roof of the left ventricle.

In congenitally malformed hearts, three other patterns may be found. These are, first, a muscular subaortic infundibulum with pulmonary-atrioventricular continuity, second, a bilaterally muscular infundibulum and, third, bilateral deficiency of the infundibulums. In the presence of a common arterial trunk, there may be a complete muscular subtruncal infundibulum, but more often there is truncal-atrioventricular valvar continuity.

Arterial valvar and truncal relationships

The final feature of consideration at the ventriculo-arterial junctions is the relationship of the arterial valves and arterial trunks. Valvar relationships are independent of both ventriculo-arterial connections and infundibular morphology. Of the many methods of description, our preference is to describe the aortic relative to the pulmonary valve as viewed from below in right-left, anteroposterior and, when necessary, superoinferior coordinates. This can be done as precisely as required. In our experience, eight coordinates combining lateral and anterior to posterior positions suffice (Fig. 6.25). When describing the relationship of the arterial trunks, it is sufficient to account for trunks that spiral round each other as they ascend, and to distinguish them from trunks that ascend in parallel fashion.

POSITION OF THE HEART

The system discussed in this chapter establishes the cardiac template. Irrespective of the internal architecture, it is well known that the heart itself can occupy many and varied positions (see Chapter 10), particularly when there are complex intracardiac malformations. To describe the position of the heart in unambiguous fashion, it is necessary to account separately for its site within the thorax, and the orientation of its apex. We describe the heart as being in the left or right side of the chest, or in the midline. Apical orientation is described as being to the left, to the middle, or to the right.

CATALOGUE OF MALFORMATIONS

Having described the template of the heart, and its position, it is finally necessary to catalogue all intracardiac malformations. In most cases, these lesions constitute the 'meat' of a given case. Any lesion, nonetheless, cannot be presumed to be the only lesion until the rest of the heart has been established as normal. It is these associated lesions which will be emphasised in subsequent chapters, taking particular note, as before, of the features of surgical significance.

References

1. Anderson RH, Ho SY. Continuing Medical Education. Sequential segmental analysis – description and categorization for the millennium. *Cardiol Young* 1997; **7**: 98–116.

2. Anderson RH, Wilcox BR. Understanding cardiac anatomy: the prerequisite for optimal cardiac surgery. *Ann Thorac Surg* 1995; **59**: 1366–1375.

3. Uemura H, Ho SY, Devine WA, Kilpatrick LL, Anderson RH. Atrial appendages and venoatrial connections in hearts with patients with visceral heterotaxy. *Ann Thorac Surg* 1995; **60**: 561–569.

4. Van Mierop LHS, Gessner IH, Schiebler GL. Asplenia and polysplenia syndromes. In: Bergsma D, ed. Birth Defects: Original Article Series, Vol VIII, No 5. *The Fourth Conference on the Clinical Delineation of Birth Defects. Part XV The Cardiovascular System.* The National Foundation March of Dimes. Baltimore: Williams and Wilkins Company, 1972: 36–44.

5. Ivemark BI. Implications of agenesis of the spleen on the pathogenesis of conotruncus anomalies in childhood. An analysis of the heart; malformations in the splenic agenesis syndrome, with 14 new cases. *Acta Paediatr Scand* 1955; **44(Suppl. 104)**: 1–110.

6. Macartney FJ, Zuberbuhler JR, Anderson RH. Morphological considerations pertaining to recognition of atrial isomerism. Consequences for sequential chamber localisation. *Br Heart J* 1980; **44**: 657–667.

7. Sharma S, Devine W, Anderson RH, Zuberbuhler JR. The determination of atrial arrangement by examination of appendage morphology in 1842 heart specimens. *Br Heart J* 1988; **60**: 227–231.

8. Huhta JC, Smallhorn JF, Macartney FJ. Two dimensional echocardiographic diagnosis of situs. *Br Heart J* 1982; **48**: 97–108.

9. Dickinson DF, Wilkinson JL, Anderson KR, Smith A, Ho SY, Anderson RH. The cardiac conduction system in situs ambiguus. *Circulation* 1979; **59**: 879–885.

10. Ho SY, Seo J-W, Brown NA, Cook AC, Fagg NLK, Anderson RH. Morphology of the sinus node in human and mouse hearts with isomerism of the atrial appendages. *Br Heart J* 1995; **74**: 437–442.

11. Van Praagh S, LaCorte M, Fellows KE, Bossina K, Busch HJ, Keck EW, Weinberg PM, Van Praagh R. Superoinferior ventricles: anatomic and angiographic findings in ten postmortem cases. In: Van Praagh R, Takao A (eds). *Etiology and Morphogenesis of Congenital Heart Disease*. New York: Futura Publishing Company Inc.1980: 317–378.

12. Anderson RH, Shinebourne EA, Gerlis LM. Criss-cross atrioventricular relationships producing paradoxical atrioventricular concordance or discordance. Their significance to nomenclature of congenital heart disease. *Circulation* 1974; **50**: 176–180.

13. Anderson RH. Criss-cross hearts revisited. *Pediatr Cardiol* 1982; **3**: 305–313.

14. Anderson RH, Smith A, Wilkinson JL. Disharmony between atrioventricular connections and segmental combinations – unusual variants of "criss-cross" hearts. *J Am Coll Cardiol* 1987; **10**: 1274–1277.

7

Lesions with normal segmental connections

SEPTAL DEFECTS

Understanding the anatomy of septal defects is greatly facilitated if the heart is thought of as having three distinct septal structures: the atrial septum, the atrioventricular septum, and the ventricular septum (Fig. 7.1).

The atrial septum is a relatively small structure comprising, for the most part, the floor of the oval fossa. It is limited superiorly and anteriorly, and posteriorly, by the rim of the fossa, this itself being formed by infolding of the adjacent right and left atrial walls. Inferiorly and anteriorly, the rim of the fossa is a true muscular septum contiguous with the atrioventricular septum, this latter structure being the superior component of the fibrous membranous septum. In the normal heart, this fibrous septum is itself contiguous with the atrial wall of the triangle of Koch (Fig. 7.2). In the past, we have described this component of the atrial wall, which overlaps the upper part of the ventricular septum between the attachments of the leaflets of the tricuspid and mitral valves, as the muscular atrioventricular septum. As we discussed in Chapter 2, in reality it is a sandwich,

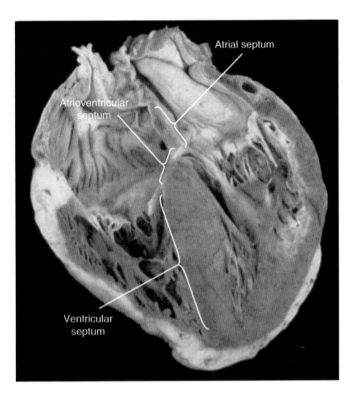

Fig. 7.1 This 'four-chamber' cut through the heart, in anatomic orientation, shows the atrial and ventricular septal components, along with the location of the muscular structures separating the cavities of right atrium and left ventricle. Previously we considered this area to be an "atrioventricular muscular septum", but we now know it to be a sandwich of fibrofatty tissue between the atrial and ventricular musculatures (see Fig. 7.3). Irrespective of such considerations, this area is deficient in the setting of deficient atrioventricular septation.

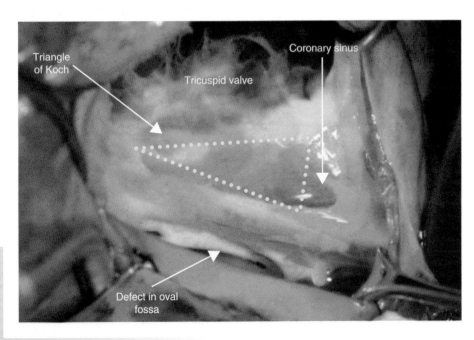

Fig. 7.2 This surgical view through a right atriotomy shows the landmarks of the triangle of Koch (triangle). This area occupies the atrial aspect of the muscular atrioventricular sandwich. Note that this patient also has a defect within the oval fossa.

since throughout this area, the adipose tissue of the inferior atrioventricular groove is incorporated between the layers of atrial and ventricular myocardium (Fig. 7.3). It is convenient, nonetheless, to consider the entire area comprising the fibrous septum and the muscular sandwich as an atrioventricular structure, since it is absent in the hearts we describe as atrioventricular septal defects.

When considering the ventricular septum, usually the surgeon views it only from its right ventricular aspect. For this reason, and other reasons discussed below, ventricular septal defects are best considered in terms of their right ventricular landmarks. The ventricular

septum is made up of a small fibrous element, the interventricular membranous septum, and a much larger muscular part. The muscular part is more complex geometrically than the other septal structures, which lie almost completely in a coronal plane. At first sight, it seems possible to divide the muscular septum into inlet, apical trabecular, and outlet components, each of these parts abutting on the membranous septum (Fig. 7.4). Closer inspection shows that such analysis is simplistic. This is because, by virtue of the deeply wedged location of the subaortic outflow tract, much of the so-called inlet septum, delimited on the right ventricular aspect by the septal

leaflet of the tricuspid valve, separates the inlet of the right ventricle from the outlet of the left (Fig. 7.5). The outlet component of the ventricular septum is also much smaller than it appears when viewed from the right ventricle. This is because most of the subpulmonary infundibulum is a free-standing muscular sleeve (Fig. 7.6). That small septal component that separates the outlets joins with the much more extensive ventriculo-infundibular fold to form the supraventricular crest (Fig. 7.7). It is the apical septum, therefore, which accounts for the greater part of the muscular ventricular septum, extending to the apex in curvilinear fashion in reflection of the fact that the banana-shaped right

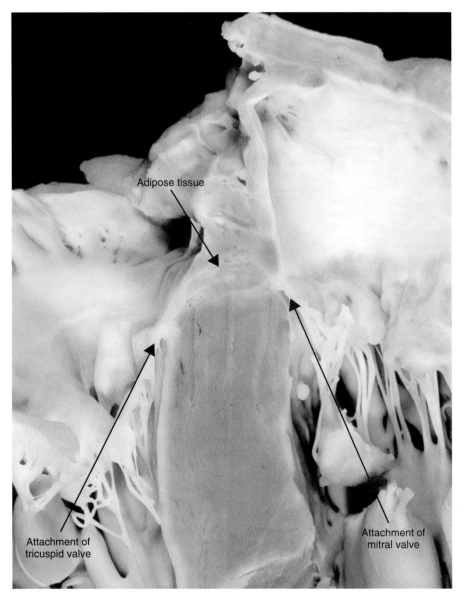

Adipose tissue

Attachment of tricuspid valve

Attachment of mitral valve

Fig. 7.3 This four-chamber section of a normal heart, shown in anatomical orientation, illustrates the differential attachments of the atrioventricular valves. Note the adipose tissue interposed between the right atrial wall and the crest of the ventricular septum, and forming the "meat" in the atrioventricular muscular sandwich.

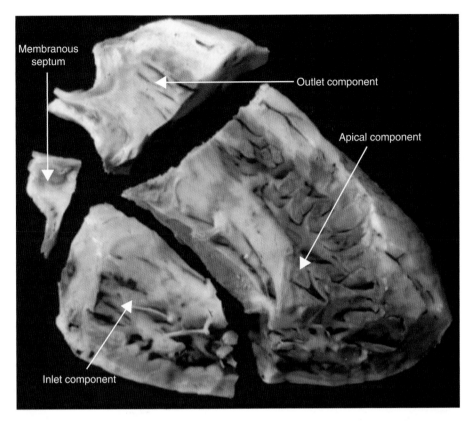

Fig. 7.4 In this dissection, seen in anatomic orientation, the ventricular septum has been separated from the remainder of the heart and is divided into fibrous and muscular parts. The muscular part is then further divided into segments corresponding to the components of the right ventricle.

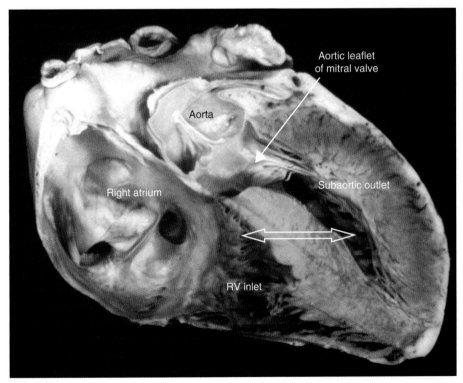

Fig. 7.5 This section, simulating the oblique subcostal echocardiographic cut, shows how the muscular septum separates the right ventricular inlet from the left ventricular outlet (double headed arrow).

ventricle wraps itself around the conical left ventricle. An important landmark for the description of defects within the ventricular septum is the septomarginal trabeculation, or septal band. This is the extensive muscular strap which overlies the right ventricular aspect of the muscular septum, with its limbs extending to the base of the heart to clasp the supraventricular crest (Fig. 7.8).

Atrial septal defects

There are several lesions which permit interatrial shunting (Fig. 7.9). Although collectively termed 'atrial septal defects',

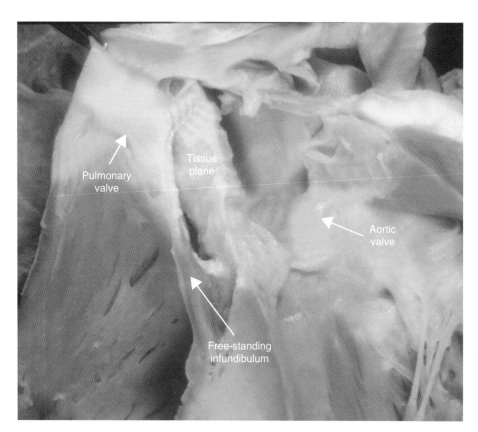

Fig. 7.6 This dissection of the ventricular outflow tracts, in anatomic orientation, shows the free-standing sleeve of infundibulum that supports the leaflets of the pulmonary valve.

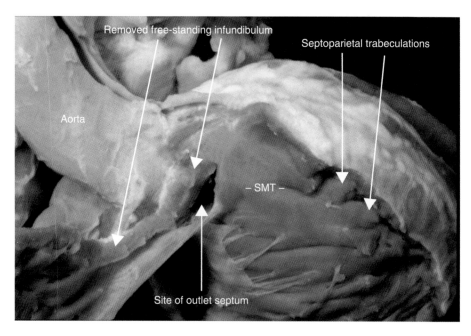

Fig. 7.7 This dissection, seen in anatomic orientation, shows how most of the supraventricular crest is formed by the ventriculo-infundibular fold. Only a small part of the subpulmonary outlet, removed in this dissection, separates the ventricular outlets. SMT – septomarginal trabeculation.

not all are within the confines of the normal atrial septum (see Fig. 2.12). The so-called 'secundum' defect, or, as we prefer to call it, the oval fossa defect, is a true deficiency of the atrial septum. The 'ostium primum' defect is due to a deficiency of the atrioventricular structures, and will be considered in the next section. Sinus venosus defects, most frequently associated with partially anomalous pulmonary venous drainage, are found at the mouths of the caval veins. Also producing interatrial shunting is the rare defect found at the mouth of the coronary sinus, mediated through a communication between the sinus itself and the cavity of the left atrium.

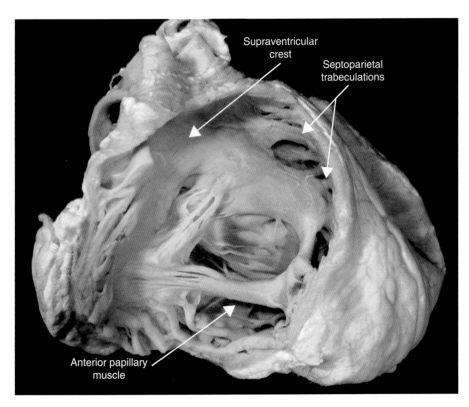

Supraventricular
crest

Septoparietal
trabeculations

Anterior papillary
muscle

Fig. 7.8 The septal surface of the right ventricle has been displayed by making a window in the anterior wall. The shows the septomarginal trabeculation, with the supraventricular crest inserting between its two limbs. From the apical part of the septomarginal trabeculation, the moderator band crosses the cavity of the ventricle to become continuous with the anterior papillary muscle, while the series of septoparietal trabeculations arise from the anterior margin of the major trabeculation.

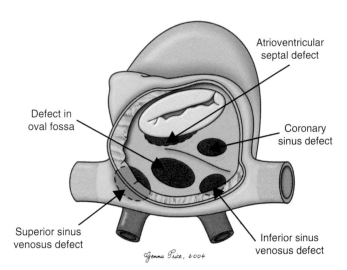

Atrioventricular
septal defect

Defect in
oval fossa

Coronary
sinus defect

Superior sinus
venosus defect

Inferior sinus
venosus defect

Gemma Price, 2004

Fig. 7.9 The cartoon shows the various holes that permit interatrial shunting. Only the hole in the oval fossa is a true deficiency of the atrial septum.

Defects within the oval fossa, or 'secundum' defects, are by far the most common. They are due to deficiency (Fig. 7.10), perforation (Fig. 7.11), or absence (Fig. 7.12) of the floor of the fossa, the latter formed by the flap–valve of the oval foramen. When the haemodynamics of the shunt across such a defect dictate surgical closure, the hole is rarely likely to be small enough to permit direct suture. If attempted, the results may so distort atrial anatomy as to result in dehiscence. Since the rims of the fossa are almost always

intact, a patch can readily be secured to its margins. It is important to remember that the superior and posterior margins are infoldings of the atrial wall (Fig. 7.13). The likeliest potential danger in this area is to the sinus nodal artery (Fig. 7.14). Sometimes this artery courses intramyocardially through the superior margin, or lies deep within the fold. Anteriorly, there is a more remote chance of damaging the aorta, which underlies the cephalad margin of the fossa, in the area called the aortic mound.

The posteroinferior edge of the fossa is deficient in some cases, and then the defect can extend into the mouth of the inferior caval vein (Fig. 7.15). It is possible, in this circumstance, to mistake a well-formed Eustachian valve for the posteroinferior margin of the defect. Because a patch attached to this valve would connect the inferior caval vein to the left atrium, it is always prudent to ensure continuity of the inferior caval vein and right atrium following placement of the patch.

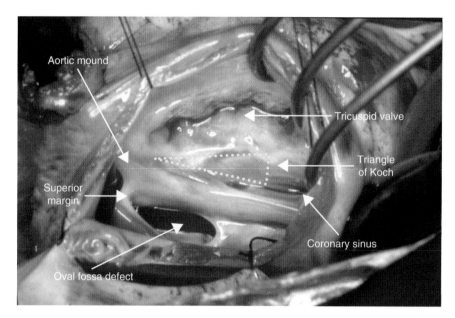

Fig. 7.10 This surgical view through a right atriotomy shows deficiency in the floor of the oval fossa. This is a true atrial septal defect.

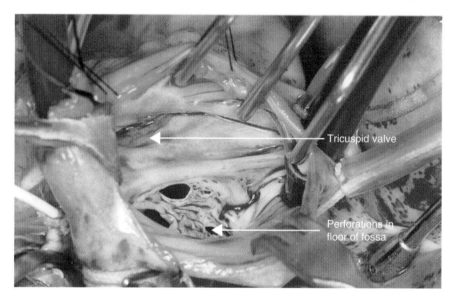

Fig. 7.11 This surgical view through a right atriotomy shows perforations in the floor of the oval fossa. This again is a true atrial septal defect.

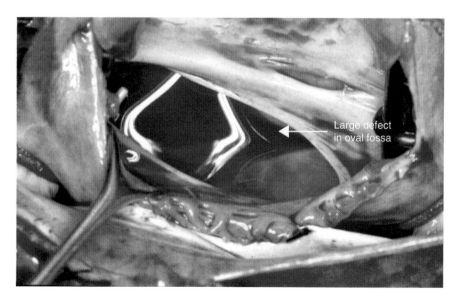

Fig. 7.12 This surgical view through a right atriotomy shows absence of the floor of the oval fossa. Once again, this is a true atrial septal defect.

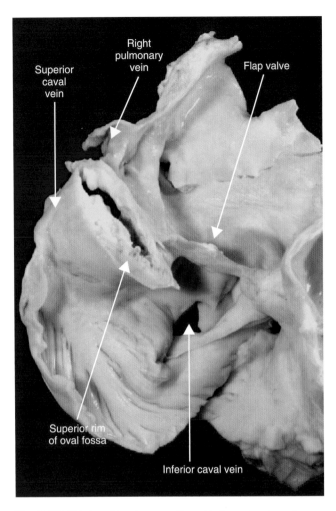

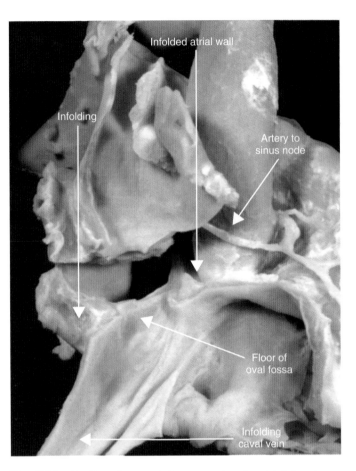

Fig. 7.13 This heart has been sectioned in four chamber plane, showing that the superior rim of the oval fossa is an infolding wall of the interatrial groove between the systemic venous sinus and the entry of the pulmonary veins into the left atrium.

Fig. 7.14 This dissection, made by transecting the atrial chambers, and illustrated in anatomic orientation, shows the relationship of artery to the sinus node to the anterosuperior rim of the oval fossa.

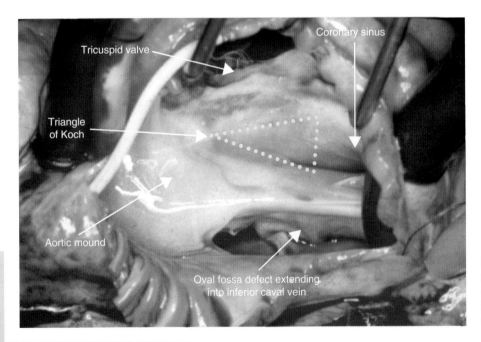

Fig. 7.15 This surgical view through a right atriotomy shows a defect within the oval fossa extending into the mouth of the inferior caval vein. Note the location of the triangle of Koch.

Sinus venosus defects are rarer than defects within the oval fossa, and present greater problems in repair. The defect adjacent to the inferior caval vein is extremely rare. It opens into the mouth of the vein posterior to the confines of the oval fossa. Usually the fossa itself is intact (Fig. 7.16), but it can be deficient or probe patent. The right inferior pulmonary vein is usually in close proximity to the interatrial defect. A defect at the mouth of the superior caval vein[1] occurs much more frequently. It, too, is outside the confines of the oval fossa[2]. It is most frequently associated with overriding of the caval vein (Fig. 7.17), but can rarely be found when the caval vein is committed exclusively to the right atrium. The defect is typically related to the orifice of the right superior pulmonary vein, which frequently drains directly into the superior caval vein, and often through more than one orifice (Figs. 7.18, 7.19). The difficulty encountered during

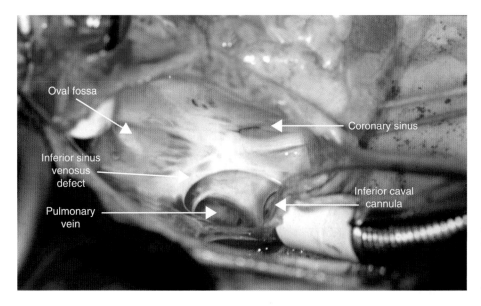

Fig. 7.16 This surgical view through a right atriotomy shows an inferior sinus venosus defect. Note that the oval fossa is intact, the inferior edge of the atrial septum being malaligned relative to the inferior caval vein.

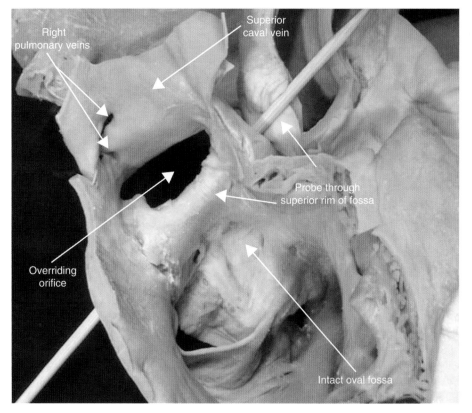

Fig. 7.17 This defect is at the mouth of the superior caval vein, which is overriding the superior rim of the oval fossa, marked by a probe passed through its fibrofatty core. Note the anomalous drainage of the right upper pulmonary veins, and the intact oval fossa. This is a typical example of the superior sinus venosus defect.

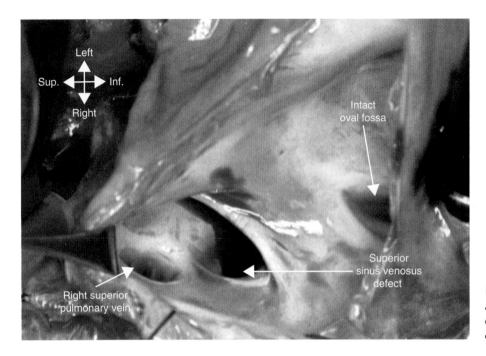

Left
Sup. Inf.
Right

Intact
oval fossa

Superior
sinus venosus
defect

Right superior
pulmonary vein

Fig. 7.18 This surgical view through a right atriotomy shows a superior sinus venosus defect, recognised because it is outside the confines of the intact oval fossa.

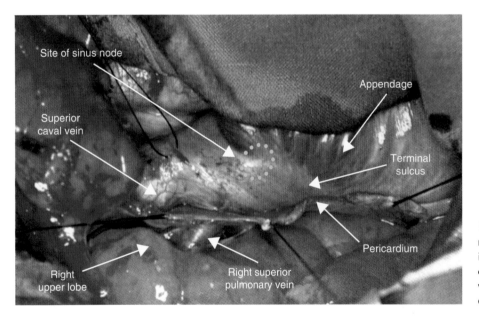

Site of sinus node

Appendage

Superior
caval vein

Terminal
sulcus

Pericardium

Right
upper lobe

Right superior
pulmonary vein

Fig. 7.19 This surgical view, through a median sternotomy of the heart shown in Fig. 7.18, illustrates the anomalous connection of the right superior pulmonary vein and the site of the sinus node (green dotted line).

surgical repair relates to the need to reconstruct the anatomy so as to reroute the venous return and, at the same time, close the interatrial communication. This must be done without obstructing venous flow or, in the case of a superior defect, damaging the sinus node. As described in Chapter 2, the sinus node is related to the anterolateral quadrant of the cavoatrial junction, and lies immediately subepicardially within the terminal groove. The sinus node should not be at risk with simple closure of the atrium

(Fig. 7.20). The problem arises should it be necessary either to suture in the area of the node when rerouting the pulmonary venous return, or if there is need to enlarge the orifice of the caval vein. The former risk can be minimised with judicious placement of the sutures. The latter problem is much greater. Because the artery to the sinus node may pass either in front of, or behind, the caval vein, the entire cavoatrial junction is a potentially dangerous area. Determining the course of the nodal artery beforehand

facilitates the execution of an operation least likely to damage the node or its artery.

Another defect which permits interatrial shunting, but which is outside the confines of the true atrial septum, is part of a constellation of lesions frequently termed 'unroofing of the coronary sinus'[3]. In this combination, a persistent left superior caval vein usually drains directly to the left atrial roof between the appendage and the left pulmonary veins (Figs. 7.21, 7.24).

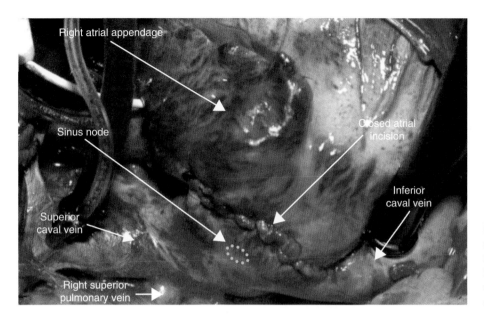

Right atrial appendage

Sinus node

Closed atrial incision

Inferior caval vein

Superior caval vein

Right superior pulmonary vein

Fig. 7.20 This view of a heart with a superior sinus venosus defect, through a median sternotomy, shows how the incision into the atrium for repair can be made without placing the sinus node (green dotted line), or its arterial supply, at risk.

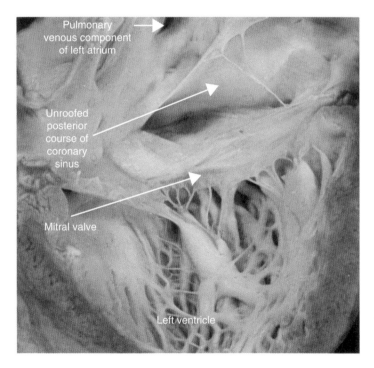

Pulmonary venous component of left atrium

Unroofed posterior course of coronary sinus

Mitral valve

Left ventricle

Fig. 7.21 The heart is shown from the left side in anatomic orientation. There is unroofing of the coronary sinus as it courses through the left atrioventricular groove, draining a persistent left superior caval vein, with filigreed remnants showing the site of the walls that initially separated the vein from the left atrium.

There is also a large hole at the expected site of the mouth of the coronary sinus (Figs. 7.22, 7.23). Often, there is evidence of the course the walls of the sinus should have taken had its course been normal through the atrioventricular groove (Fig. 7.21). Sometimes the hole can exist in isolation, without a persistent left caval vein. Surgical treatment is dictated by the presence and connections of the left superior caval vein. If it is in free communication with the right superior

caval vein, or if there is no left-sided vein, the hole at the expected site of the mouth of the coronary sinus can simply be closed and the vein, if present, ligated. If the left-sided channel has no anastomoses with the right side, it may be better to construct a channel in the posteroinferior wall of the left atrium, connecting the mouth of the left-sided vein with the interatrial communication existing at the expected orifice of the coronary sinus.

Atrioventricular septal defects

'Atrioventricular septal defect'[4] is, in our opinion, the most accurate collective term for the anomalies variously described as 'endocardial cushion defects', 'atrioventricular canal defects', and 'persistent atrioventricular canal'. This is because, in anatomic terms, the malformations are primarily due to complete absence not only of the membranous atrioventricular septum, but

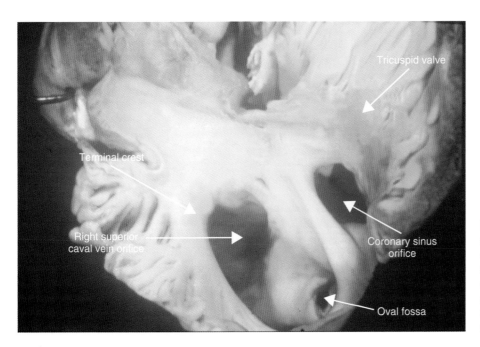

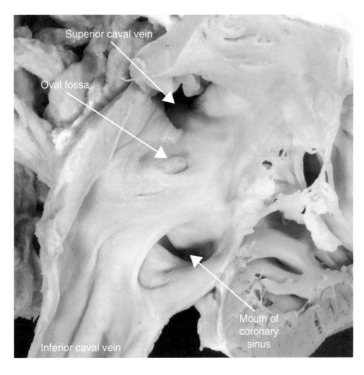

Fig. 7.22 The right atrium of the heart shown in Fig. 7.21 is shown in surgical orientation. The enlarged mouth of the coronary sinus functions as an interatrial communication outside the confines of the septum due to the absence of the walls normally separating the persistent left superior caval vein from the left atrium.

Fig. 7.23 In this heart shown in anatomic orientation, the mouth of the coronary sinus again functions as an interatrial communication.

also the overlapping region of atrial and ventricular musculatures which normally form the triangle of Koch. The structures are absent because of the pathognomonic feature of the group of hearts[5], namely a common atrioventricular junction (Fig. 7.25). The most appropriate title, therefore, would be atrioventricular septal defect with common atrioventricular junction, since very rarely a defect of the membranous atrioventricular septum can

be found in the setting of separate right and left atrioventricular junctions[6,7]. The common junction fundamentally distorts the anatomy when compared to the normally separate right and left atrioventricular junctions (Fig. 7.26).

Because of the lack of the membranous and muscular atrioventricular structures, there is no septal atrioventricular junction. Instead, the leading edges of the atrial septum and the ventricular septum,

the latter usually covered by the atrioventricular valvar leaflets, meet at the superior and inferior margins of the midpoint of the common atrioventricular junction (Fig. 7.27). This anatomy determines the anomalous disposition of the atrioventricular conduction axis. An analogue of the triangle of Koch can be seen within the leading edge of the atrial septum[8]. Because of the common atrioventricular junction, however, the

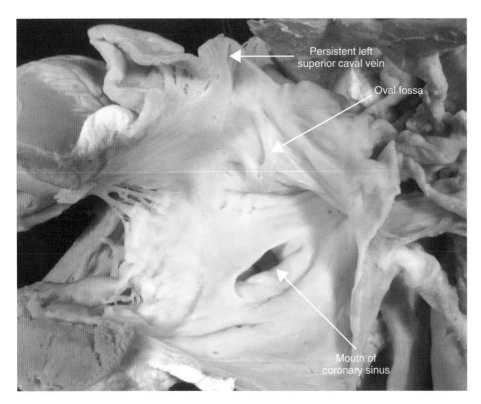

Fig. 7.24 This is the left atrium of the heart shown in Fig. 7.23. There is complete absence of any walls between the mouth of the coronary sinus and the junction of the left superior caval vein to the roof of the left atrium between the orifice of the appendage and the left pulmonary veins.

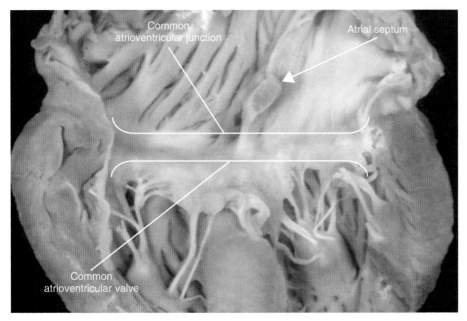

Fig. 7.25 This section, in 'four chamber' orientation, shows a common atrioventricular junction guarded by a common atrioventricular valve in a heart with deficient atrioventricular septation.

atrial septal myocardium makes contact with the ventricular myocardium only superiorly and inferiorly. Usually the atrioventricular node is displaced inferiorly, lying in a nodal triangle. The margins of this triangle, as seen by the surgeon, with the coronary sinus forming the base, are the right hand edge of the atrial septum, and the attachment of the leaflets of the effectively common atrioventricular valve (Fig. 7.28). The

atrioventricular conduction axis penetrates through the apex of this triangle. It then courses on the crest of the muscular ventricular septum, covered by the inferior bridging leaflet of the valve (see below). The distance from the base to the vertex is pertinent to surgical closure. Ideally, the surgeon wishes to place the patch so as to leave the coronary sinus draining to the systemic venous atrium. In the heart shown in Fig. 7.28, the sizable

sub-Thebesian sinus would make this feasible. In other hearts, such as the one shown in Fig. 7.29, the coronary sinus lies much closer to the apex of the nodal triangle. The distance from the base to the vertex is then such that placement of a suture line through the triangle would seriously endanger the node. In the latter situation, it would be prudent to place the patch so that the blood from the coronary sinus is left draining to the pulmonary

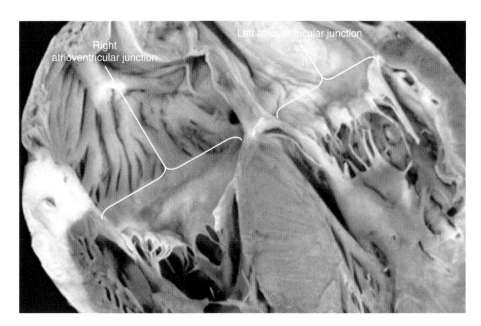

Fig. 7.26 This example of a normal heart sectioned in 'four-chamber' orientation shows the right and left atrioventricular junctions guarded by separate atrioventricular valves (compare with Fig. 7.25).

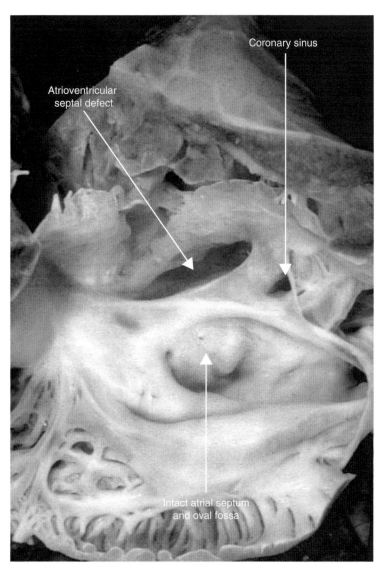

Fig. 7.27 The right side of the heart with deficient atrioventricular septation and separate right and left atrioventricular orifices (an 'ostium primum' defect) is shown in surgical orientation, the hole occupying the site of the normal atrioventricular separating structures. Note that atrial septum itself is virtually normal, and the oval fossa is intact, although the leading edge of the septum is bowed from the atrioventricular junction in the margin of the septal defect.

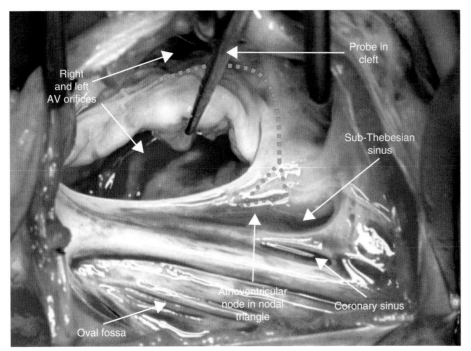

Fig. 7.28 This view through a right atriotomy shows the atrial septal surface in a heart with an atrioventricular septal defect and separate right and left atrioventricular orifices ('ostium primum' defect). Koch's triangle is well-formed, but no longer contains the atrioventricular node, which is displaced posteroinferiorly to the apex of a new nodal triangle, which contains the node (green dotted lines). Note the extensive sub-Thebesian sinus, around which the suture line can be deviated to avoid the conduction tissues.

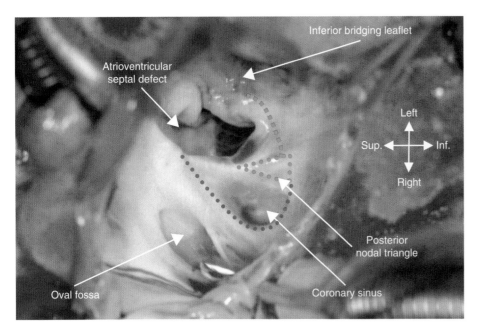

Fig. 7.29 In this heart, seen through a right atriotomy, there is little room around the coronary sinus to place a patch so as to leave the sinus draining to the right side. It is safer to deviate the suture line around the sinus (red dotted line), leaving it draining to the left atrium after correction. The danger areas for the conduction tissues are shown by the green dotted lines.

venous atrium. Occasionally, the inferior portion of the atrial septum itself is deficient. The inferior nodal triangle is then not well seen. The coronary sinus then opens more posteriorly and medially through the left atrial wall (Fig. 7.30). The conduction axis, nevertheless, is still found in its expected location at the crux of the heart[9].

The feature that distinguishes between the various forms of atrioventricular septal defects is the morphology of the leaflets of the atrioventricular valve that guards the common atrioventricular junction, together with their relationship to the septal structures bordering the defect[5]. In any heart which lacks the separating atrioventricular structures, the valve which guards the atrioventricular junction is basically a common one with five leaflets. This is most readily seen when the valve has a common orifice (Fig. 7.31).

Two of the leaflets guarding the common junction then extend across the ventricular septum, with their tension apparatus attached in both ventricles. These are the superior and inferior bridging leaflets. Two other leaflets are entirely contained within the right ventricle. There are the anterosuperior and inferior mural leaflets. The fifth leaflet is contained exclusively within the left ventricle, and is also a mural leaflet.

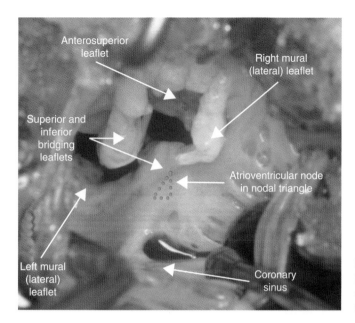

Fig. 7.30 In this atrioventricular septal defect with separate right and left valvar orifices, the atrial septum is deficient and deviated leftward away from the crux, lacking the so-called 'sinus septum'. The position of the atrioventricular node is indicated by the green dotted triangle.

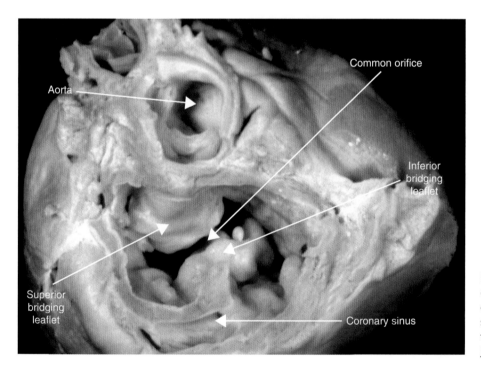

Fig. 7.31 This atrioventricular septal defect, positioned anatomically, and with a common valvar orifice, has been dissected to show the arrangement of the five leaflets that guard the common atrioventricular junction.

Although the two leaflets found within the right ventricle are comparable to similar leaflets seen in the normal heart, the left ventricular leaflets of the common atrioventricular valve (Fig. 7.32) bear no resemblance to a normal mitral valve. In the normal mitral valve, the ends of the zones of apposition between the leaflets, and the papillary muscle supporting them, are situated inferoanteriorly and superoposteriorly within the left ventricle (Fig. 7.33). With this arrangement, the extensive mural leaflet guards two–thirds of the circumference of the valvar orifice. In atrioventricular septal defects with common atrioventricular junction, in contrast, the left ventricular papillary muscles are deviated laterally, being positioned superiorly and inferiorly[10]. Because of this, the mural leaflet is relatively insignificant, and guards much less than one-third of the circumference of the left atrioventricular orifice. The left orifice is, in effect, guarded by a valve possessing three leaflets, these being the small mural leaflet, and the more extensive left ventricular components of the superior and inferior bridging leaflets. (Fig. 7.34).

It was originally suggested[11] that the common valve possessed four rather than five leaflets, with a cleft being found in the 'common anterior leaflet'. Close examination of this supposed 'cleft' (Fig. 7.35) shows that, in reality, it is a zone of apposition between the superior

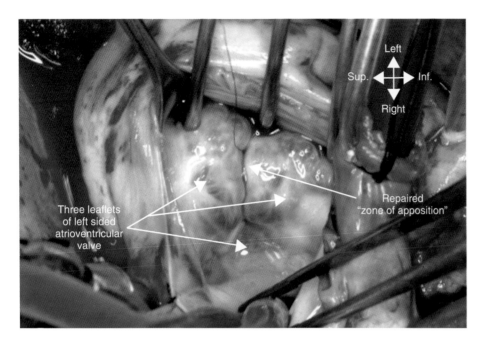

Fig. 7.32 This operative view through a right atriotomy shows the typical three-leaflet formation of the left atrioventricular valve in a heart with deficient atrioventricular septation and common atrioventricular junction. It bears no resemblance to the formation of the leaflets as seen in the normal mitral valve.

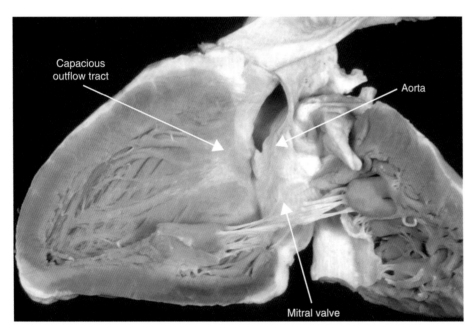

Fig. 7.33 This view of the left ventricle, taken from the apex with the chamber opened in clam-like fashion, shows the interrelationship of the normal mitral valve and the outflow tract to the aorta. Note the position of the papillary muscles supporting the zone of apposition between the leaflets of the mitral valve.

bridging leaflet and the anterosuperior leaflet of the right ventricle. The zone of apposition is supported by the medial papillary muscle of the right ventricle (Fig. 7.36). When seen from the outflow tract, in some hearts, the arrangement of the zone of apposition is virtually indistinguishable from the so-called anteroseptal commissure of the normal tricuspid valve (Fig. 7.37). This arrangement, in fact, represents minimal extension into the right ventricle of the superior bridging leaflet of a five-leaflet valve. The variability noted by Rastelli et al[11] in hearts with common valvar orifice is then readily explained on the basis of increased commitment of the superior bridging leaflet to the right ventricle, with concomitant diminution in size of the anterosuperior leaflet. The papillary muscle which supports the end of the zone of apposition itself then moves towards the right ventricular apex[12] (Fig. 7.38). A further difference between the hearts at either end of this spectrum is that, with minimal bridging, the superior bridging leaflet is usually tethered by cords to the crest of the ventricular septum. With extreme bridging, in contrast, the leaflet is almost always free-floating.

It is the morphology of the bridging leaflets that accounts for much of the remaining variability in atrioventricular septal defects. As already emphasised, the overall valvar morphology is comparable

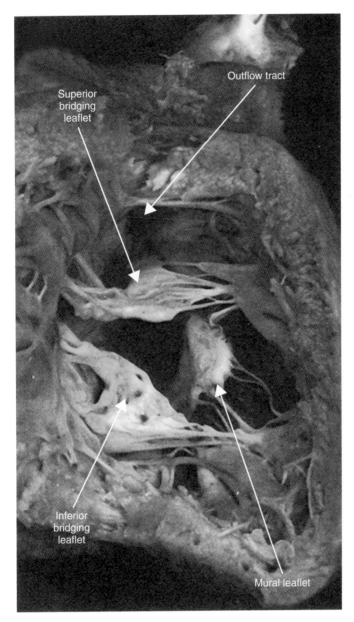

Fig. 7.34 This view of the left atrioventricular valve and the outflow tract in a heart with atrioventricular septal defect is taken in comparable fashion to the normal heart seen in Fig. 7.33. Note that the left valve in the heart with deficient atrioventricular septation has three leaflets, with papillary muscles in markedly different orientation from the normal heart.

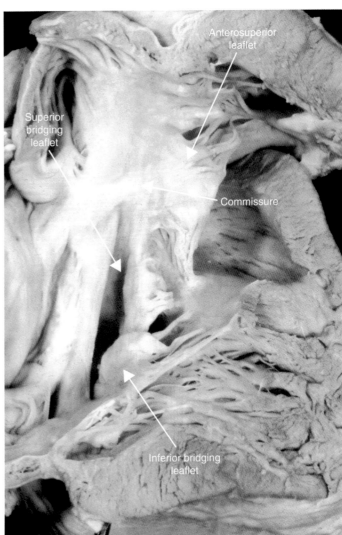

Fig. 7.35 These illustrations show the end of the zone of apposition between the superior bridging and anterosuperior leaflets of the common atrioventricular valve in an atrioventricular septal defect with common orifice. This arrangement, with minimal bridging of the superior leaflet, produces the so-called "Rastelli type A" malformation.

in all hearts with an atrioventricular septal defect and common atrioventricular junction. The variability which exists can be assessed in terms either of the relationship of the two bridging leaflets to each other, or their relationships, on the one hand, to the lower edge of the atrial septum and, on the other hand, to the crest of the muscular ventricular septum. If these two features are described

separately, there is no need to use terms such as 'complete', 'partial' and 'intermediate'. It is the use of these terms which creates most confusion in the description of the overall group of lesions.

In hearts with the so-called 'ostium primum' defect, the bridging leaflets are joined to each other along the crest of the ventricular septum by a connecting tongue of leaflet tissue (Fig. 7.39). The

'ostium primum' defect, therefore, has separate valvar orifices for the right and left ventricles. Because the heart retains its common atrioventricular junction, the left valve still possesses three leaflets, with a zone of apposition found between the left ventricular components of the superior and inferior bridging leaflets. This area is usually described as a 'cleft'. In no way, however, can it be compared

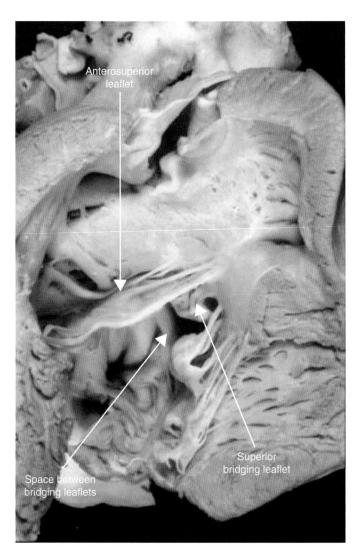

Anterosuperior leaflet

Space between bridging leaflets

Superior bridging leaflet

Fig. 7.36 These illustrations show the end of the zone of apposition between the superior bridging and anterosuperior leaflets of the common atrioventricular valve in the heart shown in Fig. 7.35 as seen from the infundibular aspect.

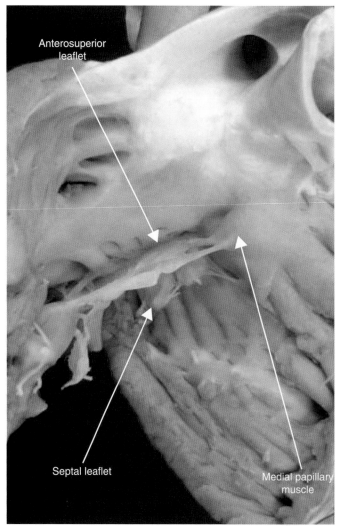

Anterosuperior leaflet

Septal leaflet

Medial papillary muscle

Fig. 7.37 The zone of apposition between the anterosuperior and septal leaflets of the tricuspid valve in the normal heart seen in comparable orientation to the heart shown in Fig. 7.35. The structures are directly comparable.

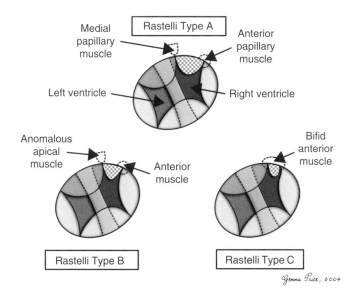

Rastelli Type A

Medial papillary muscle

Anterior papillary muscle

Left ventricle

Right ventricle

Anomalous apical muscle

Anterior muscle

Bifid anterior muscle

Rastelli Type B

Rastelli Type C

Gemma Price, 2004

Fig. 7.38 This diagram, seen in anatomic orientation as viewed from above (compare with Fig. 7.31), shows the spectrum of bridging of the superior leaflet in hearts with atrioventricular septal defect and common orifice which underlies the classification introduced by Rastelli and his colleagues. As the superior bridging leaflet (pink) extends further into the right ventricle, so there is concomitant diminution in size of the anterosuperior leaflet (pink cross-hatched), and fusion of the anterior and medial papillary muscles of the right ventricle.

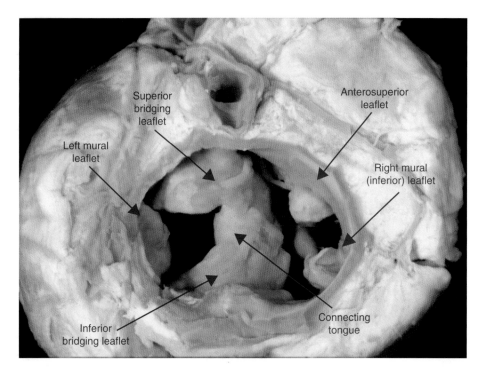

Fig. 7.39 This heart with atrioventricular septal defect and separate right and left valvar orifices is viewed in anatomical orientation from above, after removal of the atrial chambers and the arterial trunks. Note the common atrioventricular junction, albeit wth separate valvar orifices for the right and left ventricle because a tongue of leaflet tissue joins together the facing surfaces of the bridging leaflets (compare with Fig. 7.31).

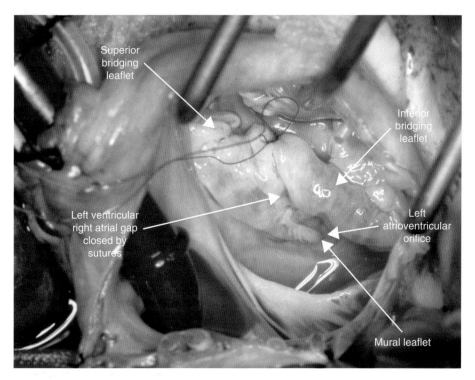

Fig. 7.40 This view through a right atriotomy shows the three-leaflet configuration of the left atrioventricular valve subsequent to repair so as to produce a competent valvar mechanism.

morphologically to the cleft that is found in the aortic leaflet of the mitral valve in hearts with normal atrioventricular septation and separate right and left atrioventricular junctions[13]!! Even though it is now accepted that usually it is necessary surgically to close part of this zone of apposition when repairing 'ostium primum' defects (Fig. 7.40), the resulting

closure does not recreate a leaflet comparable to the aortic leaflet of the normal mitral valve (Fig. 7.41).

The most important clinical feature of atrioventricular septal defects, and one which always warrants description, depends upon the relationship of the bridging leaflets to the septal structures. It is this arrangement which determines the

potential for shunting through the defect. When there is a common valvar orifice, then it is extremely rare for the leaflets to be attached directly to the crest of the ventricular septum, although the extent of their tethering by tendinous cords can vary markedly. With the bridging leaflets being unattached directly to the septums, shunting will occur at both atrial and

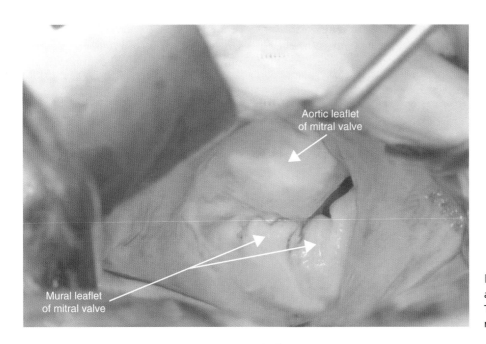

Fig. 7.41 This view through a right atriotomy shows a normal mitral valve. The structure bears no comparison to the repaired trifoliate valve shown in Fig. 7.40.

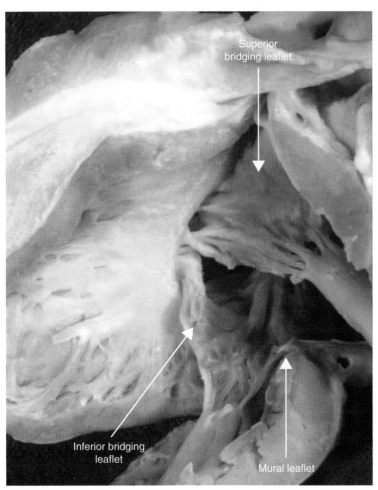

Fig. 7.42 This heart with common atrioventricular junction and separate right and left valvar orifices is shown from the left side in anatomic orientation. The bridging leaflets are firmly fused to the crest of the ventricular septum, confining shunting through the atrioventricular septal defect at atrial level ("ostium primum defect").

ventricular levels, the magnitude of the shunts depending on the prevailing haemodynamic conditions together with the extent of the tethering. If the leaflets are firmly attached to the ventricular septum, then shunting will obviously be confined at atrial level. This is the standard "ostium primum" defect, with separate right and left valvar orifices within the common junction, but with both bridging leaflets firmly fused to the crest of the ventricular septum (Fig. 7.42).

Much less frequently, the bridging leaflets can be firmly attached to the underside of the atrial septum (Fig. 7.43). This arrangement will obviously confine the potential for shunting at ventricular level, and produces the true ventricular septal defect of "atrioventricular canal" variety, since the valve guarding the common atrioventricular junction will self-evidently have characteristics of a common atrioventricular valve, rather than tricuspid and mitral valves (Figs. 7.44–7.47). The

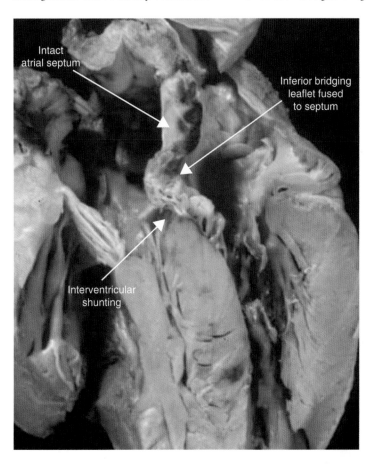

Fig. 7.43 This "four-chamber" section, seen in anatomic orientation, shows a heart with deficient atrioventricular septation and common atrioventricular junction. The inferior bridging leaflet, however, is firmly fused to the undersurface of the atrial septum, confining shunting through the atrioventricular septal defect at ventricular level.

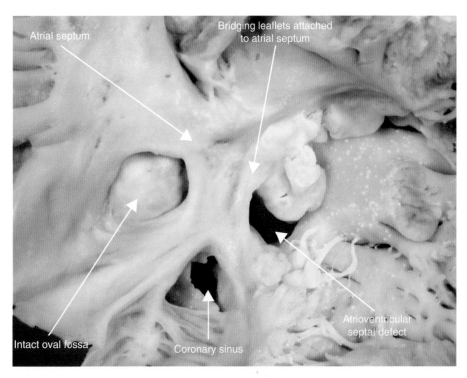

Fig. 7.44 This specimen is viewed in anatomic orientation from the right side. The defect permits shunting at ventricular level only, but the leaflets of the atrioventricular valve bridge across the crest of the ventricular septum into the left ventricle. The heart has deficient atrioventricular septation with a common atrioventricular junction.

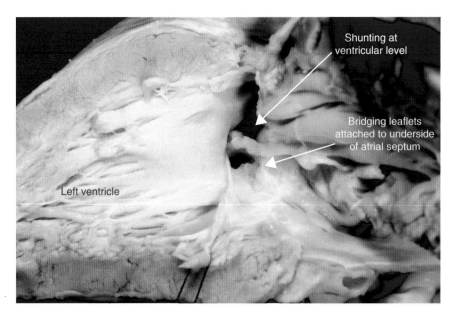

Fig. 7.45 The left-sided aspect is shown of another heart with deficient atrioventricular septation and common atrioventricular junction. This picture shows well the attachments of the bridging leaflets to the leading edge of the atrial septum, confining shunting at ventricular level.

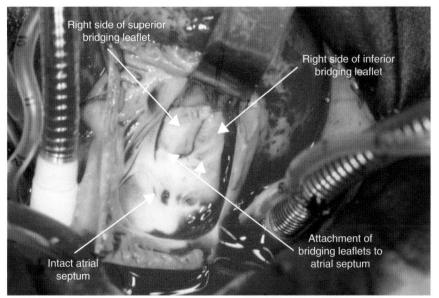

Fig. 7.46 This picture taken in the operating room shows the right atrial aspect of an atrioventricular septal defect with common atrioventricular junction in which shunting is confined at ventricular level because the bridging leaflets are firmly attached to the underside of the atrial septum.

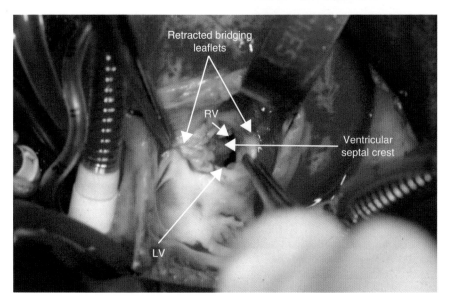

Fig. 7.47 The surgeon has separated the right ventricular components of the bridging leaflets of the heart shown in Fig. 7.46, showing the common atrioventricular junction between right (RV) and left (LV) ventricles.

potential also exists, nonetheless, for the leaflets to be free-floating even in the presence of separate valvar orifices (Fig. 7.48). As discussed, if this variability in terms of attachment of the bridging leaflets is described, together with information concerning the presence of a common valvar orifice or separate right and left orifices, then there is no need to introduce the concept of so-called intermediate or transitional variants. For example, in many patients with so-called "partial" defects, with separate right and left valvar orifices within the common junction, echo Doppler interrogation reveals the potential for interventricular shunting beneath the tongue that joins together the bridging leaflets, or else through intercordal spaces tethering the bridging leaflets themselves. We would describe such patients as having separate valvar orifices, with predominantly atrial shunting, but with the potential for minimal ventricular shunting.

It is evident from our discussion that the basic morphology of the ventricular septum is comparable in all atrioventricular septal defects[5]. It is this disposition which determines the course of the ventricular conduction pathways[8]. Although the hallmark of the malformation is the common atrioventricular junction, coupled with absence of the atrioventricular muscular and membranous separating structures, there is also hypoplasia to a greater or lesser extent of the muscular ventricular septum. The degree of hypoplasia determines how much the septum appears to be 'scooped out' (Fig. 7.49). This

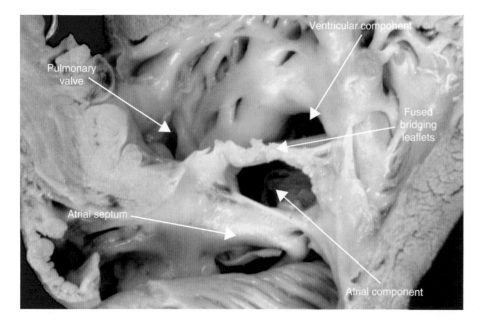

Fig. 7.48 In this atrioventricular septal defect, again with separate valvar orifices, and seen in surgical orientation, the bridging leaflets and the connecting tongue float free of both atrial and ventricular septal structures so that there are both atrial and ventricular defects.

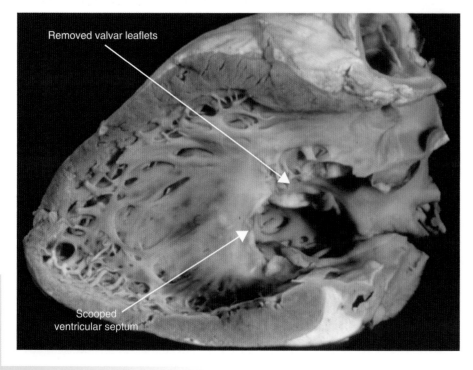

Fig. 7.49 The valvar leaflets have been removed from the ventricular mass in this heart with deficient atrioventricular septation and common atrioventricular junction, viewed from the left side in anatomic orientation. Since the leaflets have been removed, there is no way of knowing whether, originally, there was a common atrioventricular orifice, or separate valvar orifices for the right and left ventricles. Note the "scooping" of the ventricular septum, and the disproportion between inlet and outlet dimensions of the ventricular mass.

"scooping" is greater in hearts with common valvar orifice than in those with separate right and left orifices. Although the "scooping" is greater in hearts with a common valvar orifice, thus increasing the likelihood of there being a ventricular component to the defect, variability is still found among these hearts. When there is minimal scooping, it is possible to close the ventricular component of the septal defect by attaching the bridging leaflets directly to the right ventricular aspect of the ventricular septum[14]. Indeed, some have now suggested that this manoeuvre is feasible in all patients with common valvar orifice[15]. If this technique is used, care must be taken not to damage the exposed conduction tissues along the septal crest. The non-branching bundle runs down the crest of the scooped-out septum, and is covered by the inferior bridging leaflet. The inferior leaflet itself is often divided by a midline raphe immediately above the vulnerable non-branching bundle. The branching component of the conduction axis is found astride the midportion of the septal crest. This is usually covered by the connecting tongue and leaflet tissue in hearts with separate right and left valvar orifices. It is exposed in the presence of a common orifice and free-floating leaflets. The right bundle branch then runs towards the medial papillary muscle. Anterior to this point, the septum is devoid of conduction tissue (Figs. 7.50, 7.51).

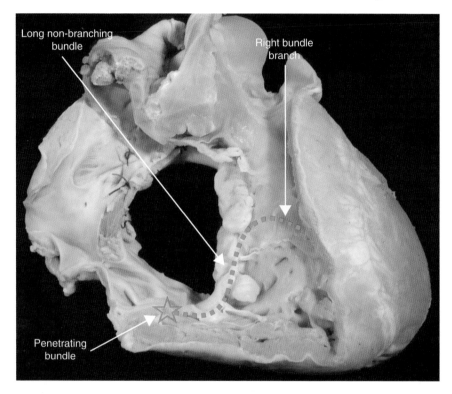

Fig. 7.50 This heart has an atrioventricular septal defect with common atrioventricular junction and shunting confined at atrial level, in other words an "ostium primum" defect. The disposition of the atrioventricular conduction axis (green) has been superimposed on the picture.

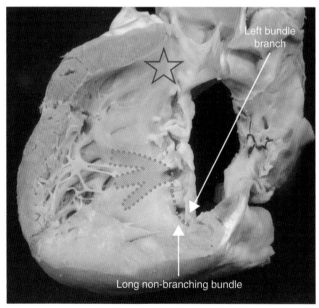

Fig. 7.51 This photograph shows the left ventricular aspect of the heart illustrated in Fig. 7.50, again with the location of the atrioventricular conduction axis (green) superimposed on the picture. Note that the left ventricular outflow tract (red star) is distant from the conduction tissues.

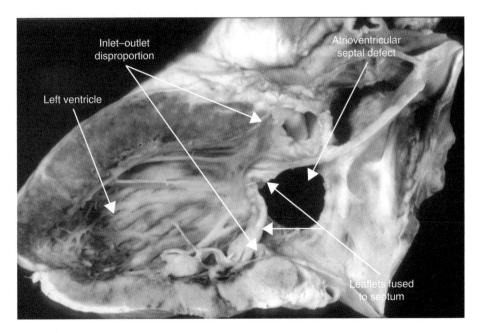

Fig. 7.52 This heart, shown in anatomical orientation from the left side, has been dissected to show the extent of the narrowed outflow tract in an atrioventricular septal defect with separate right and left atrioventricular valves, and with the potential only for atrial shunting. Because the superior bridging leaflet is firmly attached to the crest of the ventricular septum, the outflow tract has considerable length.

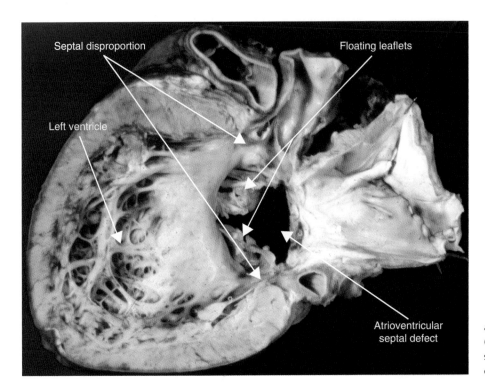

Fig. 7.53 In this heart, again shown in anatomical orientation from the left side (compare with Fig. 7.52), the outflow tract is seen to be much shorter in the presence of a common atrioventricular valvar orifice.

Although not readily evident to the surgeon during operation, the left ventricular outflow tract in atrioventricular septal defects is intrinsically narrow[16]. It is much longer in hearts with separate orifices because of the attachment of the superior bridging leaflet to the ventricular septal crest (compare Figs. 7.52 & 7.53). This makes the area prone to postoperative obstruction, and surgical enlargement may be necessary. The obstruction may be due either to naturally occurring lesions[17], or to injudicious placement of a prosthesis used to replace the left atrioventricular valve. If a prosthesis must be employed, the anatomy dictates insertion of a model with low profile, or else resection of the shelf which exists between the hingepoint of the superior bridging leaflet and the attachment of the aortic valve[18]. It is also possible, in hearts with separate valvar orifices, to liberate the superior bridging leaflet from the septal crest. A gusset can then be inserted so as to enlarge the outflow tract (Figs. 7.54 & 7.55).

There is also variability in the commitment of the common atrioventricular junction to the ventricular mass. Usually it is shared equally, giving a

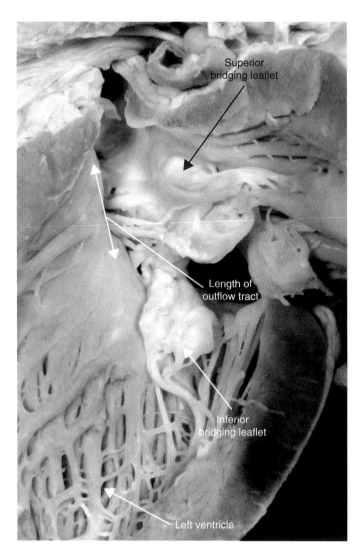

Fig. 7.54 This heart has an atrioventricular septal defect with common atrioventricular orifice, but with the superior bridging leaflet tethered across the subaortic outflow tract. It is photographed in anatomic orientation from the left side.

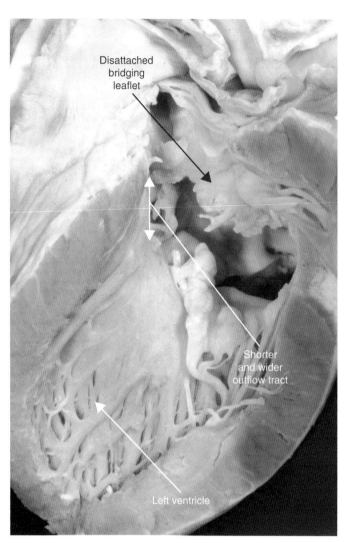

Fig. 7.55 An incision has been made in the superior bridging leaflet of the heart shown in Fig. 7.54, at the same time detaching the leaflet from the crest of the ventricular septum. The incision makes it possible to insert a patch so as to widen the outflow tract.

balanced arrangement. Should the common junction favour one or other ventricle, producing so-called right or left ventricular dominance, the other ventricle is often severely hypoplastic. This can have a major influence on the outcome of surgery, and should always be assessed preoperatively.

Malalignment can also be found between the atrial septum and the muscular ventricular septum (Fig. 7.56). This produces an arrangement analogous to straddling of the tricuspid valve[19] (see below). When the atrial and ventricular septal structures are malaligned, the connecting atrioventricular node is no

longer to be found at the crux. Instead, it is found where the ventricular septum meets the atrioventricular junction. This particular arrangement must be identified preoperatively, since it can be exceedingly difficult to recognise during surgery. If unrecognised, it is likely that a standard repair will damage the conduction axis. Septal malalignment, therefore, should be excluded in all cases of atrioventricular septal defect with left ventricular dominance. This arrangement should also be distinguished from those hearts in which the atrial septum is absent, and the coronary sinus terminates in the left atrium (see Fig. 7.30).

Ventricular septal defects

When faced with a clinically significant ventricular septal defect, the primary concern of the surgeon is whether it is possible to effect a safe and secure closure. The important anatomical considerations relate to the location of the defect within the ventricular septum. It is this feature that determines the proximity of the defect to the atrioventricular conduction axis, and to the leaflets of the atrioventricular and arterial valves. The categorization of ventricular septal defects proposed by Soto et al[20] was designed to focus the attention of the surgeon on these

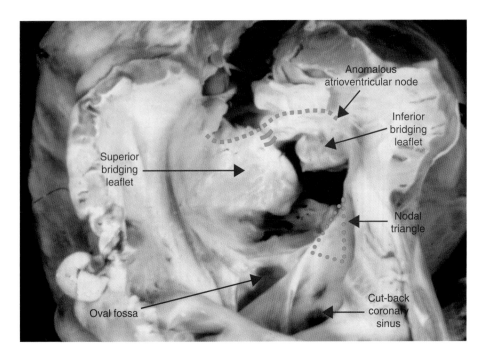

Fig. 7.56 In this specimen, viewed in surgical orientation, there is gross malalignment between the muscular ventricular septum and the atrial septum. As a consequence, the atrioventricular conduction axis (green dotted line) originates from an anomalous node in the posterior aspect of the atrioventricular junction, rather than from the apex of the nodal triangle (green dotted triangle).

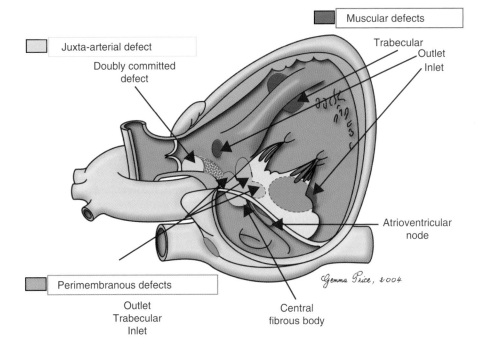

Fig. 7.57 This cartoon, shown in surgical orientation, illustrates the categorization used for differentiation of the various types of ventricular septal defect.

pertinent features. Thus, Soto and his colleagues suggested that defects could be defined according to whether they were embedded in the musculature of the septum, were bordered directly by fibrous continuity between the atrioventricular valves and an arterial valve, or were bordered directly by fibrous continuity between the leaflets of the aortic and pulmonary valves (Fig. 7.57). When defects fall in the third group, they are located, of necessity, between the outflow tracts of the ventricles. Defects within the other groups, however, can be further described according to whether they open primarily to the inlet, to the apical, or to the outlet components of the right ventricle.

The essence of the largest group is that a part of the central fibrous body, specifically the area of fibrous continuity between the leaflets of the mitral, aortic, and tricuspid valves, forms a direct part of the rim of the defect. This fibrous area incorporates the atrioventricular component of the membranous septum remains, which retains its integrity, being an integral part of the central fibrous body. The defects, therefore, are perimembranous (Fig. 7.58). Furthermore, a remnant of the interventricular component of the membranous septum is frequently

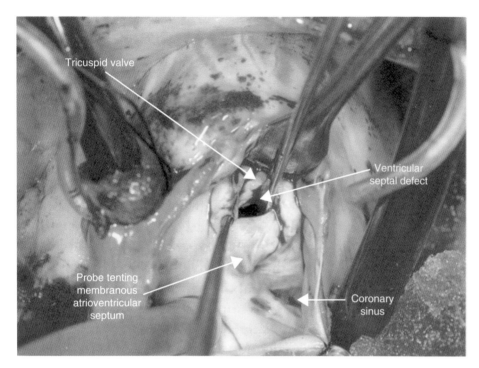

Fig. 7.58 This view, through a right atriotomy with retraction of the leaflets of the tricuspid valve, shows the fibrous tissue of the atrioventricular septum lifted by the nerve hook that forms a direct border of those defects we categorise as being perimembranous.

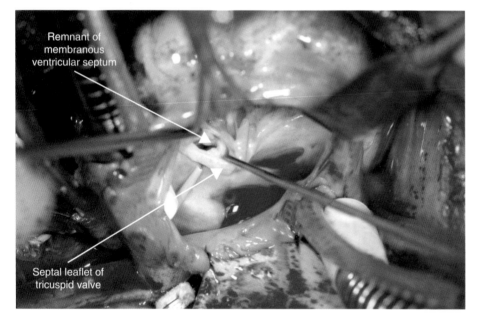

Fig. 7.59 In this heart, viewed through a right atriotomy and through the orifice of the tricuspid valve, there is a remnant of the interventricular membranous septum in the posteroinferior margin of the perimembranous defect.

found as a fold of fibrous tissue in the posteroinferior margin of the defect (Fig. 7.59).

The defect itself results from a deficiency of the muscular ventricular septum, this lack of tissue providing a perimeter for the space around the components of the central fibrous body. Indeed, defects requiring surgical closure will always be considerably larger than the area occupied by the interventricular

membranous septum of the normal heart. The degree of septal deficiency has important consequences for the disposition of the axis of atrioventricular conduction tissue[21]. As described in Chapter 5, the axis penetrates through the atrioventricular membranous septum to reach the crest of the muscular septum. In the normal heart, with intact septal structures, it is then sandwiched between the muscular septum and the

interventricular component of the membranous septum (Fig. 7.60). In perimembranous defects, in the setting of concordant atrioventricular connections, the axis penetrates through the area of continuity between the leaflets of the aortic and tricuspid valves to reach the crest of the muscular septum (Fig. 7.61). When a remnant of the interventricular membranous septum is present, it lies immediately on top of the atrioventricular

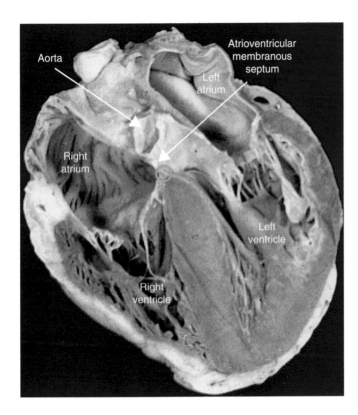

Fig. 7.60 This 'four-chamber' section, shown in anatomic orientation, reveals the position of the penetrating atrioventricular bundle (green circle) in the normal heart.

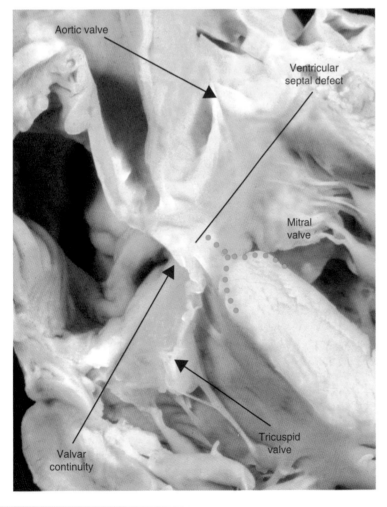

Fig. 7.61 This 'four-chamber' section, again seen in anatomic orientation, shows the position of the penetrating atrioventricular bundle (green dots) in a heart with a perimembranous ventricular septal defect.

bundle (Fig. 7.61). If such a remnant is seen at operation (Fig. 7.59), and is substantial, it may safely be used for anchorage of superficial stitches.

The location of the medial papillary muscle, together with the apex of the triangle of Koch, provides the guide for predicting the location of the conduction axis in all types of perimembranous defects. The only exceptions are those associated with straddling and overriding of the tricuspid valve[22]. The proximity of the conduction tissues to the leaflets of the aortic and atrioventricular valves, however, varies depending upon the precise area of deficiency of the muscular septum. It is likely that all parts are deficient to a certain extent. It can usually

be determined, nonetheless, which part is most affected.

When a perimembranous defect extends to open mostly into the inlet of the right ventricle, its atrial margin, as viewed through the tricuspid valve, is an extensive area of fibrous continuity between the leaflets of the mitral, aortic, and tricuspid valves (Fig. 7.62). The apex of the triangle of Koch is usually deviated towards the coronary sinus. It is then to the right hand of the surgeon working through the atrium. The axis of atrioventricular conduction tissue penetrates through this corner of the defect. Usually, the non-branching and branching bundles are carried on the left ventricular aspect of the muscular septum

as they descend the right hand margin of the defect. The right bundle branch then courses intramyocardially, surfacing beneath the medial papillary muscle, which is usually at the left hand margin of the defect. The non-coronary leaflet of the aortic valve is more to the left, and usually distant from the rim of the defect, although it often maintains fibrous continuity with the septal leaflet of the tricuspid valve (Fig. 7.63).

When a perimembranous defect is located so as to open mostly into the trabecular part of the septum, its orientation is more towards the ventricular apex. Such defects, when large, also open to the inlet and outlet components as well, and are said to be confluent. The triangle

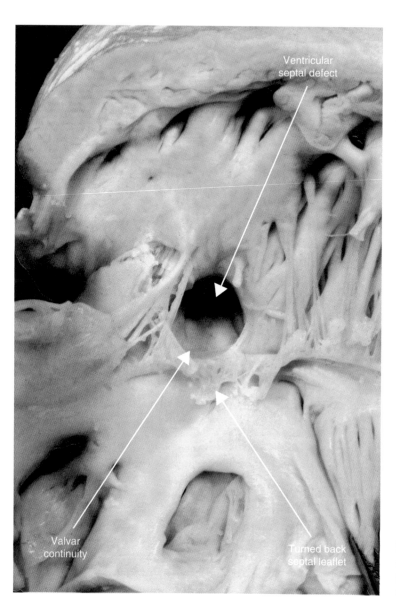

Ventricular septal defect

Valvar continuity

Turned back septal leaflet

Fig. 7.62 This perimembranous defect, shown in surgical orientation, opens primarily into the inlet of the right ventricle. The septal leaflet of the tricuspid valve has been retracted.

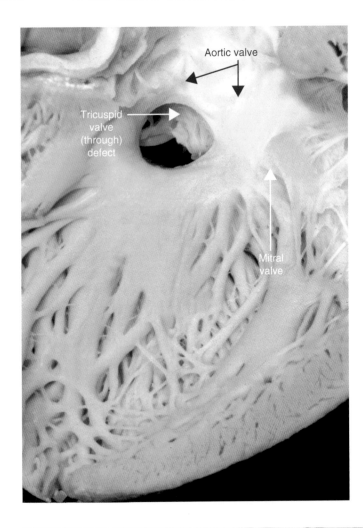

Fig. 7.63 This illustration, seen in anatomical orientation, shows the left ventricular aspect of the perimembranous defect that opened primarily to the inlet of the right ventricle shown in Fig. 7.62.

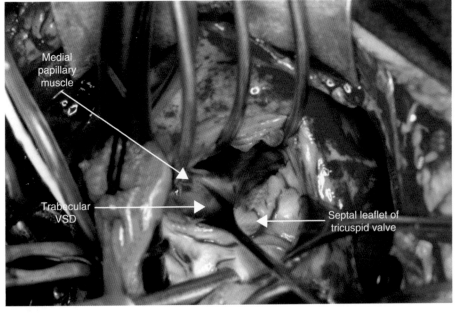

Fig. 7.64 In this heart, viewed through a right atriotomy and via the orifice of the tricuspid valve, the perimembranous defect (VSD) opens mostly towards the apex of the right ventricle – a so-called trabecular defect. Note the insertion of the medial papillary muscle toward the apex of the defect.

of Koch is not deviated as far towards the coronary sinus in such defects, but the right hand rim is still the major area at risk (Fig. 7.64). The medial papillary muscle tends to be at the apex of such defects, and the non-coronary leaflet of the aortic valve is more closely related to the atrial margin. The septal leaflet of the tricuspid valve is often cleft at the defect, an arrangement which may permit shunting from left ventricle to right atrium[6]. If the cleft in the septal leaflet of the tricuspid valve requires surgical closure, it should be remembered that the penetrating atrioventricular bundle is located at its apex.

The third type of perimembranous defect extends mostly so as to open into the outlet of the right ventricle. The outlet septum, along with the free-standing subpulmonary infundibulum, can then be recognised separating the leaflets of the aortic and pulmonary valves, being malaligned relative to the rest of the septum (Fig. 7.65). In this setting, the aortic valve overrides the crest of the muscular ventricular septum (Fig. 7.66). The medial papillary muscle is on the right hand margin of the defect, and the

axis of atrioventricular conduction tissue is more distant from the edge, being carried well down on the left surface of the ventricular septum. The non-coronary and right coronary leaflets of the aortic valve are much more closely related to the left hand margin (Fig. 7.67).

The essential feature of muscular defects is that they are entirely enclosed within the muscular part of the ventricular septum. As with perimembranous defects, they can be located so as to open to the inlet, apical, or outlet parts of the right ventricle, but will be embedded within the muscular components of the septum. Thus, the septal musculature will interpose between the edges of the

defect and the attachments of the leaflets of the valves. When a muscular defect opens to the inlet of the right ventricle (Fig. 7.68), it is inferior to the axis of conduction tissue. When viewed by the surgeon through the tricuspid valve (Figs. 7.69 & 7.70), the conduction axis is located on the left hand margin of the defect. The proximity of the axis to the edge depends upon the adjacency of the defect to the intact membranous septum. The upper margin of the muscular septum separates the septal leaflet of the tricuspid valve from the mitral valve. Its size will determine whether it is suitable to be an anchorage for sutures.

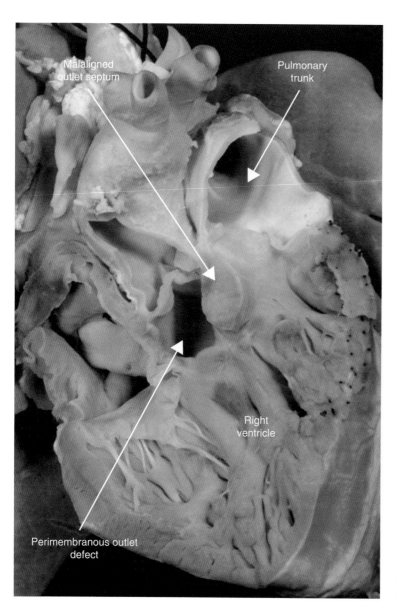

Malaligned outlet septum

Pulmonary trunk

Right ventricle

Perimembranous outlet defect

Fig. 7.65 This heart, shown in anatomical orientation, has been sectioned to replicate the subcostal oblique long axis echocardiographic projection. The perimembranous defect opens towards the outlet of the right ventricle, with the muscular outlet septum itself being malaligned and attached within the right ventricle.

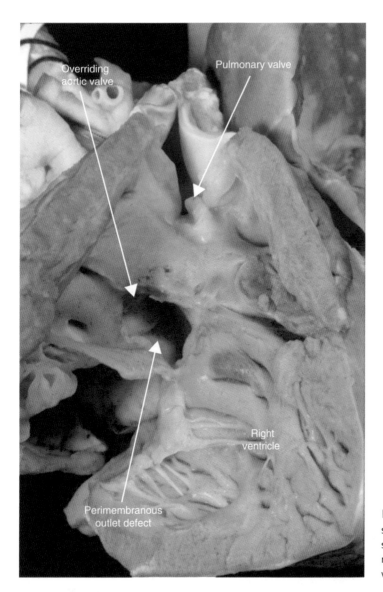

Overriding
aortic valve

Pulmonary valve

Right
ventricle

Perimembranous
outlet defect

Fig. 7.66 This is the heart shown in Fig. 7.65 prior to making the section to correlate with the echocardiographic plane. As can be seen, the ventricular septal defect opens to the outlet of the right ventricle, with the aortic valve overriding the crest of the ventricular septum.

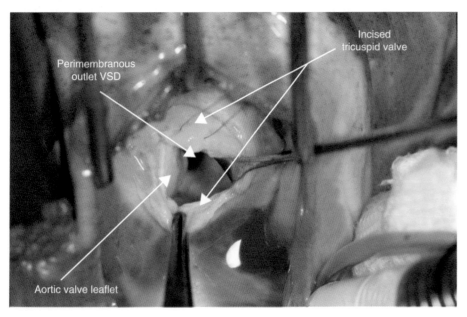

Perimembranous
outlet VSD

Incised
tricuspid valve

Aortic valve leaflet

Fig. 7.67 This view is through a right atriotomy, subsequent to making an incision at the junction of the septal and anterosuperior leaflets of the tricuspid valve. It shows a perimembranous defect opening to the outlet of the right ventricle. Note the relationship of the leaflets of the aortic valve to the left hand margin of the defect.

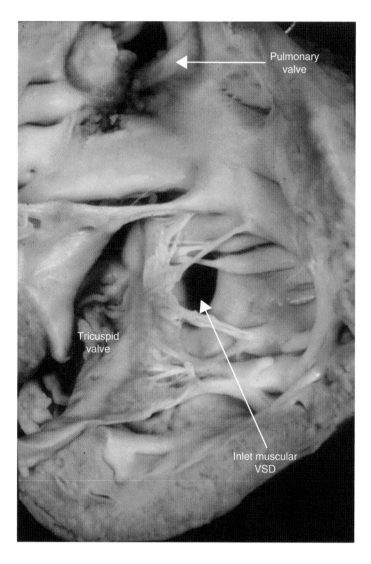

Fig. 7.68 This heart, photographed from the right side in anatomic orientation, has a muscular ventricular septal defect opening to the inlet of the right ventricle.

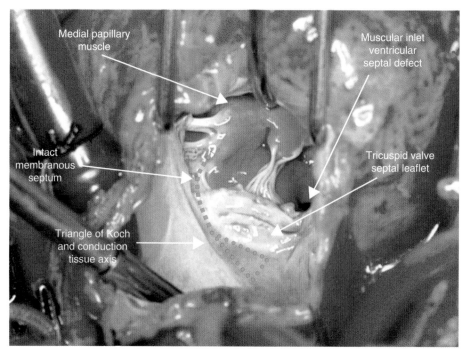

Fig. 7.69 This view through a right atriotomy and across the orifice of the tricuspid valve show a muscular defect opening to the inlet of the right ventricle. Note that the atrioventricular conduction axis, superimposed in green dots on the photograph, courses to the left hand of the surgeon relative to the defect.

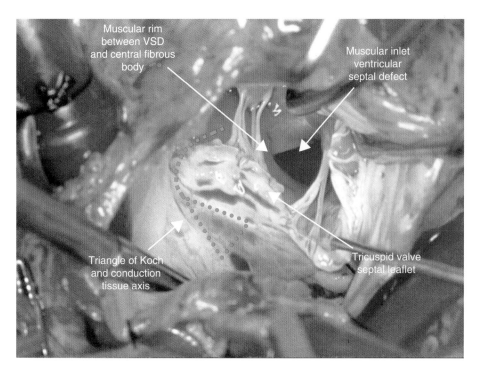

Muscular rim between VSD and central fibrous body

Muscular inlet ventricular septal defect

Triangle of Koch and conduction tissue axis

Tricuspid valve septal leaflet

Fig. 7.70 In this view of the heart shown in Fig. 7.69, reflection of the septal leaflet of the tricuspid valve shows the muscle bar separating the upper margin of the defect from the hingepoint of the valvar leaflet. The conduction tissues are depicted with green dots.

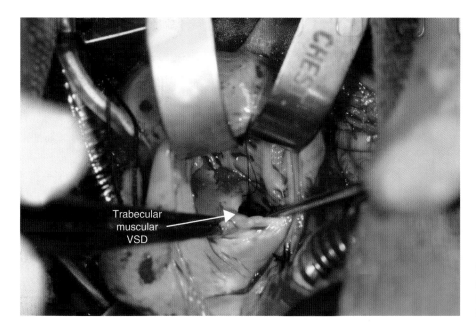

Trabecular muscular VSD

Fig. 7.71 This view through a right atriotomy and the tricuspid valve shows a muscular defect opening into the apical trabecular component of the right ventricle.

Defects opening through the apical part of the septum can be single and large (Fig. 7.71), double and large, or multiple (Fig. 7.72). They are unrelated to the proximal parts of the conduction tissue axis, but may be related to ramifications of the distal bundle branches. The right ventricular aspect of these defects is frequently obscured by the coarse apical trabeculations. Indeed, multiple small defects may not be visible through a right ventriculotomy. The defect is much more readily identified from the left ventricular aspect. This demonstrates that, often times the defect is a solitary hole (Fig. 7.73). The multiple right ventricular openings (Fig. 7.71) simply reflect crossing of the solitary defect by the right ventricular apical trabeculations[23].

Muscular defects opening to the outlet of the right ventricle are relatively rare in patients with concordant atrioventricular and ventriculo-arterial connections. When found, they are usually small (Fig. 7.74). On initial inspection, the endocardium may appear to be heaped up at the edges to produce a fibrous rim (Fig. 7.75). Close inspection will show whether the posterior limb of the septomarginal trabeculation is fused with the ventriculo-infundibular fold to form a muscular posteroinferior rim to the defect. When present, the fusion of these muscle bars separates

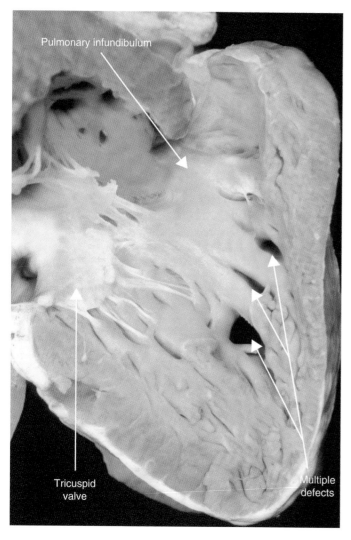

Fig. 7.72 In this heart, viewed in anatomical orientation, it seems that there are three muscular defects opening anteriorly into the apical trabecular component of the right ventricle.

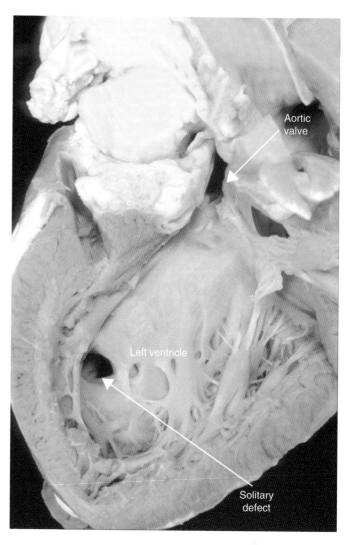

Fig. 7.73 The left ventricular view, seen in anatomical orientation, shows the left ventricular aspect of the heart illustrated in Fig. 7.72. In reality, there is a solitary defect in the muscular septum but it is crossed by trabeculations on the right side, giving the spurious impression of multiple defects.

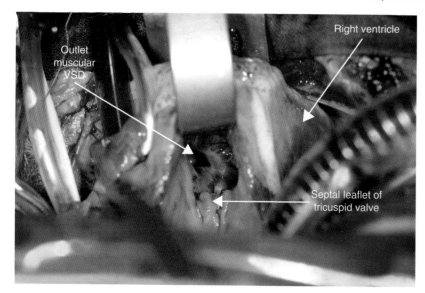

Fig. 7.74 This defect is seen through a right atriotomy with the tricuspid valve retracted. It shows a muscular defect opening into the outlet of the right ventricle.

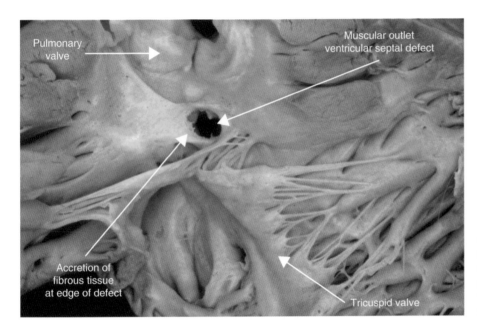

Pulmonary valve

Muscular outlet ventricular septal defect

Accretion of fibrous tissue at edge of defect

Tricuspid valve

Fig. 7.75 The heart is photographed in anatomical orientation, showing a muscular defect opening to the outlet of the right ventricle, comparable to the surgical picture shown in Fig. 7.74. Note the accretion of fibrous tissue at the edges of the defect, reducing its size.

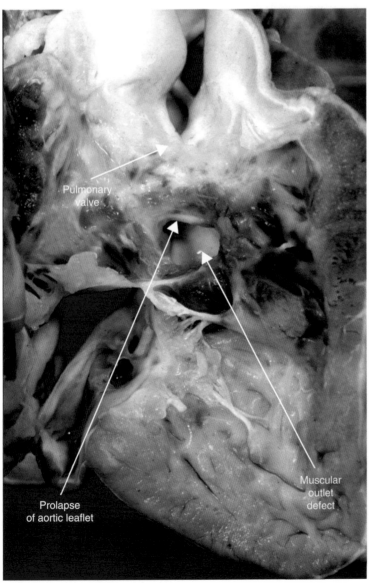

Pulmonary valve

Prolapse of aortic leaflet

Muscular outlet defect

Fig. 7.76 In this heart, viewed in anatomical orientation, the right coronary leaflet of the aortic valve prolapses minimally through a muscular defect opening to the outlet of the right ventricle.

the edge of the defect from the axis of atrioventricular conduction tissue. The superior rim is the muscular outlet septum, combined with the free-standing subpulmonary infundibulum. These tissues separate the leaflets of the pulmonary valve from the right coronary leaflet of the aortic valve, the latter attached to its left ventricular surface. If this superior muscular rim is attenuated, then the leaflet of the aortic valve may prolapse through the defect (Fig. 7.76).

The third type of ventricular septal defect is the one which is doubly committed and juxta-arterial. The phenotypic feature of this defect is absence of both the muscular outlet septum, and the posterior aspect of the free-standing subpulmonary infundibulum. Because of the absence of these structures, the facing leaflets of the aortic and pulmonary valves are in fibrous continuity, producing a fibrous raphe which forms the superior rim of the defect (Fig. 7.77). The leaflets can be attached at the same level, albeit that in some hearts part of the aortic sinus may interpose between them, producing valvar offsetting. In either event, sutures can be secured in the region of fibrous continuity. The doubly committed defect can also be found with overriding of the orifice of the aortic valve (Fig. 7.78). In most instances, the inferior rim of the defect is similar to that found in the muscular defect which opens to the outlet part of the right ventricle, the posterior limb of the septomarginal trabeculation fusing with the ventriculo-infundibular fold (Figs. 7.77, 7.79). When present, this muscular rim buttresses the axis of atrioventricular conduction tissue away from the edge of the defect. Occasionally, however, the muscular bundles do not fuse. The defect then extends to be bordered by fibrous continuity between the leaflets of the aortic and tricuspid valves, making it perimembranous as well as doubly committed. The conduction axis is then much closer to its inferior corner (Fig. 7.80).

Although the descriptions thus far relate to ventricular septal defects in hearts with concordant atrioventricular and ventriculo-arterial connections, this topology, and the guidance it gives to the site of the conduction axis, is also valid for hearts with concordant atrioventricular connections but abnormal ventriculo-arterial connections (see Chapter 8). The only exception is the defect found in presence of an overriding and straddling tricuspid valve (see below).

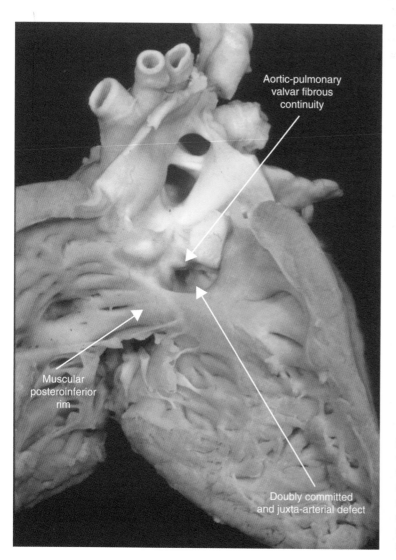

Aortic-pulmonary valvar fibrous continuity

Muscular posteroinferior rim

Doubly committed and juxta-arterial defect

Fig. 7.77 In this heart, the defect opening to the outlet of the right ventricle is doubly committed and juxta-arterial, due to complete failure of formation of the muscular subpulmonary infundibulum. The roof of the defect is made up of fibrous continuity between the leaflets of the aortic and pulmonary valves. Note the extensive muscular posteroinferior rim to the defect that protects the atrioventricular conduction axis.

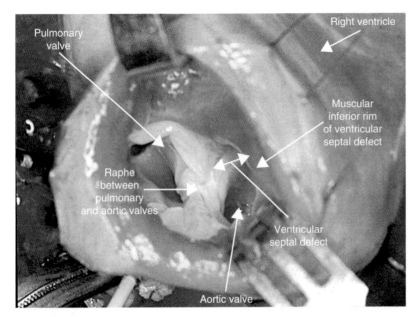

Fig. 7.78 This operative view, taken via a median sternotomy and an incision in the infundibulum of the right ventricle, shows the features of a doubly committed and juxta-arterial ventricular septal defect. In this patient, as in the specimen shown in Fig. 7.77, a muscular rim interposes between the leaflets of the aortic and tricuspid valves, protecting the conduction tissue axis.

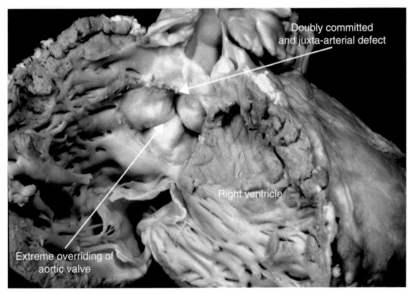

Fig. 7.79 This heart, photographed in anatomic orientation, also has a doubly committed and juxta-arterial ventricular septal defect opening to the outlet of the right ventricle in absence of formation of the muscular subpulmonary infundibulum, but note the extensive overriding of the orifice of the aortic valve.

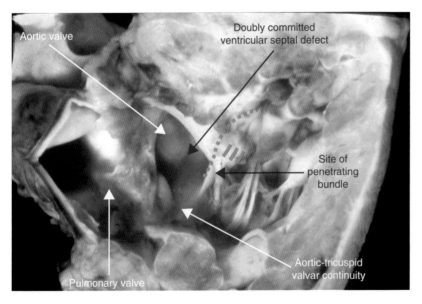

Fig. 7.80 This doubly committed and juxta-arterial ventricular septal defect, shown in surgical orientation, extends so that its posteroinferior margin in formed by fibrous continuity between the leaflets of the aortic and tricuspid valves (perimembranous). Note the proximity of the conduction axis, superimposed on the photograph in green dots, to the margin of the defect.

MALFORMATIONS OF THE ATRIOVENTRICULAR VALVES

The pathological lesions which affect atrioventricular valves, both acquired and congenital, are legion. Not all are amenable to surgical repair. We will concentrate on features of immediate surgical relevance.

The anatomy of atrioventricular valves themselves indicates that problems may be encountered at the atrioventricular junction, or the 'annulus', in the leaflets, or in the tension apparatus. Sometimes all the components of the valve, along with the entire atrioventricular connection, are totally absent. This produces the commonest variant of atrioventricular valvar atresia, which is discussed in

Chapter 8. The lesions to be considered in this section can affect either the morphologically tricuspid or mitral valves. Because the tricuspid valve usually functions in an environment of low pressure, the lesions are more frequently manifest when affecting the mitral valve. Each lesion will be dealt with in turn, indicating its proclivity towards one or the other valve.

Of considerable surgical significance is overriding of the atrioventricular junction. This means that the valvar orifice is connected to both ventricles astride a septal defect. Almost always, this is associated with straddling of the valvar tension apparatus, with the tendinous cords attached across the defect (Fig. 7.81). Although it is the site of insertion of

the tension apparatus across the septum that determines the surgical options, the degree of override is also important. Overriding usually indicates septal malalignment, with major consequences in terms of arrangement of the conduction tissues. Straddling and overriding can affect either valve, and can occur in various segmental combinations[22]. Straddling in the setting of double inlet ventricle, and with discordant atrioventricular connections, is considered in Chapter 8. Here, the concern is with straddling valves co-existing with concordant atrioventricular connections.

When the mitral valve straddles, it does so through a ventricular septal defect that opens to the outlet of the right ventricle. The muscular ventricular septum is then

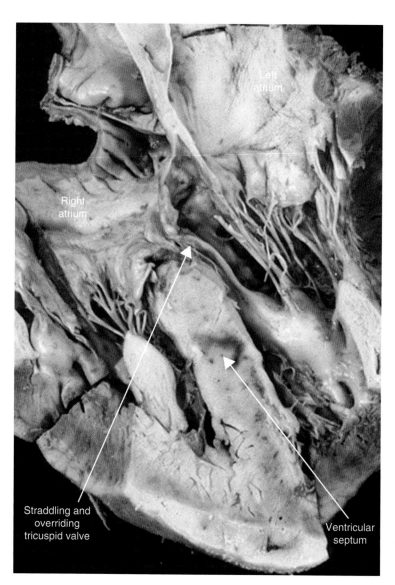

Fig. 7.81 This heart has been sectioned to replicate the "four-chamber" echocardiographic view, and is shown in anatomic orientation. There is overriding of the orifice of the tricuspid valve, and straddling of its tension apparatus. Note the gross malalignment between the atrial and ventricular septal structures.

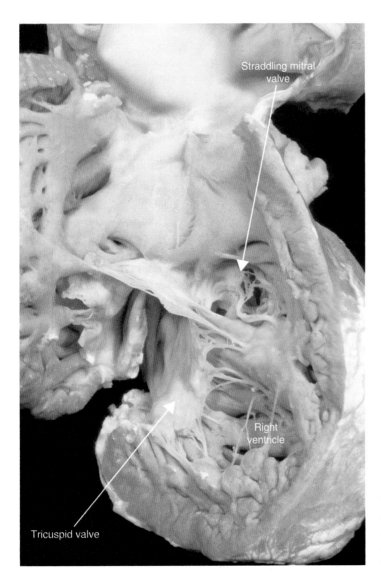

Straddling mitral valve

Right ventricle

Tricuspid valve

Fig. 7.82 This heart has concordant atrioventricular and discordant ventriculo-arterial connections. It is viewed in anatomical orientation, showing straddling of the tension apparatus of the mitral valve through a defect opening to the outlet of the right ventricle.

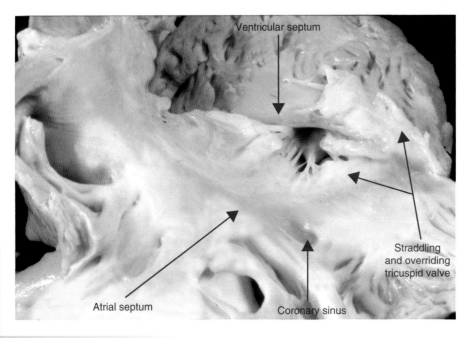

Ventricular septum

Atrial septum

Coronary sinus

Straddling and overriding tricuspid valve

Fig. 7.83 This heart is photographed in surgical orientation, showing the right atrial aspect of straddling and overriding of the tricuspid valve in the setting of basically concordant atrioventricular connections.

normally related to the atrial septum at the crux (Fig. 7.82). With this arrangement, the conduction tissue is normally disposed. The superior papillary muscle of the mitral valve is usually abnormally attached within the right ventricle, arising from the septomarginal trabeculation alongside, but separate from, the anterior papillary muscle of the tricuspid valve. This arrangement, seen most typically with either discordant ventriculo-arterial connections or double outlet right ventricle with subpulmonary defect, the so-called Taussig-Bing malformation, can seriously compromise surgical repair.

Straddling of the tricuspid valve is found more frequently with a ventricular septal defect opening to the inlet of the right ventricle (Fig. 7.83), or with tetralogy of Fallot (Fig. 7.81). It may also be found with abnormal ventriculo-arterial connections (Fig. 7.84). The phenotypic feature is that the muscular ventricular septum does not extend to the crux (Fig. 7.85). The septal defect exists because of malalignment between the atrial and ventricular septal structures. The conduction axis originates not from the normal atrioventricular node, but from an anomalous node in the posterolateral margin of the right atrioventricular junction (Fig. 7.86). This node is found at the point where the muscular septum comes into contact with the junction. The septal leaflet of the tricuspid valve is usually tethered to the enlarged posteromedial papillary muscle of the mitral valve. A 'mini-septation' procedure is often necessary for complete ventricular repair, which carries a high risk of producing heart block[24]. Alternatively, a patch can be placed by sewing the stitches exclusively in the straddling leaflet of the tricuspid valve (Figs. 7.87 & 7.88).

Dilation of the atrioventricular junction occurs almost exclusively as an acquired lesion. A dilated mitral valvar orifice is most frequently secondary to myocarditis. When surgical narrowing of the orifice is indicated, often it can be accomplished using various annuloplasty techniques, without resorting to replacement of the valve. Dilation of the tricuspid valvar orifice is seen most frequently as a result of right heart failure.

More of a challenge surgically is the dilation that accompanies Ebstein's malformation[25]. The crucial feature of this anomaly is the attachment of the hingepoint of the septal and mural leaflets of the tricuspid valve towards the junction of the inlet and apical trabecular components of the right ventricle, rather than at the atrioventricular junction (Fig. 7.89). The anterosuperior leaflet is less affected in terms of its junctional attachment, but shows important variations in its distal attachments[26]. These can be focal (Fig. 7.90). In more severe cases, the leading edge of the leaflet is attached in linear fashion, severely restricting antegrade flow into the pulmonary trunk (Fig. 7.91). In the most severe form, the anterosuperior leaflet completely blocks this junction, producing an imperforate Ebstein's malformation, which presents as tricuspid atresia (see Chapter 8).

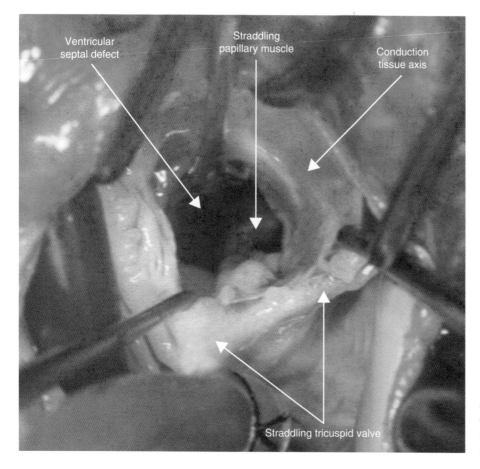

Fig. 7.84 This heart with straddling and overriding of the tricuspid valve with basically concordant atrioventricular connections is photographed in the operating room through a right atriotomy (compare with Fig. 7.83).

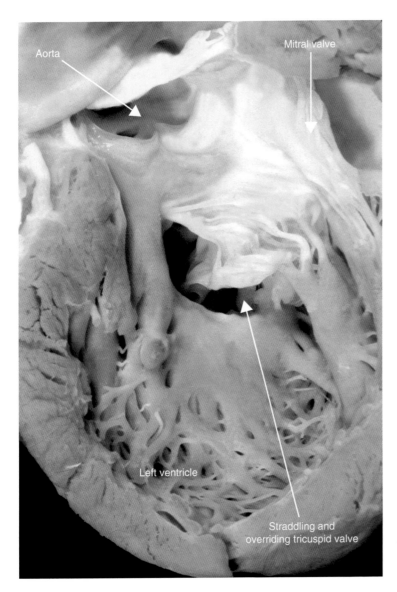

Aorta

Mitral valve

Left ventricle

Straddling and overriding tricuspid valve

Fig. 7.85 This picture, taken in anatomic orientation, shows the left ventricular aspect of the heart shown in Fig. 7.83. Note the straddling part of the right atrioventricular valve, and the malalignment of the ventricular septum.

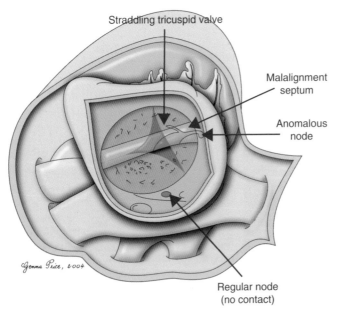

Straddling tricuspid valve

Malalignment septum

Anomalous node

Regular node (no contact)

Gemma Price, 2004

Fig. 7.86 This cartoon shows the anomalous location of the atrioventricular conduction axis as seen by the surgeon operating through a right atriotomy in the setting of straddling and overriding of the tricuspid valve.

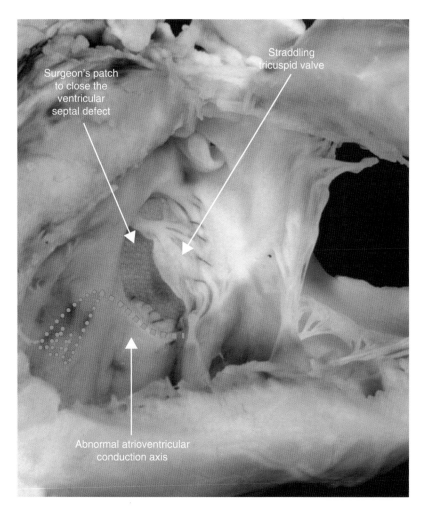

Surgeon's patch to close the ventricular septal defect

Straddling tricuspid valve

Abnormal atrioventricular conduction axis

Fig. 7.87 In this heart with straddling and overriding of the tricuspid valve, shown here from the left ventricle in anatomic orientation, the surgeon placed a patch to close the malalignment ventricular septal defect, keeping his sutures in the leaflets of the overriding valve, and avoiding the abnormally located atrioventricular conduction axis (superimposed in green on the photograph).

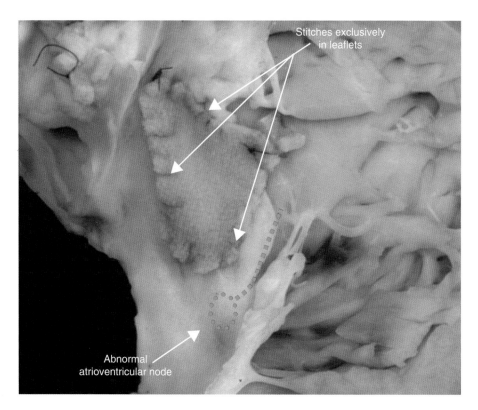

Stitches exclusively in leaflets

Abnormal atrioventricular node

Fig. 7.88 The right atrial aspect of the heart shown in Fig. 7.87, photographed in anatomical orientation, shows that the surgeon has successfully closed the hole between the ventricles, and at the same time avoided the atrioventricular conduction axis. The site of the abnormal atrioventricular node is superimposed in green dots on the photograph.

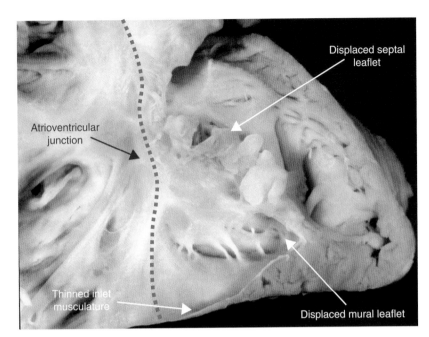

Fig. 7.89 This heart is photographed from the right side in anatomical orientation. The hinge lines of the septal and mural leaflets of the tricuspid valve are within the right ventricle, away from the atrioventricular junction shown by the red dotted line. This feature, usually described as 'downwards displacement', is the hallmark of Ebstein's malformation. Note also the marked dysplasia of the septal leaflet.

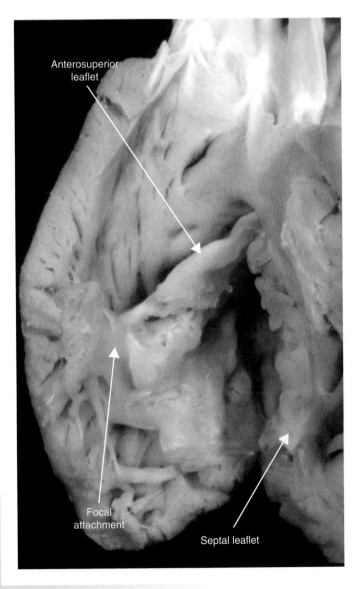

Fig. 7.90 This picture, photographed in anatomical orientation from the right ventricle, shows the ventricular aspect of the heart shown in Fig. 7.89. The anterosuperior leaflet of the abnormal tricuspid valve is tethered in focal fashion, with normal attachments to the medial and anterior papillary muscles.

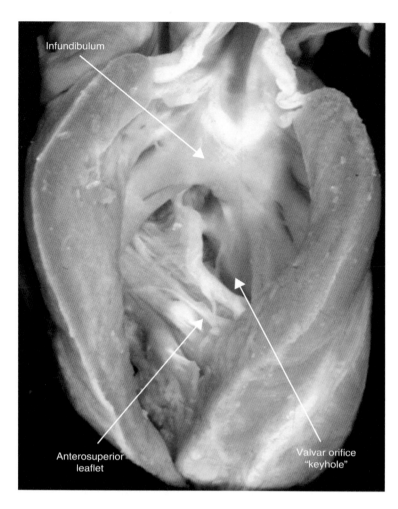

Infundibulum

Anterosuperior
leaflet

Valvar orifice
"keyhole"

Fig. 7.91 This heart also has Ebstein's malformation, and is again photographed in anatomic orientation to show the ventricular aspect of the tricuspid valve. In this example, the anterosuperior leaflet has grossly abnormal linear attachments towards the apex of the right ventricle. The valvar orifice is now a "keyhole" opening towards the subpulmonary infundibulum.

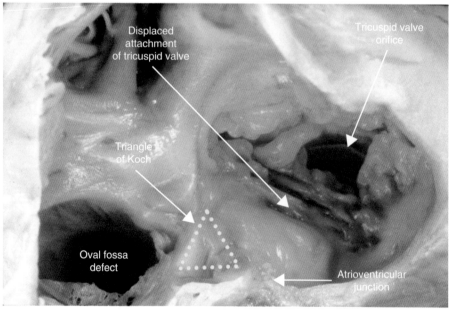

Displaced
attachment
of tricuspid valve

Tricuspid valve
orifice

Triangle
of Koch

Oval fossa
defect

Atrioventricular
junction

Fig. 7.92 This heart with Ebsteins' malformation, viewed in surgical orientation as seen from the right atrium, shows how the triangle of Koch (yellow dots) remains the guide to the atrial components of the atrioventricular conduction tissue axis, despite the abnormal attachments of the septal leaflet.

Ebstein's malformation requires surgical treatment when there is significant dilation of the true atrioventricular junction, and when the wall of the inlet component of the right ventricle is both dilated and thinned[27]. Reparative operations require placement of sutures in the area of thinning. Particular care should be taken to avoid the right coronary artery and its branches. In the septal area, the triangle of Koch remains the guide to the atrioventricular conduction axis (Fig. 7.92).

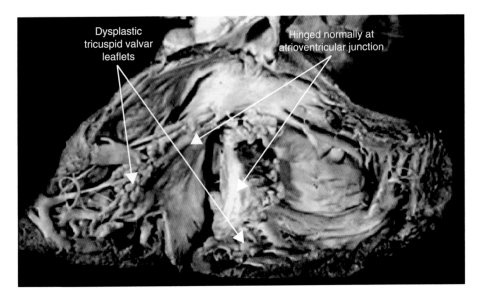

Fig. 7.93 The right ventricle in this heart is opened in clam-like fashion. The tricuspid valve, although grossly dysplastic, has normal junctional attachments. This is not Ebstein's malformation.

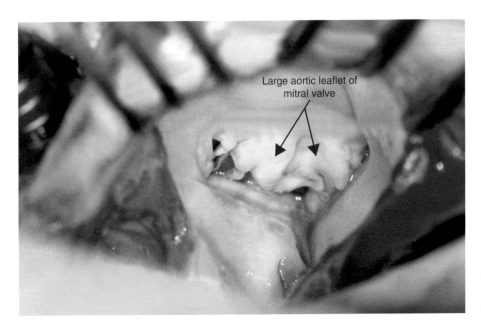

Fig. 7.94 This surgical view of the mitral valve, taken through the dome of the left atrium, shows prolapse of the aortic leaflet.

Ebstein's malformation involving the left-sided morphologically tricuspid valve in congenitally corrected transposition is discussed in Chapter 8. Rarely, an Ebstein-like lesion can involve the normally located morphologically mitral valve[28,29].

Malformations of the leaflets can be summarised in terms of dysplasia, prolapse, and clefts. The morphology of the dysplastic process is thickening and 'heaping up' of the substance of the leaflet, usually with obliteration of the intercordal spaces. A dysplastic valve may pose a significant surgical problem. It is frequently seen with atresia of the outflow

tract, and is an integral part of Ebstein's malformation[30]. Isolated dysplasia is exceedingly rare except in neonatal life[31], when it is often a fatal lesion (Fig. 7.93).

Prolapse occurs more frequently, and usually involves the mitral valve (Fig. 7.94). It is usually associated with deficiency of the tension apparatus[32], particularly elongation of the tendinous cords (Fig. 7.95). It can be repaired by valvar replacement, or by various techniques including cordal shortening (Fig. 7.96) and insertion of annular rings (Fig. 7.97).

Simply reconstituting its edges can repair the true cleft of the aortic leaflet of

the mitral valve. Such an "isolated" cleft of the aortic leaflet (Fig. 7.98) should be distinguished from the lesion usually described as a 'cleft' in the setting of atrioventricular septal defects[13]. The latter structure (Fig. 7.99) is no more than the zone of apposition between the left ventricular components of the bridging leaflets which guard the left side of the common atrioventricular junction.

We have already discussed some of the abnormalities of the tension apparatus that accompany malformations of the junction or leaflets, such as straddling

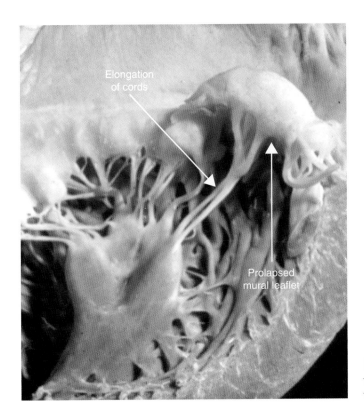

Elongation
of cords

Prolapsed
mural leaflet

Fig. 7.95 In this specimen, photographed in anatomic orientation, there is gross elongation of the cords supporting the middle scallop of the mural leaflet of the mitral valve, which is prolapsed.

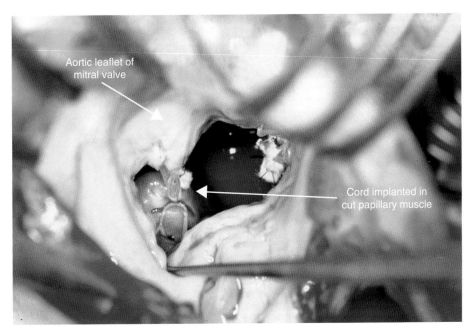

Aortic leaflet of
mitral valve

Cord implanted in
cut papillary muscle

Fig. 7.96 As shown in Fig. 7.95, when the leaflets of the mitral valve are prolapsed, then the cords supporting them are usually elongated. This view shows how the surgeon has shortened the elongated cords.

papillary muscles. Of those which remain, the so-called 'parachute' deformity is the most worrisome lesion of the tension apparatus, apart from exceptionally rare anomalies such as arcade lesions[33]. Some confusion exists about the definition of a 'parachute' valve. Some would define it as fusion of the papillary muscle groups (Fig. 7.100) so that all the cords insert into a common muscle mass[34]. Others, following the original description of Shone et al[35], define a parachute lesion of the mitral valve as gross hypoplasia of one end of the zone of apposition between leaflets, together with absence of its supporting papillary muscle. Irrespective of how the lesion is defined, surgical reconstruction is difficult, and valvar replacement is likely to be necessary[36]. Parachute deformity of the mitral valve may be further complicated by other lesions, such as supravalvar left atrial stenosing ring, and coarctation of the aorta[35]. Parachute malformation of the tricuspid valve can occur, but is rarely of clinical significance[37].

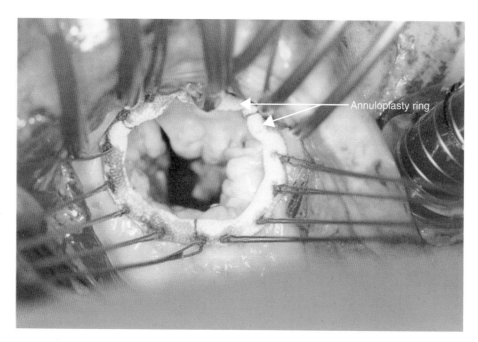

Fig. 7.97 Having shortened the cords of the prolapsed mitral valve, as shown in Fig. 7.96, the surgeon has completed the repair by inserting an annular ring to support the atrioventricular junction, which has been reduced by annuloplasty.

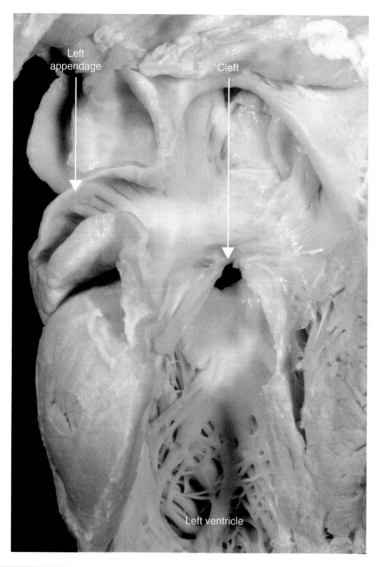

Fig. 7.98 This specimen, seen from the inlet aspect of the left ventricle in anatomical orientation, has a cleft in the aortic leaflet of an otherwise normally structured mitral valve. This lesion should be distinguished from the space between the left ventricular bridging leaflets, or the so-called 'cleft', found in the left atrioventricular valve of hearts with deficient atrioventricular septation and common atrioventricular junction (see Fig. 7.99).

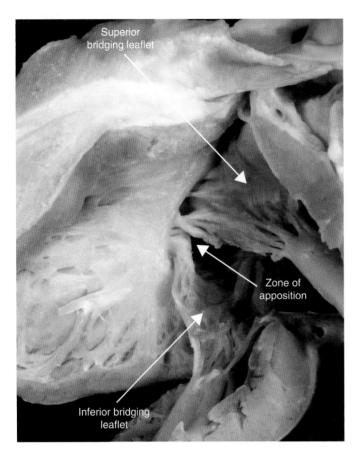

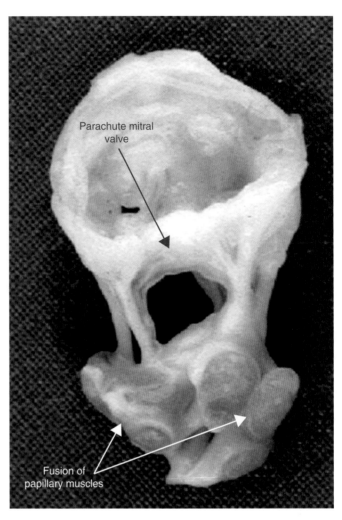

Fig. 7.99 This heart with deficient atrioventricular septation, common atrioventricular junction, and shunting exclusively at ventricular level, the so-called "ostium primum" defect, is photographed from the left side in anatomic orientation. Note the difference between the zone of apposition between the left ventricular components of the bridging leaflets, the so-called "cleft", and the true cleft of the aortic leaflet of an otherwise normal mitral valve shown in Fig. 7.98.

Fig. 7.100 This specimen, removed at surgery, shows the so-called "parachute" arrangement of the mitral valve. There is fusion of the papillary muscles, along with thickening and fusion of the tendinous cords.

MALFORMATIONS OF THE ARTERIAL VALVES AND OUTFLOW TRACTS

In this section, we consider the surgical aspects of subvalvar obstruction of the ventricular outflow tracts, valvar stenosis, and atresia of the outflow. In the normally connected heart, obstruction in the left ventricular outflow tract produces subaortic stenosis. It must then be remembered that the same anatomic lesions will produce subpulmonary obstruction in the patient with discordant ventriculo-arterial connections. Similarly, obstruction of the right ventricular outflow tract produces subpulmonary obstruction in the heart with normal

segmental connections, but subaortic stenosis when the ventriculo-arterial connections are discordant. When both outflow tracts are connected to the same ventricle, the anatomical problems are more discrete. These are considered separately in Chapter 8.

Stenosis of the aortic valve can occur at valvar, subvalvar, and supravalvar levels. Aortic regurgitation is ultimately a valvar problem, and the perivalvar anatomy is often of great importance. To understand fully the substrates for stenosis and regurgitation across the arterial valves, it is essential to have a firm grasp of the arrangement of the valvar leaflets at the ventriculo-arterial junction. As described in Chapters 2 and 3, the arterial valves do

not possess an 'annulus' in the sense of a circular ring of collagen that supports the leaflets in the fashion of a circle. The only ring within the valvar complex, aside from the sinutubular junction, is the circular area over which the fibrous wall of the great arterial trunk is supported by the underlying ventricular structures[38]. These are partly muscular and partly fibrous in the left ventricle (Fig. 7.101), but exclusively muscular at the right ventriculo-arterial junction (Fig. 7.102). The attachments of the leaflets are thus arranged as half moons, with the bases of the leaflets attached to ventricular muscle, but the apex of the leaflets attached to the fibrous wall of the arterial trunk at the sinutubular junction. When seen in closed

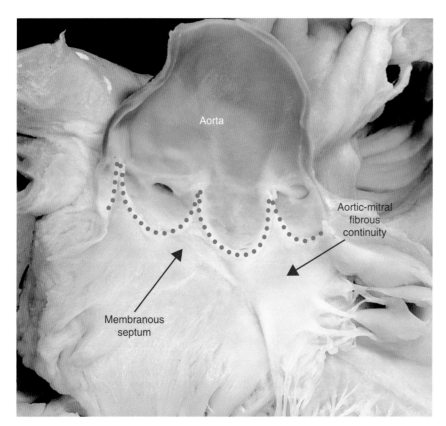

Fig. 7.101 The aortic outflow tract has been spread open and is photographed from the ventricular aspect in anatomic orientation. The arterial valvar leaflets are attached in semilunar fashion, (red dotted line), taking their origin in part from fibrous tissue, and in part from the muscular ventricular septum.

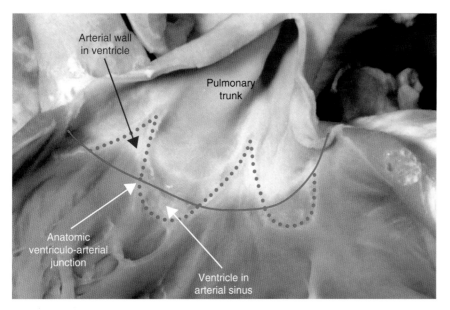

Fig. 7.102 In this anatomic specimen, the subpulmonary infundibulum has been opened and photographed in anatomical orientation having removed the leaflets of the pulmonary valve. Note that the semilunar attachments of the leaflets (dotted red line) cross the circular anatomic ventriculo-arterial junction (solid red line). This is more obvious than in the subaortic outflow tract (see Fig. 7.101), but the basic arrangement is comparable.

position, the three leaflets then coapt snugly along their zones of apposition, which extend from the circumferential margins of the arterial wall to the centre of the valve (Fig. 7.103). It is on the basis of perturbation of this coaptation of the leaflets under pressure of the diastolic column of blood that stenosis or regurgitation occurs within the valvar complex.

Valvar aortic stenosis may occur with unicuspid, bicuspid, tricuspid and, rarely, even quadricuspid valves. Dysplastic lesions are also seen in the aortic valve, but only rarely can surgery provide the answer to this problem. The unicuspid valve has two raphes at the ends of abortive zones of apposition (Fig. 7.104). The leaflets are also abnormally attached in linear rather than semilunar fashion (Fig. 7.105). Little

can be done other than an attempt to open the valve as much as possible, short of producing severe regurgitation. Attempts to open the rudimentary raphe invariably result in prolapse of the leaflets and regurgitation.

A valve with two effective leaflets is most frequently seen in the adult patient. Perhaps this is because such a bicuspid valve, in itself, is not usually intrinsically

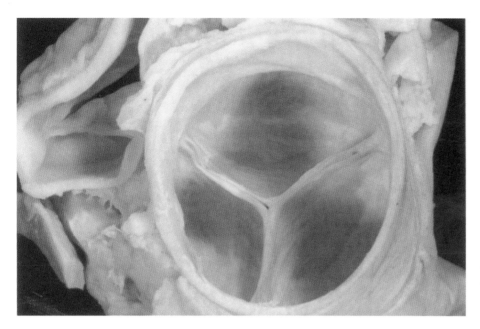

Fig. 7.103 In this specimen, the aortic valve is photographed from above in its closed position. The three zones of apposition between the leaflets extend from the sinutubular junction at the periphery to the centre of the valvar orifice. The leaflets are closed by the hydrostatic pressure of the column of blood they support.

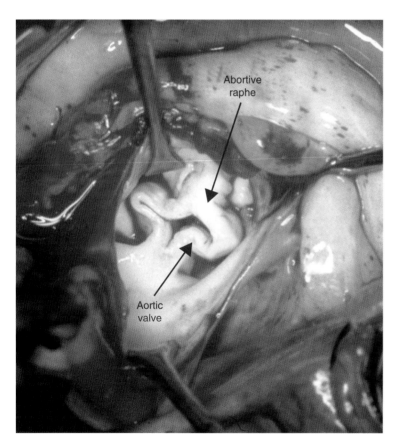

Abortive raphe

Aortic valve

Fig. 7.104 This view of an abnormal aortic valve seen through an aortotomy shows the so-called unicuspid and unicommissural arrangement. Fusion of two of the putative zones of apposition during development leaves the persisting zone of apposition as the eccentric valvar orifice.

stenotic. It is only with the effects of time and turbulence that these valves typically become manifestly obstructive. If the valvar morphology has not been totally obscured by calcific deposits, a bicuspid valve seen at operation will take one of two forms. Occasionally the two leaflets are of equal size, the solitary zone of apposition between them bisecting the aortic root (Fig. 7.106). This type is frequently found in patients with coarctation of the aorta. In the other form, the leaflets are unequal, with the large, or conjoined, leaflet often exhibiting an eccentrically-placed raphe (Fig. 7.107), or with a raphe bisecting the conjoined leaflets (Fig. 7.108). Both coronary arteries may arise from the sinuses of the conjoined leaflet, but they may also be positioned so that one coronary artery arises from the conjoined sinuses, and the other from the third

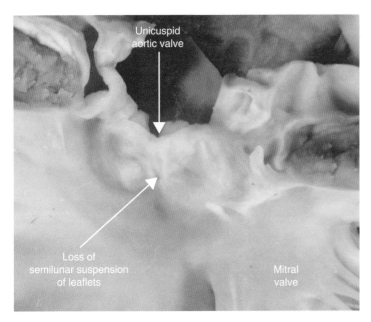

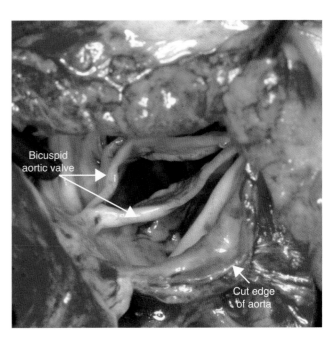

Fig. 7.105 This picture of the aortic valve, taken in a specimen having opened the left ventricular outflow tract, shows the unicuspid and unicommissural arrangement as shown in Fig. 7.104. There is loss of the semilunar suspension of the leaflets, so that paradoxically they are attached in true annular fashion. The solitary zone of apposition points backwards towards the mitral valve.

Fig. 7.106 This picture, taken in the operating room through an aortotomy, shows an aortic valve with two leaflets of comparable size.

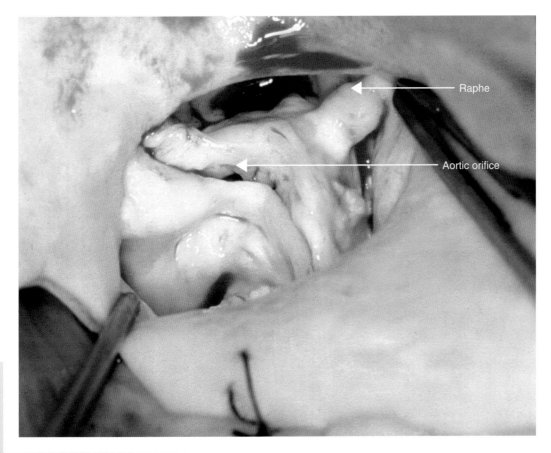

Fig. 7.107 This picture, again taken in the operating room through an aortotomy, show a bicuspid aortic valve with a raphe in one of the leaflets.

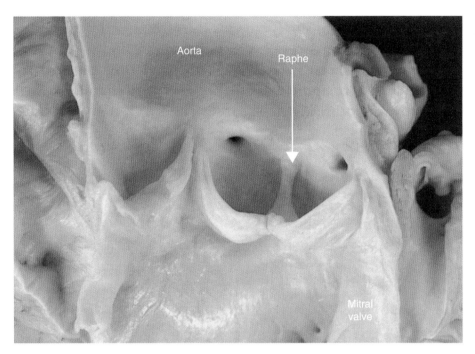

Fig. 7.108 In this specimen, the aortic valve is photographed from behind in anatomic orientation having opened the left ventricular outflow tract through the mitral valve. The two leaflets arising from the sinuses giving rise to the coronary arteries have fused, with the line of fusion represented by the raphe.

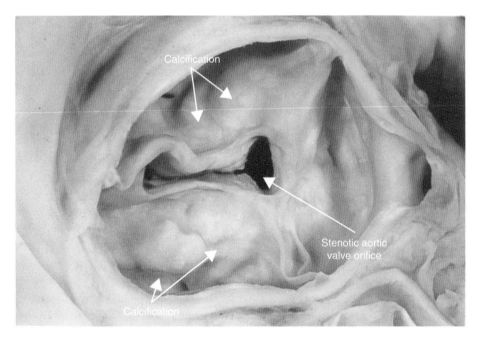

Fig. 7.109 This abnormal aortic valve, photographed from the aortic aspect, has fusion of two of the zones of apposition between the leaflets, with calcification also present. This is the typical substrate of aortic stenosis as seen in the elderly.

sinus[39]. If valves with two effective leaflets are seen before they become rigid and distorted by calcification, some relief from the stenosis can be obtained by careful enlargement of the ends of the solitary zone of apposition.

Aortic stenosis does occur in patients with valves having three leaflets, but is not usually seen until later in life. A possible cause of such stenosis is the unequal size

of the leaflets in the normal aortic valve. This, coupled with the high pressure in the aortic root, may lead to the development of calcification and stenosis in the elderly (Fig. 7.109)[40].

Subvalvar stenosis may be fibrous, fibromuscular, or muscular, reflecting the fact that the left ventricular outflow tract is partly muscular and partly fibrous. The muscular portion comprises the

ventriculo–infundibular fold anterolaterally, the small outlet component of the muscular septum anteriorly, and the upper edge of the apical part of the muscular septum posteriorly. The fibrous part comprises the central fibrous body, the area of continuity between the leaflets of the aortic and mitral valves, and the left fibrous trigone. Subvalvar stenoses may also be either fixed or dynamic in nature.

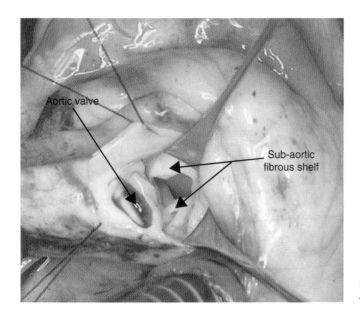

Fig. 7.110 This view, taken in the operating room through the aortic valve, shows a circular fibrous shelf producing subaortic stenosis.

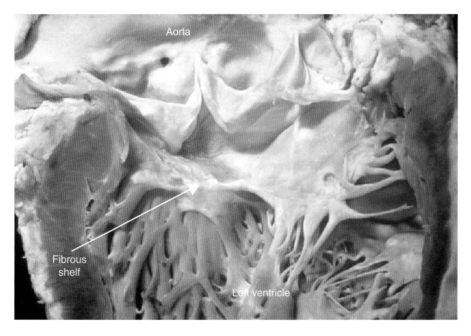

Fig. 7.111 This specimen is opened anteriorly through the subaortic outflow tract, and is photographed in anatomical orientation. Note the extensive shelf-like lesion producing subvalvar stenosis, and extending onto the aortic leaflet of the mitral valve.

Of the variants producing fixed stenosis, a subvalvar fibrous shelf is perhaps most easily approached surgically. It appears circular when viewed through the usually normal aortic valve. Indeed, it can be circular (Fig. 7.110). This is not always the case. A relatively thin shelf of tissue sometimes runs from beneath the non-coronary leaflet of the aortic valve, over the site of the penetrating bundle, to the septal musculature, finally coursing over the ventriculo–infundibular fold to involve the aortic leaflet of the mitral valve (Fig. 7.111). If dissection is performed carefully[41], a circumferential lesion can

be completely removed (Fig. 7.112), taking particular care where the shelf intimately overlies the conduction tissues. Too vigorous an attack on the side of the mitral valve may lead to detachment of that structure. In cases where the ventricular septum appears to be playing a part in causing the stenosis, it may be prudent to remove a segment of muscle (Fig. 7.113).

In cases where complete removal proves difficult, interruption of the fibrous shelf in the safe area over the ventriculo–infundibular fold will result in a safe and satisfactory relief of the

stenosis. The same rules apply when resecting the variant of aortic stenosis producing a fibromuscular tunnel. Surgical correction, however, may be less successful than with a simple shelf, since the tunnel extends farther into the left ventricle, making the obstruction it produces more difficult to relieve.

A rather rare form of fixed subaortic obstruction is produced by hypertrophy of the usually inconspicuous anterolateral muscle bundle[42]. This muscle runs down the outflow tract from the ventriculo–infundibular fold to the ventricular septum. In its course over the parietal

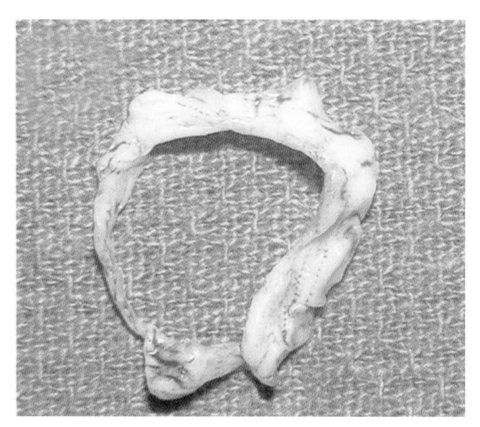

Fig. 7.112 This specimen is the subaortic shelf shown in Fig. 7.110 subsequent to its surgical removal. Note the horseshoe configuration.

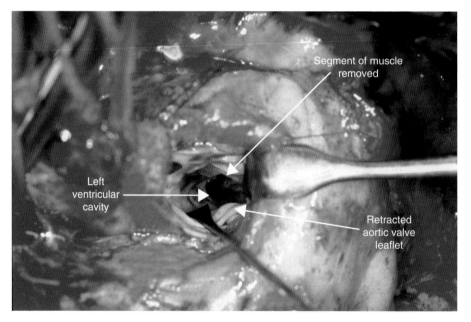

Segment of muscle removed

Left ventricular cavity

Retracted aortic valve leaflet

Fig. 7.113 This view taken in the operating room through the aorta shows how a segment of ventricular muscle can safely be removed to relieve shelf-like fibrous obstruction of the left ventricular outflow tract.

wall, it would not be expected to involve the conduction tissues.

Anomalous attachment of the left atrioventricular valve can also cause fixed obstruction, as can a deviated muscular outlet septum. The former is usually seen with atrioventricular septal defect. The latter occurs only in the presence of a ventricular septal defect (Fig. 7.114).

The final fixed type of subaortic obstruction is produced by so-called 'tissue tags'. These can herniate from any adjacent fibrous tissue structure, but are exceedingly rare as an isolated lesion in the normally connected heart[43]. They can produce significant obstruction of the left ventricular outflow tract in hearts with an atrioventricular septal defect (Fig. 7.115), or with discordant ventriculo-arterial connections.

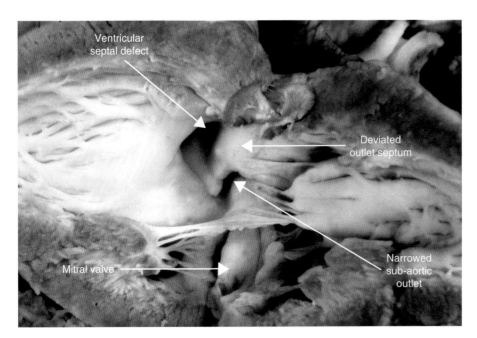

Fig. 7.114 This anatomic specimen shows the left ventricle opened in clam-like fashion, and viewed from the apex of the left ventricle. There is fixed subaortic obstruction produced by posterior deviation of the muscular outlet septum through a ventricular septal defect.

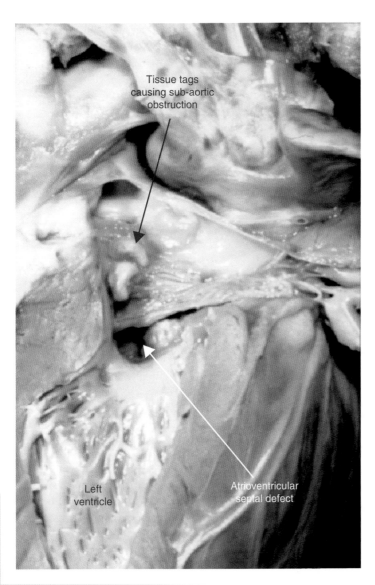

Fig. 7.115 This heart is opened through the subaortic outflow tract, and photographed in anatomic orientation. There is an atrioventricular septal defect with common atrioventricular junction, with subaortic obstruction due to tissue tags.

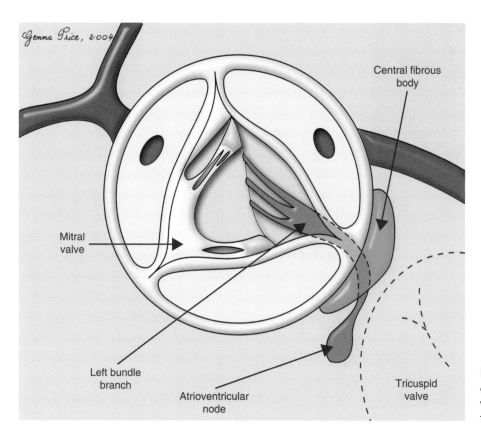

Gemma Price, 2004

Central fibrous body

Mitral valve

Left bundle branch

Atrioventricular node

Tricuspid valve

Fig. 7.116 The cartoon shows the location of the atrioventricular conduction axis as it would be visualised by the surgeon working through the aortic valve.

Dynamic subvalvar obstruction is a result of thickening of the septal musculature abutting the aortic leaflet of the mitral valve during ventricular systole. This usually creates a ridge of thickened endocardium easily seen through the aortic valve. If an operation becomes necessary, resection of this muscle bundle, as advocated by Morrow et al[44], offers satisfactory relief of the obstruction. Again the surgeon must scrupulously avoid the conduction tissue as it emerges beneath the zone of apposition between the right and non-coronary leaflets and descends on the muscular ventricular septum (Fig. 7.116).

Supravalvar aortic stenosis is said to occur as one of three types: the hourglass, membranous, and more diffuse tubular deformities. All forms are rare. Fortunately, the severe tubular type is extremely unusual. Two problems are shared by all three varieties because of narrowing of the aorta at the junction of the sinuses with the ascending tubular aorta[45]. First, the aortic sinuses, which usually contain the coronary arteries, may be converted into high pressure zones, in which the arteries provide the only run-off other than through the distal stenosis. This can produce marked dilation of both the sinuses and the coronary arteries. Second, the circumferential narrowing at the sinutubular junction (Fig. 7.117) tends to tether the three aortic leaflets at the ends of their zones of apposition in such a way that it is rarely enough to perform a simple 'aortoplasty'[46]. If possible, all three sinuses should be opened to release the tethering of the leaflets. This can be accomplished by resecting the thickened sinutubular junction, and inserting pericardial patches in each sinus (Figs. 7.118–7.123).

Aortic valvar insufficiency may be due to congenital malformation of the valve (Fig. 7.124), its supporting structures (Fig. 7.125), or both. It may also be secondary to an infectious process in the aortic root (Fig. 7.126), or to 'degenerative' disease. Occasionally, aortic insufficiency may be due to trauma. Its frequent association with the doubly committed and juxta-arterial ventricular septal defect suggests that deficiency in the structures supporting the leaflets plays

some role in these problems. Prolapse of the leaflets, and insufficiency, may occur with other types of ventricular septal defect (Fig. 7.127). Prolapse can be found even when the ventricular septum is intact, the latter situation usually being associated with a bicuspid aortic valve.

The critical importance of the anatomy of this region is perhaps best demonstrated by the problems exhibited by patients with endocarditis of the aortic valve[47]. Because the valve is the 'keystone' to all the other valves and chambers of the heart (Fig. 7.128), an eroding abscess in the aortic root may lead to formation of a fistula involving any of these adjacent structures. The patient may present with findings of left heart failure, left-to-right shunting, complete heart block, or any combination of these, in addition to the usual signs of sepsis. Surgical management clearly requires a detailed knowledge of this area, since the surgeon may be faced with virtual disruption of the ventriculo-arterial connection[48]. A very similar problem can occur when the aortic root, or the fibrous coronet, is severely

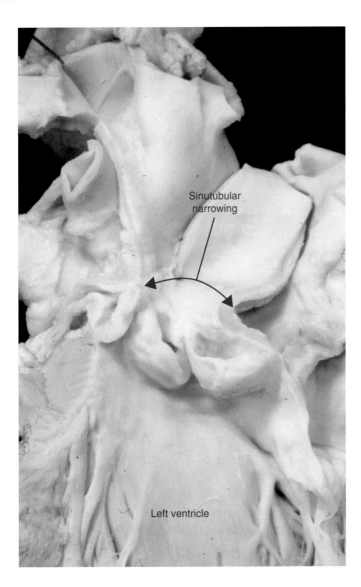

Sinutubular
narrowing

Left ventricle

Fig. 7.117 In this specimen, photographed in anatomic orientation, there is severe narrowing at the level of the sinutubular junction. Although usually termed "supravalvar", the obstruction involves the attachment of the valvar leaflets at the sinutubular junction.

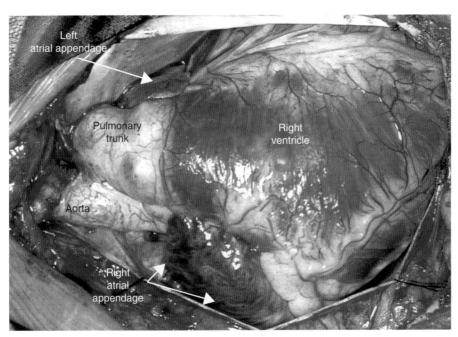

Left
atrial appendage

Pulmonary
trunk

Right
ventricle

Aorta

Right
atrial
appendage

Fig. 7.118 This picture taken in the operating room through a median sternotomy shows the small aortic root in comparison with the normally sized pulmonary trunk in a patient with supravalvar aortic stenosis.

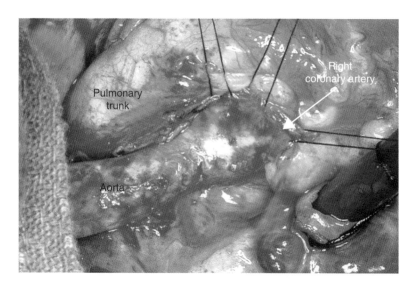

Fig. 7.119 Further dissection in the patient shown in Fig. 7.118 reveals the supravalvar constriction.

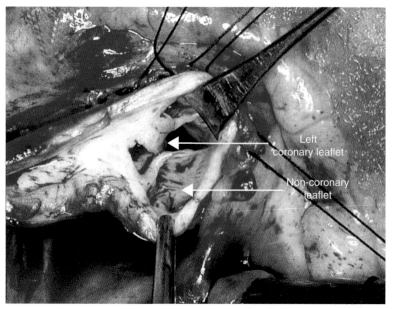

Fig. 7.120 In this patient with supravalvar aortic stenosis, the surgeon has made an extensive vertical excision into the non-coronary sinus, revealing the marked constriction at the sinutubular junction, with a particularly narrow left coronary sinus.

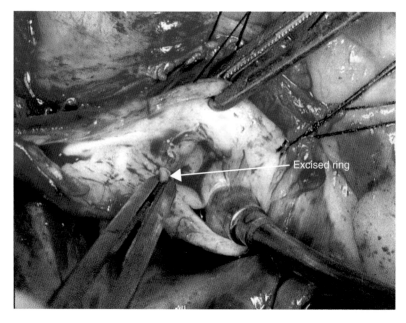

Fig. 7.121 This operative view in the patient with supravalvar aortic stenosis shows how it is possible to excise the thickened sinutubular junction, releasing the attachments of the left coronary leaflet to allow full excursion.

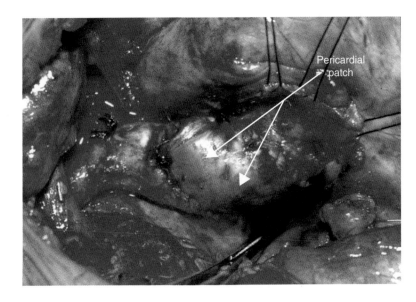

Fig. 7.122 In the same patient with supravalvar aortic stenosis as shown in the previous illustrations, insertion of a helical pericardial patch has enlarged the ascending aorta.

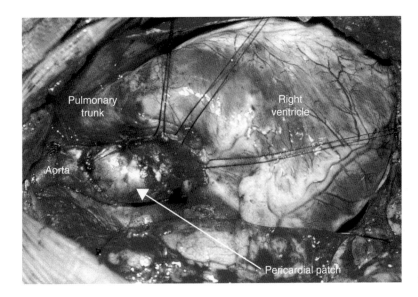

Fig. 7.123 Subsequent to the operative repair, the aorta is now approximately the same size as the pulmonary trunk (compare with Fig. 7.117).

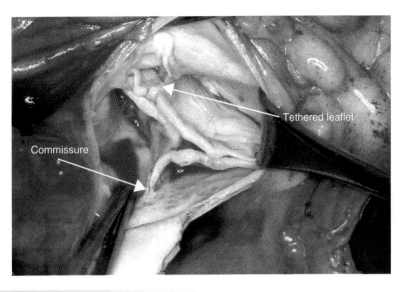

Fig. 7.124 This operative view of the aortic valve, taken through an aortotomy, shows a regurgitant valve as the consequence of tethering of one of its leaflets.

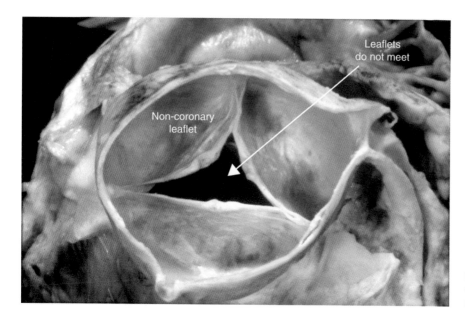

Fig. 7.125 This anatomic specimen is photographed from above, showing regurgitant of the aortic valve because of dilation of the sinutubular junction.

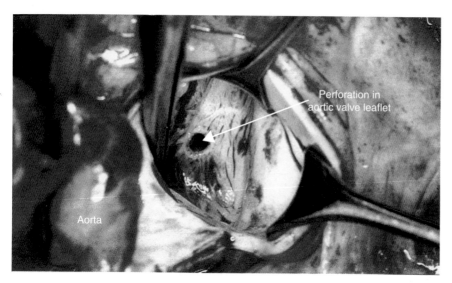

Fig. 7.126 This operative view, taken through an aortotomy, shows a perforation in one leaflet of a bicuspid aortic valve due to infective endocarditis.

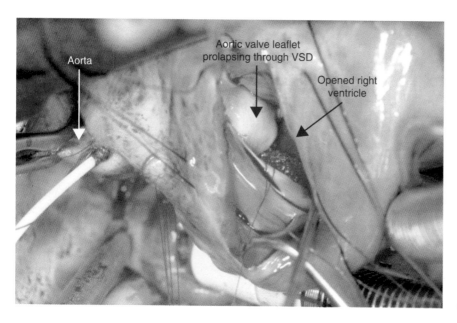

Fig. 7.127 This operative view, seen through a right ventriculotomy, shows prolapse of the leaflets of the aortic valve in the setting of a perimembranous ventricular septal defect opening to the outlet of the right ventricle.

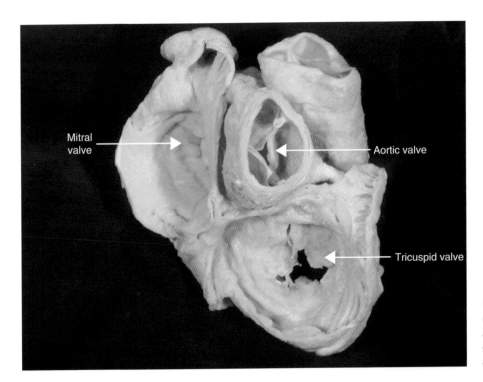

Fig. 7.128 The short axis of the ventricular mass has been displayed by removing the atrial musculature and the arterial trunks, showing the "keystone" location of the centrally positioned aortic valve.

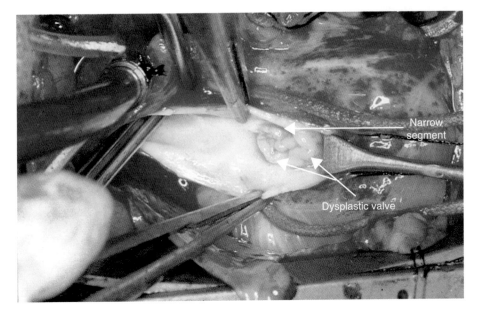

Fig. 7.129 This operative view, taken through an incision in the pulmonary trunk, shows gross dysplasia of the leaflets of the pulmonary valve.

damaged by dissection or marked degeneration of its fibrous structure.

As with aortic stenosis, stenosis of the right ventricular outflow can occur at the valvar, supravalvar or subvalvar levels. The latter is discussed in association with tetralogy of Fallot (see below). Dysplasia of the valvar leaflets is most often seen as marked distortion and thickening, although three discrete leaflets can sometimes be recognised (Fig. 7.129). It can be associated with insufficiency as well as stenosis.

Isolated pulmonary stenosis is typically found in the form of a dome-shaped valve with three well-developed but fused commissures[38] (Fig. 7.130). In some cases, the leaflets are attached to the wall of the pulmonary trunk along the peripheral ends of the zones of apposition between them, leaving only a restricted central opening (Fig. 7.131), and a narrowed arterial root. These areas of tethering can be dissected from the arterial wall and incised, resulting in a particularly satisfactory relief of the obstruction (Figs.

7.132–137). The effectiveness of surgery is best measured six to nine months after operation, since significant secondary muscular obstruction at the subvalvar level may maintain a pressure gradient across the outflow tract. This muscular hypertrophy will almost always regress with time[48]. Despite the excellent results of surgery, treatment of congenital pulmonary valvar stenosis has largely become the province of the interventional cardiologist. It is doubtful, however, whether inflation of a balloon will ever

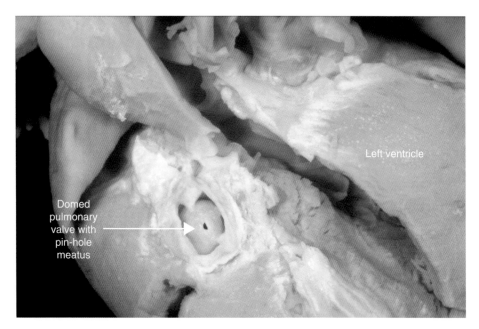

Domed pulmonary valve with pin-hole meatus

Left ventricle

Fig. 7.130 This pulmonary valve is viewed from above in anatomic orientation. There is gross fusion of the zones of apposition between the leaflets, leaving a domed membrane with a central orifice the size of a pinhole.

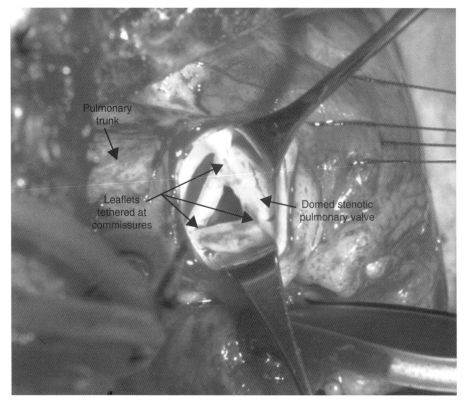

Pulmonary trunk

Leaflets tethered at commissures

Domed stenotic pulmonary valve

Fig. 7.131 This operative view, taken through an incision in the pulmonary trunk, shows a pulmonary valve with fusion of the zones of apposition between the leaflets, and tethering of the fused leaflets to the wall of the pulmonary trunk.

rival the anatomic precision illustrated in Figures 7.132 through 7.137.

Supravalvar stenosis usually takes the form of a waist-like narrowing of the pulmonary trunk just distal to the valve (Fig. 7.138), though it may occur at the sinutubular junction, or anywhere at one or more locations within the pulmonary arterial tree. Narrowing has also been reported within collateral arteries supplying the lung directly from the aorta in cases of tetralogy of Fallot with pulmonary atresia[49]. Very rarely, the obstructions may be membrane-like, but the usual lesion is more akin to a segment of tubular hypoplasia. These lesions, if anatomically accessible, are amenable to enlargement using a simple patch.

One form of obstruction of the right ventricular outflow tract is so clearly demarcated that it constitutes an entity in its own right, namely tetralogy of Fallot. Its anatomical hallmark is anterosuperior deviation of the insertion of the muscular outlet septum, combined with muscular subpulmonary obstruction due to hypertrophy of septoparietal trabeculations[50]. In the normal heart (Fig. 7.139), the outlet part of the muscular ventricular outlet septum is inconspicuous,

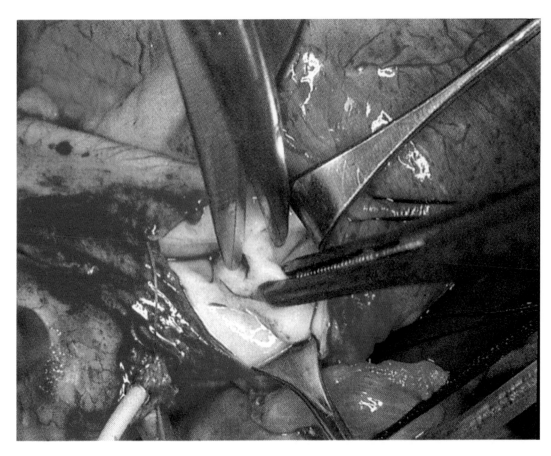

Figs. 7.132–137 This series of operative illustrations, taken through an incision in the pulmonary trunk, shows how the surgeon is able to separate the fused zones of apposition between the leaflets, and also resect the attachments of the fused zones from the sinutubular junction, restoring the function of the valve. It is unlikely that the interventionist can match the accuracy of this repair by blowing up a balloon.

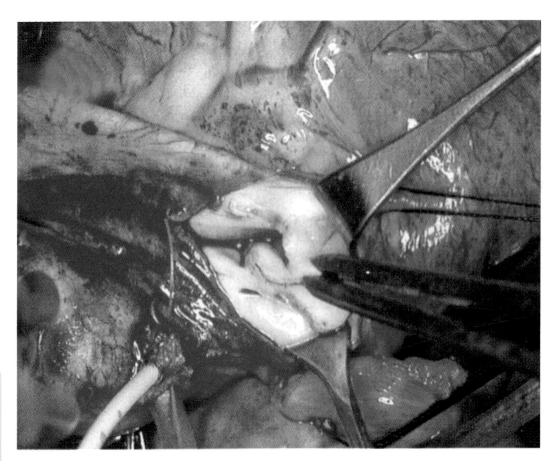

Fig. 7.133

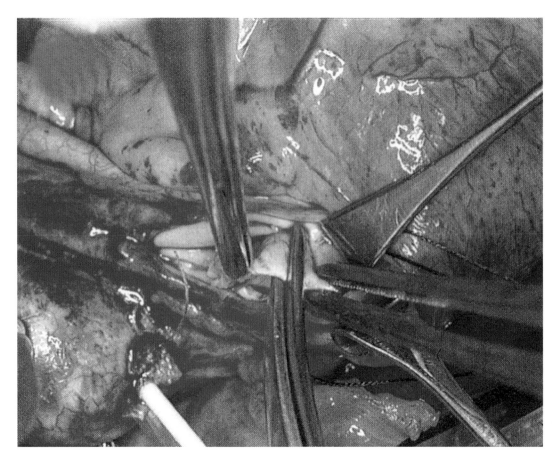

Fig. 7.134

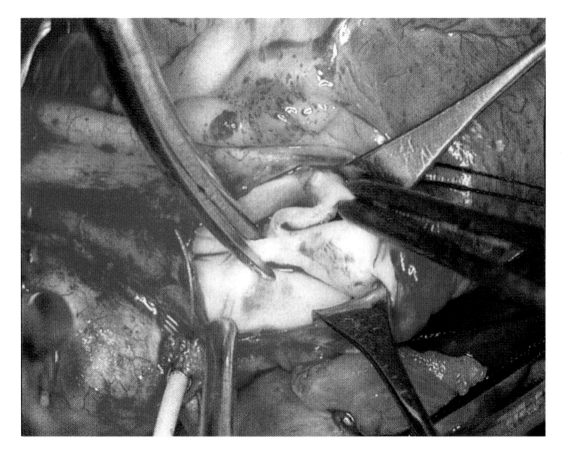

Fig. 7.135

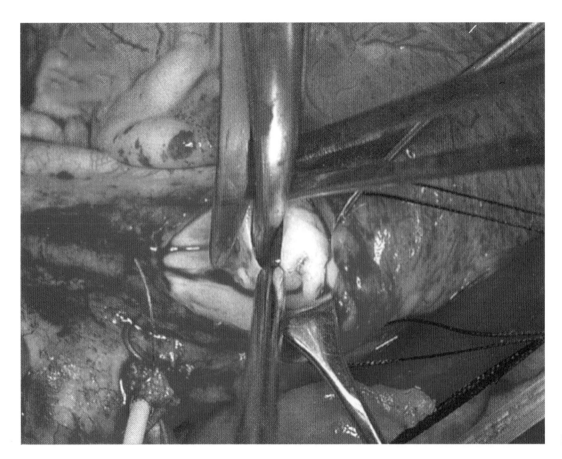

Fig. 7.136

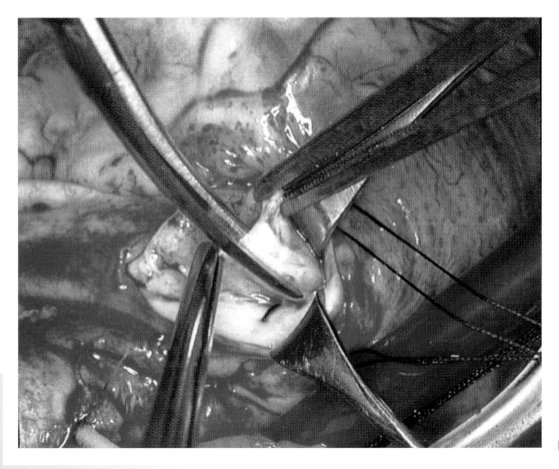

Fig. 7.137

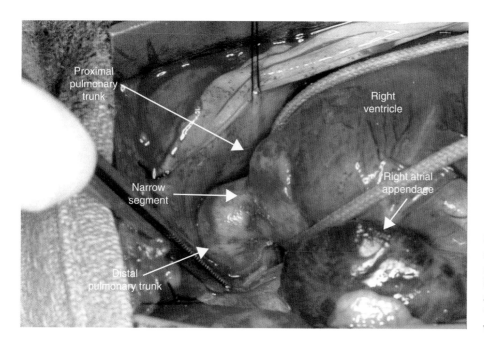

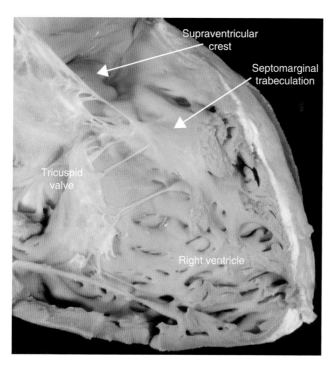

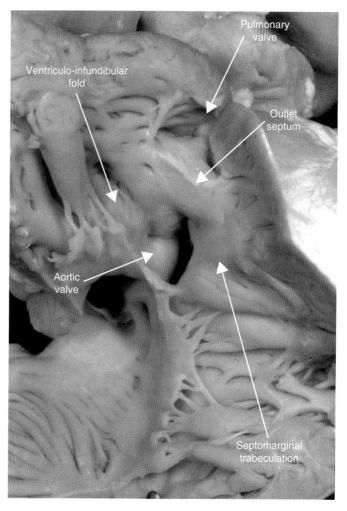

Fig. 7.138 This view, taken through a median sternotomy shows waist-like narrowing of the pulmonary trunk at the level of the sinutubular junction, the arrangement usually described as "supravalvar" narrowing. The abnormal valve in this heart was shown in Fig. 7.131.

Fig. 7.139 The normal right ventricle is photographed in anatomical orientation, showing the septal aspect. Note that the supraventricular crest inserts between the limbs of the septomarginal trabeculation. Although there is a small part of the "outlet septum" buried within the supraventricular crest, it is not possible, in the normal heart, to distinguish where the septum finishes and where the musculature becomes that of the parietal ventricular wall.

Fig. 7.140 This view of the outlet of the right ventricle in tetralogy of Fallot, in anatomic orientation, shows the divorce of the various muscular structures making up the normal outflow tract.

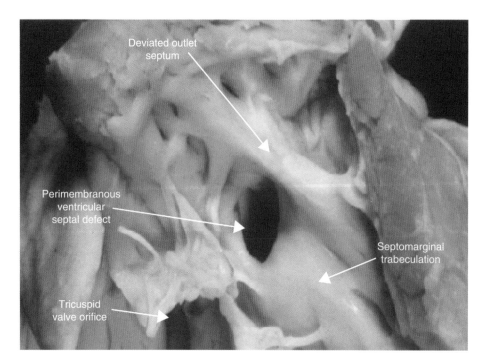

Fig. 7.141 This view of an anatomic specimen, photographed in anatomic orientation, shows a ventricular septal defect in tetralogy of Fallot with the posteroinferior border formed by fibrous continuity between the leaflets of the aortic and tricuspid valves, making the defect perimembranous.

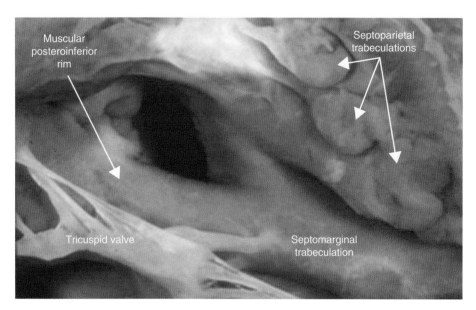

Fig. 7.142 In this specimen with tetralogy of Fallot, photographed in anatomic orientation, the defect as seen from the right ventricle has exclusively muscular borders.

being firmly anchored between the limbs of the septomarginal trabeculation, where it is fused with the much more extensive ventriculo–infundibular fold to form the supraventricular crest. It is the alignment of the outlet part of the muscular septum and the ventriculo–infundibular fold which produces the normal supraventricular crest, itself in continuity with the septomarginal trabeculation, or "septal band".

In tetralogy of Fallot, the outlet part of the septum is malaligned anterocephalad to the anterior limb of the septomarginal

trabeculation. In a single stroke, this deviation divorces the outlet septum from the ventriculo–infundibular fold. The deviated position of the septum, combined with hypertrophy of the septoparietal trabeculations, then serves to narrow the subpulmonary outflow tract. At the same time, it leaves an interventricular communication that is overridden by the leaflets of the aortic valve (Fig. 7.140).

The interventricular communication, therefore, is positioned beneath the ventricular outlets in association with malalignment of the muscular outlet

septum. There can be fibrous continuity in the posteroinferior quadrant of the defect between the leaflets of the aortic and tricuspid valves. This makes the defect perimembranous (Fig. 7.141). Alternatively, the posteroinferior rim can be muscular[51] (Fig. 7.142). These features have the same implications for disposition of the axis of atrioventricular conduction tissue as they do in isolated ventricular septal defects (see Chapter 7). When the posteroinferior margin is formed by an area of continuity between the leaflets of the aortic, tricuspid, and

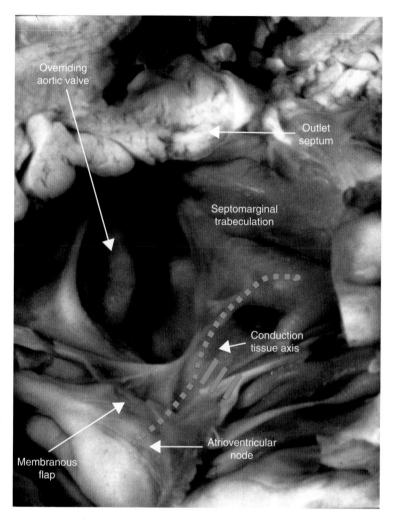

Overriding aortic valve

Outlet septum

Septomarginal trabeculation

Conduction tissue axis

Membranous flap

Atrioventricular node

Fig. 7.143 This anatomical specimen with tetralogy of Fallot, photographed in anatomical orientation, has been prepared by removal of the septal leaflet of the tricuspid valve. It shows the so-called membranous flap, and the relationships of the atrioventricular conduction tissue axis (superimposed in green) to a perimembranous ventricular septal defect.

mitral valves, the atrioventricular conduction axis penetrates beneath the atrioventricular membranous component of this fibrous area (Fig. 7.143). Often this is overlain by the so-called membranous flap, or pseudoflaps derived from the tricuspid valve[52]. Usually, in tetralogy, the non-branching and the branching components of the atrioventricular bundle are carried down the left ventricular side of the septum, being positioned some distance from the septal crest. In a minority of cases, the bundle can branch directly astride the septum[53,54]. It can then be traumatised (Fig. 7.144) by sutures placed directly through the septal crest (Fig. 7.145).

The cases in which the posterior limb of the septomarginal trabeculation has fused with the ventriculo–infundibular fold superior to an intact interventricular membranous septum (Fig. 7.142), thus

protecting the atrioventricular conduction tissues, account for about one-fifth of the overall population with this lesion. When seen, superficial sutures can be placed along the entire muscular margin of the right ventricular aspect of these defects without fear of traumatizing the conduction axis.

In rare cases, more frequently encountered in Asia or South America[55,56], the outlet septum is completely absent, along with the posterior aspect of the free-standing subpulmonary infundibulum. The defect then becomes doubly committed and juxta-arterial (Fig. 7.146). The significant surgical feature in these cases is again the relationship of the conduction axis in the inferior border of the defect, which may be either muscular or perimembranous.

While it is clearly important to close securely the right ventricular margin of the interventricular communication in

patients with tetralogy, patching the aorta into the left ventricle, probably the most important feature for a successful surgical outcome is relief of the subpulmonary obstruction. One of the major determinants of this success is the size of the pulmonary trunk. Tables are available for preoperative evaluation to select those hearts which can be successfully corrected without incising across the ventriculo–arterial junction[57,58]. An understanding of the precise anatomy of the subpulmonary outflow tract is also vital if the surgeon is to plan accurately a reproducible operation for successful relief of the muscular obstruction. This is the consequence of formation of a constrictive muscular ring at the mouth of the subpulmonary infundibulum, with its parietal segment produced by hypertrophy of free-standing septoparietal trabeculations. Knowledge of this feature is important to the surgeon when deciding

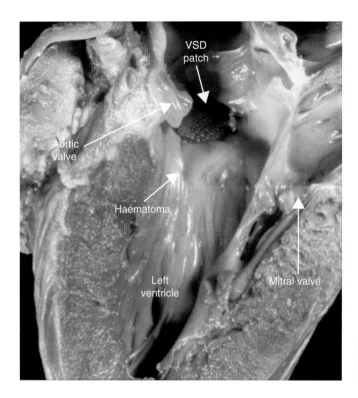

Fig. 7.144 In this heart, viewed in anatomical orientation from the left ventricle, the defect in a patient with tetralogy of Fallot was repaired by placing sutures directly through the septal crest.

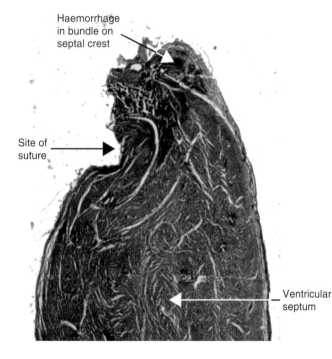

Fig. 7.145 In the patient with tetralogy of Fallot shown in Fig. 7.144, the atrioventricular conduction tissue axis unfortunately branched directly astride the septum. As shown by this histological section, the bundle was traumatised by the sutures securing the patch.

which muscle to resect in order to widen the narrowed outflow tract. The major limiting structure is always the hypertrophied septal insertion of the outlet septum, which can be incised without fear of damaging vital structures. At the same time, any free-standing septoparietal trabeculations should be identified and removed (Figs. 7.147,

7.148) since they, too, never contain vital structures. The body of the outlet septum usually contributes to obstruction, and it is tempting also to resect this structure. Excessive resection, however, may lead to damage to the leaflets of the aortic valve arising from its left ventricular aspect.

It is also usual to resect the parietal insertion of the outlet septum (Fig. 7.149).

This fuses with the ventriculo-infundibular fold, which is the inner curvature of the heart. Care must be taken in this area not to perforate through to the right-sided atrioventricular groove. Dissection, or injudicious placement of sutures, in this region can damage the right coronary artery[59]. It is very unusual for the septomarginal trabeculation itself

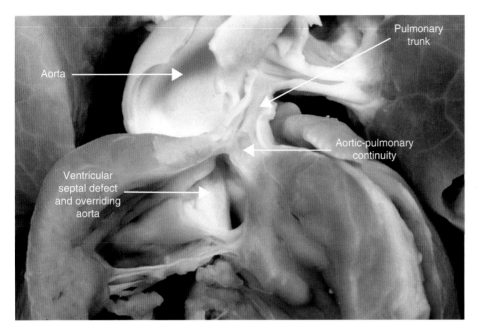

Fig. 7.146 This specimen, viewed in anatomic orientation from the apex of the right ventricle, shows tetralogy of Fallot with a doubly committed and juxta-arterial defect due to failure of formation of the muscular subpulmonary infundibulum. Note the fibrous continuity between the leaflets of the aortic and pulmonary valves.

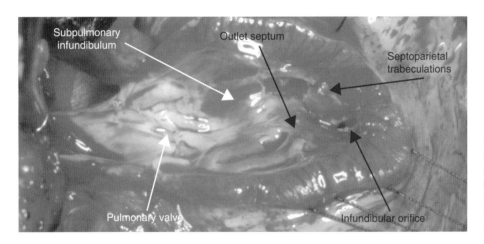

Fig. 7.147 This view taken in the operating room through a right infundibulotomy shows the stenotic orifice of the subpulmonary infundibulum in tetralogy of Fallot. The stenosis is formed in part by the hypertrophied outlet septum, but to the other side by septoparietal trabeculations.

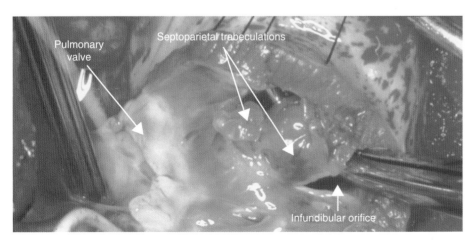

Fig. 7.148 The septoparietal trabeculations shown in Fig. 7.147 have been liberated, and can now be excised.

to contribute to the subpulmonary obstruction. Thus, it is usually unnecessary to resect its limbs. Its body, and the moderator band, nonetheless, may be hypertrophied, particularly when the latter structure has a high take-off. Severe hypertrophy produces a two-chambered right ventricle[60]. The intervening muscle bay may then require resection (Fig. 7.150). The anterior papillary muscle of the tricuspid valve often arises from the inlet aspect of the obstructing

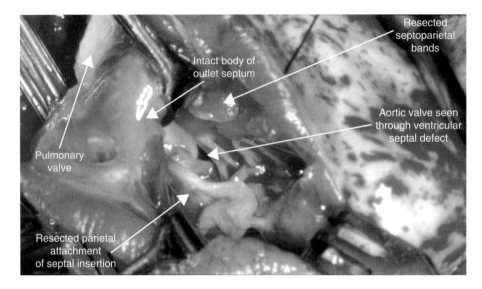

Resected septoparietal bands

Intact body of outlet septum

Aortic valve seen through ventricular septal defect

Pulmonary valve

Resected parietal attachment of septal insertion

Fig. 7.149 The obstruction shown in Fig. 7.147 is completely relieved by the resection of the parietal extension of the outlet septum.

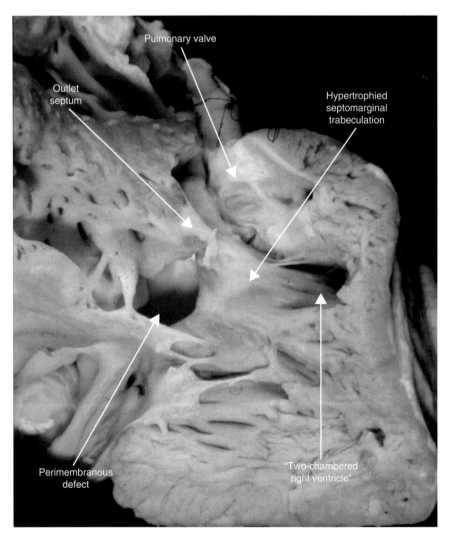

Pulmonary valve

Outlet septum

Hypertrophied septomarginal trabeculation

Perimembranous defect

"Two-chambered right ventricle"

Fig. 7.150 The right ventricle in this specimen of tetralogy of Fallot is shown in anatomic orientation. The body of the septomarginal trabeculation is hypertrophied, separating the apical trabecular component into two parts. This is so-called "two-chambered right ventricle".

shelf. Care must be taken, therefore, not to damage this muscle during resection.

The final variable in tetralogy of Fallot is the connection of the leaflets of the overriding aortic valve. This varies from the aorta being connected mostly to the left ventricle, making the ventriculo-arterial connection concordant, to its being connected mostly to the right ventricle, and hence producing a double outlet connection. The degree of override should not markedly affect the surgical procedure.

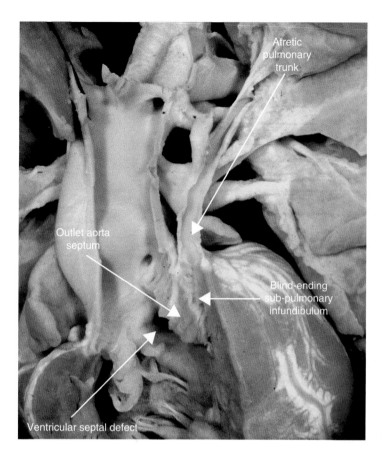

Fig. 7.151 This specimen of tetralogy with pulmonary atresia, viewed in anatomical orientation, has confluent pulmonary arteries supplied by an arterial duct.

With greater commitment of the aorta to the right ventricle, nonetheless, the placement of the patch tunnelling the aorta to the left ventricle becomes more important. The 'internal conduit' constructed from the left ventricle to the aorta may further complicate relief of the obstruction to the right ventricular outflow tract, since it is always necessary to ensure an adequate outlet from the left ventricle.

Although the primary obstruction in tetralogy is at infundibular level, the pulmonary valve is frequently stenotic. This must be relieved during operative repair. The sequels of postoperative pulmonary regurgitation are only now becoming evident. It could be that, in the long term, they will be just as troublesome as residual pulmonary stenosis, and less easy to relieve.

The most common type of pulmonary atresia with ventricular septal defect is, in essence, tetralogy of Fallot with valvar or infundibular pulmonary atresia. This is the most appropriate descriptor[61]. The ventricular anatomy includes deviation of the muscular outlet septum sufficient to block completely the subpulmonary infundibulum (Fig. 7.151). The anatomy of the interventricular communication can vary as in tetralogy, but the intracardiac anatomy is of relatively minor surgical significance. The feature which dominates the surgical options is the morphology of the pulmonary arteries. Exceedingly rarely, the pulmonary arteries may be supplied through a so-called persistent fifth arch[62], an aortopulmonary window, or coronary arterial fistulas[63]. In most instances, nonetheless, the lungs are supplied either through a persistent arterial duct (Fig. 7.152), or through major aortopulmonary collateral arteries[64]. Only very rarely will a duct and collateral arteries supply the same lung, although these two sources of flow can supply separate lungs (Fig. 7.153). When a duct is present, and the pulmonary arteries are confluent, the arteries supply the entirety of the lung parenchyma (Fig. 7.152), although they may be variably developed. The degree of hypoplasia determines whether total correction is feasible.

When the right and left pulmonary arteries are not confluent, or when major aortopulmonary collateral arteries are present, the situation is more complex. Non-confluent pulmonary arteries can be supplied independently by bilateral ducts, or one lung can be supplied by a duct and the other through collateral arteries (Fig. 7.153). It is more usual for collateral arteries to supply both lungs with no duct being present.

Well-developed confluent pulmonary arteries usually coexist within the pericardial sac even when there are collateral arteries (Fig. 7.154). It is important to establish how much of the pulmonary parenchyma is connected to the intrapericardial pulmonary arteries, and how much is supplied directly by collateral arteries. It is known that collateral arteries can anastomose with the pulmonary arteries at the hilum, or extend into the parenchyma to supply lobar or segmental arteries directly. Intersegmental anastomoses also occur. The object of preoperative evaluation, therefore, should be to establish precisely how much of each lung is supplied by the intrapericardial pulmonary arteries[64], since this is the ultimate determinant of the success of any

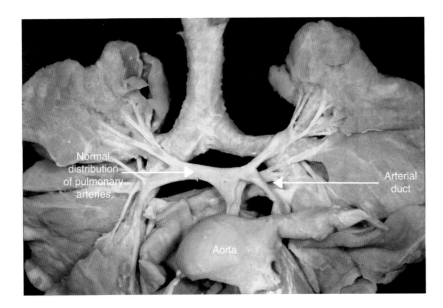

Fig. 7.152 As shown by this dissection, the pulmonary arteries in the heart shown in Fig. 7.151 have a normal segmental distribution.

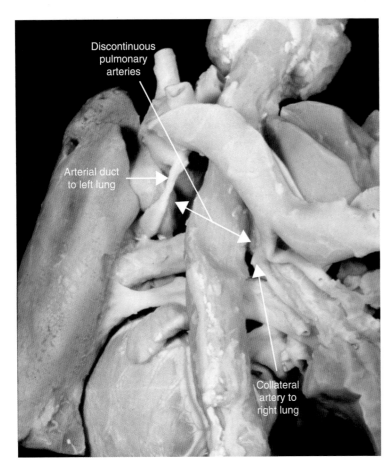

Fig. 7.153 In this specimen of tetralogy with pulmonary atresia, viewed from behind, the pulmonary arteries are discontinuous, the left being supplied through a ligamentous arterial duct, and the right lung through systemic-to-pulmonary collateral arteries.

attempted total correction. Cases can be found with supply exclusively from collateral arteries. In this setting, the arterial trunk is best described as a solitary structure (see below).

In contrast to tetralogy with pulmonary atresia, where initial survival is good, and the results of surgery are continually improving, pulmonary atresia with intact septum has a grave prognosis. The results of attempted corrective surgery are still disappointingly poor. The anatomy of the lesion itself accounts for the dismal outcome[65–67]. The atresia can be due either to an imperforate pulmonary valvar membrane (Fig. 7.155), or to muscular infundibular atresia. In the latter situation, the pulmonary trunk is blind-ending with no vestiges of leaflets of the pulmonary valve (Fig. 7.156). The cavities of the outlet and trabecular components

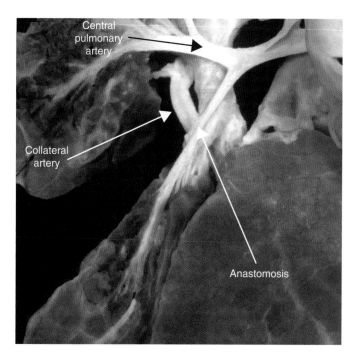

Fig. 7.154 This dissection of a heart with tetralogy and pulmonary atresia, shown in anatomical orientation, illustrates how true intrapericardial pulmonary arteries usually co-exist with systemic-to-pulmonary collateral arteries, a systemic-to-pulmonary collateral artery anastomosing with well-formed intrapericardial pulmonary arteries to supply the right lung.

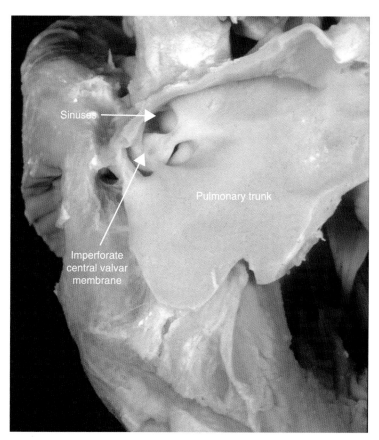

Fig. 7.155 This dissection of the ventriculopulmonary junction in a specimen with pulmonary atresia and intact ventricular septum, viewed from above, shows an imperforate pulmonary valvar membrane.

parts of the right ventricle are more-or-less completely obliterated by gross hypertrophy of the ventricular wall. In consequence, the cavity is effectively represented only by the hypoplastic inlet portion (Fig. 7.157). This cavity is unlikely ever to perform a useful function, particularly when fistulous communications extend to the coronary arteries. The right ventricle should probably be disregarded when deciding surgical treatment. When there is a pulmonary valve present, but its leaflets are imperforate, a spectrum is seen in terms of the size of the right ventricular cavity[68]. In some hearts, hypertrophy of the right ventricular myocardium obliterates the apical trabecular part of

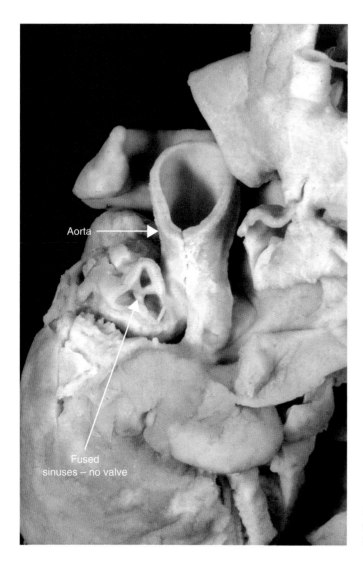

Aorta

Fused
sinuses – no valve

Fig. 7.156 In this specimen with pulmonary atresia and intact ventricular septum, there is no evidence of valvar tissue in the blind-ending pulmonary root (compare with Fig. 7.156).

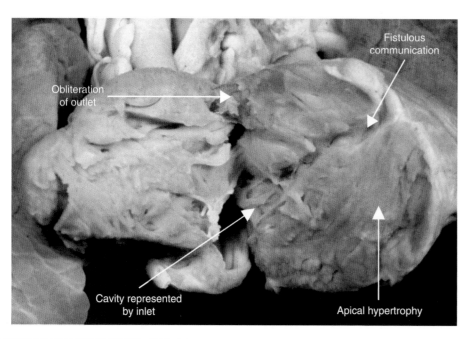

Fistulous
communication

Obliteration
of outlet

Cavity represented
by inlet

Apical hypertrophy

Fig. 7.157 In this specimen with pulmonary atresia and intact ventricular septum, viewed anatomically, the cavity of the right ventricle is represented by virtually the inlet component alone, due to gross hypertrophy of the walls of the apical trabecular and outlet components. Note the fistulous communication extending through the wall to the anterior interventricular coronary artery.

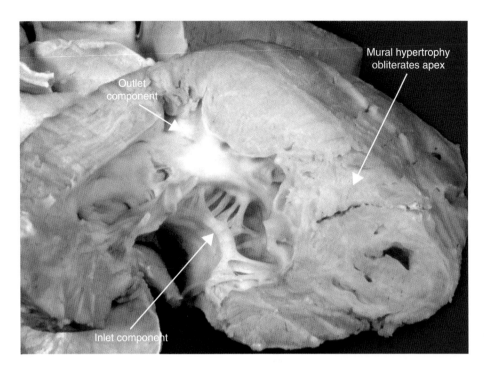

Fig. 7.158 In this heart, the mural hypertrophy has virtually obliterated the apical trabecular component of the cavity, while leaving narrowed inlet and outlet components.

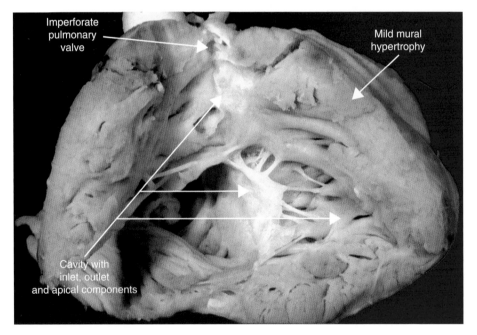

Fig. 7.159 In contrast, in this specimen with the most favourable variant of pulmonary atresia with an intact ventricular septum, the valve is imperforate but the mural hypertrophy has barely obliterated any of the cavity.

the cavity (Fig. 7.158). It is questionable if these ventricles will ever grow and become useful, although attempts have been made to resect apical trabeculations and "rehabilitate" the ventricle[69]. In the most favourable situation, the cavity is less hypoplastic and has well-developed inlet, apical, and outlet components (Fig. 7.159). These cases are those which are most amenable to total operative correction, although increasingly they are treated by the interventional

cardiologist, who will perforate the valvar membrane before dilating it with balloons.

Whatever the intracardiac anatomy, it is rare that one finds the thread-like pulmonary arteries seen so frequently with tetralogy and pulmonary atresia. Furthermore, the flow of pulmonary blood is almost always duct-dependent. With prostaglandins now available to improve ductal flow, the pulmonary arteries are almost always of sufficient

size to permit construction of a systemic-pulmonary shunt. Other options, such as the need for pulmonary valvotomy, should be decided after assessment of the precise anatomy of the individual case.

Pulmonary valvar insufficiency may be congenital or acquired, the latter usually secondary to surgical intervention or pulmonary hypertension. Congenital pulmonary valvar insufficiency may be associated with marked deformity of the

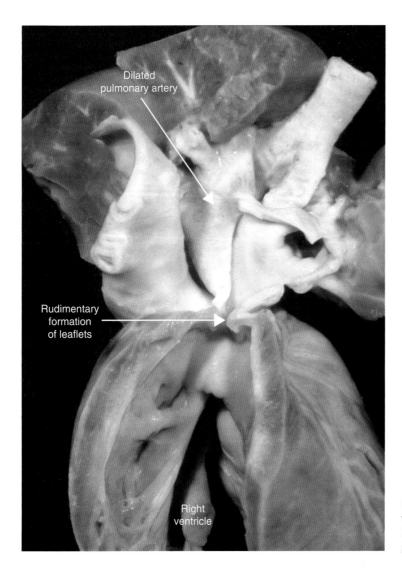

Dilated
pulmonary artery

Rudimentary
formation
of leaflets

Right
ventricle

Fig. 7.160 In this specimen, seen in anatomical orientation, with tetralogy of Fallot and rudimentary formation of the leaflets of the pulmonary valve, there is gross dilation of the pulmonary trunk and arteries.

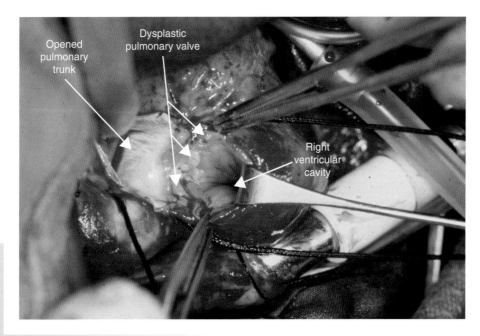

Opened
pulmonary
trunk

Dysplastic
pulmonary valve

Right
ventricular
cavity

Fig. 7.161 This operative view shows the right ventriculo-pulmonary arterial junction with the markedly malformed pulmonary valvar tissue in a patient with tetralogy of Fallot.

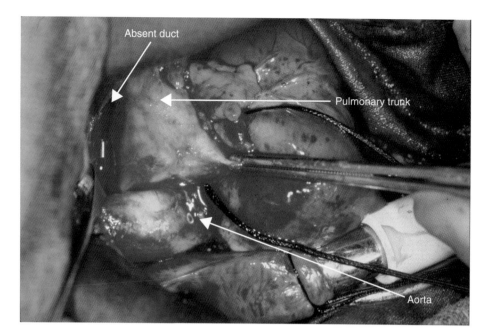

Absent duct

Pulmonary trunk

Aorta

Fig. 7.162 This operative view shows the grossly enlarged pulmonary trunk of the patient illustrated in Fig. 7.161. Note the absence of an arterial duct or ligament.

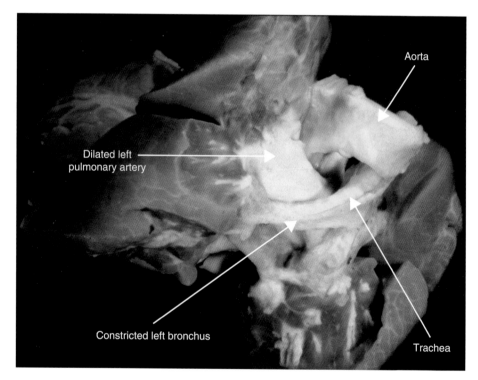

Aorta

Dilated left pulmonary artery

Constricted left bronchus

Trachea

Fig. 7.163 This view of the hilum of the left lung of the patient seen in Fig. 7.160, viewed from behind, shows the obstruction produced by the gross dilation of the left pulmonary artery as it crosses the bronchus.

valvar tissue, as in valvar dysplasia, or with absence of the valvar tissue altogether. Rudimentary leaflets may be seen with an intact ventricular septum[70,71], or in combination with a ventricular septal defect (Fig. 7.160). Absence of the leaflets of the pulmonary valve is also found in combination with tetralogy of Fallot[72] (Fig. 7.161).

While gross pulmonary valvar insufficiency may be relatively well-tolerated by the right heart, it can result in marked enlargement of the pulmonary trunk and arteries, and is usually associated with absence of the arterial duct[71] (Fig. 7.162). Indeed, compromise of the tracheobronchial tree by these grossly enlarged vessels (Figs. 7.163,

7.164) results in most patients presenting with symptoms of respiratory distress. Because only a limited number of cases have come to surgical correction, the efficacy of replacement of the valve with or without arterial plication has not been proved. Fortunately, so-called absence of the pulmonary valvar leaflets is a rare condition.

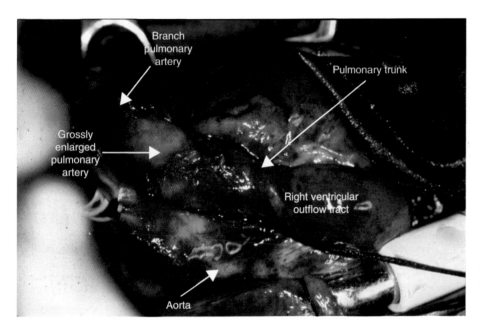

Branch pulmonary artery
Pulmonary trunk
Grossly enlarged pulmonary artery
Right ventricular outflow tract
Aorta

Fig. 7.164 This operative view of the patient shown in Fig. 7.161 shows the grossly enlarged left pulmonary artery. On bypass, the left pulmonary artery is seen to be as large as the aorta.

References

1. Ettedgui JA, Siewers RD, Anderson RH, Zuberbuhler JR. Diagnostic echocardiographic features of the sinus venous defect. *Br Heart J* 1990; **64**: 329–331.

2. Al Zaghal AM, Li J, Anderson RH, Lincoln C, Shore DF, Rigby ML. Anatomic criteria for the diagnosis of sinus venosus defects. *Heart* 1997; **78**: 298–304.

3. Knauth A, McCarthy KP, Webb S, Ho SY, Allwork SP, Cook AC, Anderson RH. Interatrial communication through the mouth of the coronary sinus defect. *Cardiol Young* 2002; **12**: 364–372.

4. Becker AE, Anderson RH: Atrioventricular septal defects. What's in a name? *J Thorac Cardiovasc Surg* 1982; **83**: 461–469.

5. Anderson RH, Ho SY, Falcao S, Daliento L, Rigby ML. The diagnostic features of atrioventricular septal defect with common atrioventricular junction. *Cardiol Young* 1998; **8**: 33–49.

6. Gerbode F, Hultgren H, Melrose D, Osborn J. Syndrome of left ventricular-right atrial shunt, successful surgical repair of defect in five cases with observation of bradycardia on closure. *Ann Surg* 1958; **148**: 433–446.

7. McKay R, Battistessa SA, Wilkinson JL, Wright JP. A communication from the left ventricle to the right atrium: a defect in the central fibrous body. *Int J Cardiol* 1989; **23**: 117–123.

8. Thiene G, Wenink ACG, Frescura C, Wilkinson JL, Gallucci V, Ho SY, Mazzucco A, Anderson RH. The surgical anatomy of the conduction tissues in atrioventricular defects. *J Thorac Cardiovasc Surg* 1981; **82**: 928–937.

9. Wilcox BR, Anderson RH, Henry GW, Mattos SS. Unusual opening of coronary sinus in atrioventricular septal defects. *Ann Thorac Surg* 1990; **50**: 767–770.

10. Penkoske PA, Neches WH, Anderson RH, Zuberbuhler JR. Further observations on the morphology of atrioventricular septal defects. *J Thorac Cardiovasc Surg* 1985; **90**: 611–622.

11. Rastelli GC, Kirklin JW, Titus JL:. Anatomic observations on complete form of persistent common atrioventricular canal with special reference to atrioventricular valves. *Proc Staff Meet Mayo Clin* 1966; **41**: 296–308.

12. Piccoli GP, Wilkinson JL, Macartney FJ, Gerlis LM, Anderson RH. Morphology and classification of complete atrioventricular defects. *Br Heart J* 1979; **42**: 633–639.

13. Sigfússon G, Ettedgui JA, Silverman NH, Anderson RH. Is a cleft in the anterior leaflet of an otherwise normal mitral valve an atrioventricular canal malformation? *J Am Coll Cardiol* 1995; **26**: 508–515.

14. Wilcox BR, Jones DR, Frantz EG, Brink LW, Henry GW, Mill MR, Anderson RH. An anatomically sound, simplified approach to repair of "complete" atrioventricular septal defect. *Ann Thorac Surg* 1997; **64**: 487–494.

15. Nicholson IA, Nunn GR, Sholler GF, Hawker RE, Cooper SG, Lau RM, Cohn SL. Simplified single patch technique for the repair of atrioventricular septal defect. *J Thorac Cardiovasc Surg* 1999; **118**: 642–646.

16. Ebels T, Anderson RH, Devine WA, Debich DE, Penkoske PA, Zuberbuhler JR. Anomalies of the left atrioventricular valve and related ventricular septal morphology in atrioventricular septal defects. *J Thorac Cardiovasc Surg* 1990; **99**: 299–307.

17. Piccoli GP, Ho SY, Wilkinson JL, Macartney FJ, Gerlis LM, Anderson RH. Left sided obstructive lesions in atrioventricular septal defects. *J Thorac Cardiovasc Surg* 1982; **83**: 453–460.

18. Ebels T, Ho SY, Anderson RH, Meijboom EJ, Eigelaar A. The surgical anatomy of the left ventricular outflow tract in atrioventricular septal defect. *Ann Thorac Surg* 1986; **41**: 483–488.

19. Pillai R, Ho SY, Anderson RH, Shinebourne EA, Lincoln C. Malalignment of the interventricular septum with atrioventricular septal defect: its implications concerning conduction tissue disposition. *Thorac Cardiovasc Surgeon* 1984; **32**: 1–3.

20. Soto B, Becker AE, Moulaert AJ, Lie JT, Anderson RH. Classification of ventricular septal defects. *Br Heart J* 1980; **43**: 332–343.

21. Milo S, Ho SY, Wilkinson JL, Anderson RH. The surgical anatomy and atrioventricular conduction tissues of hearts with isolated ventricular septal defects. *J Thorac Cardiovasc Surg* 1980; **79**: 244–255.

22. Milo S, Ho SY, Macartney FJ, Wilkinson JL, Becker AE, Wenink ACG, Gittenberger-de Groot AC, Anderson RH. Straddling and overriding atrioventricular valves morphology and classification. *Am J Cardiol* 1979; **44**: 1122–1134.

23. Tsang VT, Hsai T-Y, Yates R, Anderson RH. Surgical repair of multiple defects within the apical part of the muscular ventricular septum. *Ann Thorac Surg* 2002; **73**: 58–62.

24. Pacifico AD, Soto B, Bargeron LMJ: Surgical treatment of straddling tricuspid valves. *Circulation* 1979; **60**: 655–664.

25. Chauvaud SM, Mihaileanu SA, Gaer JAR, Carpentier AC. Surgical treatment of Ebstein's malformation – the 'Hôpital Broussais' experience. *Cardiol Young* 1996; **6**: 4–11.

26. Leung MP, Baker EJ, Anderson RH, Zuberbuhler JR. Cineangiographic spectrum of Ebstein's malformation: its relevance to clinical presentation and outcome. *J Am Coll Cardiol* 1988; **11**: 154–161.

27. Schreiber C, Cook A, Ho SY, Augustin N, Anderson RH. Morphologic spectrum of Ebstein's malformation: revisitation relative to surgical repair. *J Thorac Cardiovasc Surg* 1999; **117**: 148–155.

28. Ruschhaupt DG, Bharati S, Lev M: Mitral valve malformation of Ebstein type in absence of corrected transposition. *Am J Cardiol* 1976; **38**: 109–112.

29. Leung M, Rigby ML, Anderson RH, Wyse RKH, Macartney FJ. Reversed off-setting of the septal attachments of the atrioventricular valves and Ebstein's malformation of the morphologically mitral valve. *Br Heart J* 1987; **57**: 184–187.

30. Becker AE, Becker MJ, Edwards JE. Pathologic spectrum of dysplasia of the tricuspid valve, features in common with Ebstein's malformation. *Arch Pathol* 1971; **91**: 167–178.

31. Oberhoffer R, Cook AC, Lang D, Sharland G, Allan LD, Fagg NLK, Anderson RH. Correlation between echocardiographic and morphological investigations of lesions of the tricuspid valve diagnosed during fetal life. *Br Heart J* 1992; **68**: 580–585.

32. Van der Bel-Kahn J, Duren DR, Becker AE. Isolated mitral valve prolapse: chordal architecture as an anatomic basis in older patients. *J Am Coll Cardiol* 1985; **5**: 1335–1340.

33. Layman TE, Edwards JE: Anomalous mitral arcade: A type of congenital mitral insufficiency. *Circulation* 1967; **35**: 389–395.

34. Rosenquist GC: Congenital mitral valve disease associated with coarctation of the aorta. A spectrum that includes parachute deformity of the mitral valve. *Circulation* 1974; **49**: 985–993.

35. Shone JD, Sellers RD, Anderson RC, Adams P, Lillehei CW, Edwards JE. The developmental complex of "parachute mitral valve", supravalvular ring of left atrium, subaortic stenosis, and coarctation of the aorta. *Am J Cardiol* 1963; **11**: 714–725.

36. Chauvaud S, Mihaileanu S, Gaer JAR, Carpentier A. Surgical treatment of congenital mitral valve stenosis. "The Hôpital Broussais" experience. *Cardiol Young* 1997; **7**: 15–21.

37. Milo S, Stark J, Macartney FJ, Anderson RH. Parachute deformity of the tricuspid valve (case report). *Thorax* 1979; **34**: 543–546.

38. Stamm C, Anderson RH, Ho SY. Clinical anatomy of the normal pulmonary root compared with that in isolated pulmonary valvular stenosis. *J Am Coll Cardiol* 1998; **31**: 1420–1425.

39. Angelini A, Ho SY, Anderson RH, Devine WA, Zuberbuhler JR, Becker AE, Davies MJ. The morphology of the normal aortic valve as compared with the aortic valve having two leaflets. *J Thorac Cardiovasc Surg* 1989; **98**: 362–367.

40. Vollebergh FEMG, Becker AE. Minor congenital variations in cusp size in tricuspid aortic valves. Possible link with isolated aortic stenosis. *Br Heart J* 1977; **39**: 1006–1011.

41. McKay R, Ross DN. Technique for the relief of discrete subaortic stenosis. *J Thorac Cardiovasc Surg* 1982; **84**: 917–920.

42. Moulaert AJ, Oppenheimer-Dekker A. Anterolateral muscle bundle of the left ventricle, bulboventricular flange and subaortic stenosis. *Am J Cardiol* 1976; **37**: 78–81.

43. Anderson RH, Lenox CC, Zuberbuhler JR. Morphology of ventricular septal defect associated with coarctation of the aorta. *Br Heart J* 1983; **50**: 176–181.

44. Morrow AG. Hypertrophic subaortic stenosis: operative methods utilised to relieve left ventricular outflow obstruction. *J Thorac Cardiovasc Surg* 1978; **76**: 423–430.

45. Stamm C, Li J, Ho SY, Redington AN, Anderson RH. The aortic root in supravalvar aortic stenosis: the potential surgical relevance of morphologic findings. *J Thorac Cardiovasc Surg* 1997; **114**: 16–24.

46. Doty DB, Polansky DB, Jenson CB. Supravalvular aortic stenosis. Repair by extended aortoplasty. *J Thorac Cardiovasc Surg* 1977; **74**: 362–371.

47. Frantz PJ, Murray GF, Wilcox BR. Surgical management of left ventricular-aortic discontinuity complicating bacterial endocarditis. *Ann Thorac Surg* 1980; **29**: 1–7.

48. Gilbert JW, Morrow AG, Talbert JW. The surgical significance of hypertrophic infundibular obstruction accompanying valvar pulmonary stenosis. *J Thorac Cardiovasc Surg* 1963; **46**: 457–467.

49. Haworth SG, Macartney FJ. Growth and development of pulmonary circulation in pulmonary atresia with ventricular septal defect and major aortopulmonary collateral arteries. *Br Heart J* 1980; **44**: 14–24.

50. Anderson RH, Tynan M. Tetralogy of Fallot – a centennial review. *Int J Cardiol* 1988; **21**: 219–232.

51. Anderson RH, Allwork SP, Ho SY, Lenox CC, Zuberbuhler JR. Surgical anatomy of tetralogy of Fallot. *J Thorac Cardiovasc Surg* 1981; **81**: 887–896.

52. Suzuki A, Ho SY, Anderson RH, Deanfield JE. Further morphologic studies on tetralogy of Fallot, with particular emphasis on the prevalence and structure of the membranous flap. *J Thorac Cardiovasc Surg* 1990; **99**: 528–535.

53. Titus JL, Daugherty GW, Edwards JE. Anatomy of the atrioventricular conduction system in ventricular septal defect. *Circulation* 1963; **28**: 72–81.

54. Anderson RH, Monro JL, Ho SY, Smith A, Deverall PB. Les voies de conduction auriculo-ventriculaires dans le tetralogie de Fallot. *Coeur* 1977; **8**: 793–807.

55. Ando M. Subpulmonary ventricular septal defect with pulmonary stenosis. Letter to Editor. *Circulation* 1974; **50**: 412.

56. Neirotti R, Galindez E, Kreutzer G, Coronel AR, Pedrini M, Becu L. Tetralogy of Fallot with sub-pulmonary ventricular septal defect. *Ann Thorac Surg* 1978; **25**: 51–56.

57. Blackstone EH, Kirklin JW, Bertranou EG, Labrosse CJ, Soto B, Bargeron LMJr. Preoperative prediction from cineangiograms of post-repair right ventricular pressure in tetralogy of Fallot. *J Thorac Cardiovasc Surg* 1979; **78**: 542–552.

58. Kirklin JW, Blackstone EH, Pacifico AD, Brown RN, Bargeron LMJr. Routine primary repair versus two-stage repair of tetralogy of Fallot. *Circulation* 1979; **60**: 373–385.

59. McFadden PM, Culpepper WS, Ochsner J. Iatrogenic right ventricular failure in tetralogy of Fallot repairs: reappraisal of a distressing problem. *Ann Thorac Surg* 1982; **33**: 400–402.

60. Alva C, Ho SY, Lincoln CR, Rigby ML, Wright A, Anderson RH. The nature of the obstructive muscular bundles in double-chambered right ventricle. *J Thorac Cardiovasc Surg* 1999; **117**: 1180–1189.

61. Alfieri OA, Blackstone EH, Kirklin JW, Pacifico AD, Brown RN, Bargeron LMJr. Surgical treatment of tetralogy of Fallot with pulmonary atresia. *J Thorac Cardiovasc Surg* 1978; **76**: 321–335.

62. Macartney FJ, Scott O, Deverall PB. Haemodynamic and anatomical characteristics of pulmonary blood supply in pulmonary atresia with ventricular septal defect – including a case of persistent fifth aortic arch. *Br Heart J* 1974; **36**: 1049–1060.

63. Pahl E, Fong L, Anderson RH, Park SC, Zuberbuhler. Fistulous communications between a solitary coronary artery and the pulmonary arteries as the primary source of pulmonary blood supply in tetralogy of Fallot with pulmonary valve atresia. *Am J Cardiol* 1989; **63**: 140–143.

64. Rossi RN, Hislop A, Anderson RH, Maymone Martins F, Cook AC. Systemic-to-pulmonary blood supply in tetralogy of Fallot with pulmonary atresia. *Cardiol Young* 2002; **12**: 373–388.

65. Freedom RM, Dische MR, Rowe RD. The tricuspid valve in pulmonary atresia with intact ventricular septum. A morphological study of 60 cases. *Arch Pathol Lab Med* 1978; **102**: 28–31.

66. Zuberbuhler JR, Anderson RH. Morphological variations in pulmonary atresia with intact ventricular septum. *Br Heart J* 1979; **41**: 281–288.

67. Anderson RH, Anderson C, Zuberbuhler JR. Further morphologic studies on hearts with pulmonary atresia and intact ventricular septum. *Cardiol Young* 1991; **1**: 105–114.

68. Bull C, de Leval MR, Mercanti C, Macartney FJ, Anderson RH. Pulmonary atresia with intact ventricular septum: a revised classification. *Circulation* 1982; **66**: 266–271.

69. Pawade A, Capuani A, Penny DJ, Karl TR, Mee RB. Pulmonary atresia with intact ventricular septum: surgical management based on right ventricular infundibulum. *J Card Surg* 1993; **8**: 371–383.

70. Smith RD, DuShane JW, Edwards JE. Congenital insufficiency of the pulmonary valve: including a case of fetal cardiac failure. *Circulation* 1959; **20**: 554–560.

71. Macartney FJ, Miller GAH. Congenital absence of the pulmonary valve. *Br Heart J* 1970; **32**: 483–490.

72. Emmanouilides GC, Thanopoulos B, Siassi B, Fishbein M. Agenesis of ductus arteriosus associated with the syndrome of tetralogy of Fallot and absent pulmonary valve. *Am J Cardiol* 1976; **37**: 403–409.

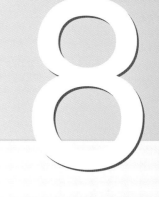

Lesions in hearts with abnormal segmental connections

In the previous chapter, we paid attention to those hearts in which the associated cardiac malformation existed in the setting of normal connections between the cardiac segments. All those associated lesions, of course, can also be found in hearts with abnormal segmental connections. It is these abnormal connections which will be our focus in this chapter. We will also emphasise those associated anomalies that are particularly frequent with a given abnormal segmental arrangement.

DOUBLE INLET VENTRICLE

Over the years, hearts with double inlet ventricle have represented one of the greater challenges to surgical correction. They have also posed significant problems in adequate description and categorisation. Thus, even now, the lesions are often described in terms of 'single ventricles' or 'univentricular hearts'. This

is despite the fact that almost all hearts with double inlet atrioventricular connection have two chambers within the ventricular mass, one being large and the other small[1-3]. We will describe here the relevant anatomic characteristics of all those hearts unified by the presence of the double inlet connection, irrespective of whether or not they have one or two ventricles. In the past, we became involved with ongoing debates as to whether both chambers found within the ventricular mass deserved ventricular status[4,5]. Such semantic arguments regarding the standing of a ventricular chamber may have tended to obscure many of their important morphological features. Suffice it to say that we no longer seek to deny any chamber its ventricular recognition as long as it possesses a characteristic and recognisable apical component. The significant point is that the combination of one big and one small ventricle produces a functionally univentricular arrangement

whenever the small chamber is incapable of pumping in isolation to the pulmonary or systemic circuits. Thus, many other lesions, in addition to double inlet ventricle, fall into the group of those producing functionally univentricular hearts.

Concentrating first on double inlet atrioventricular connection, this arrangement exists whenever the greater part of both atrioventricular junctions, those of the right-sided and left-sided atrial chambers, are connected to the same ventricle. The connections thus formed are usually guarded by two separate atrioventricular valves, one for each atrium (Fig. 8.1). Double inlet also exists when the two atrial chambers are connected to the same ventricle through a common valve (Fig. 8.2). Double inlet can also be found in the presence of overriding and straddling atrioventricular valves, but only when the degree of overriding is such as to leave the greater part of both junctions

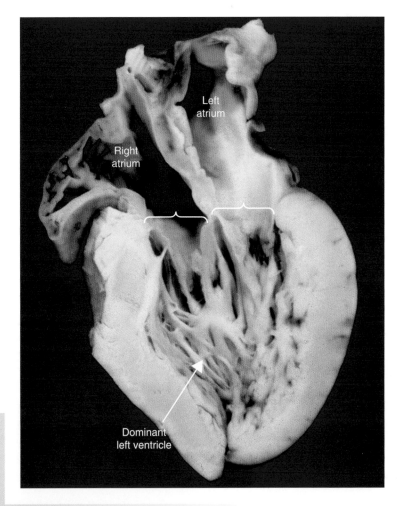

Left atrium

Right atrium

Dominant left ventricle

Fig. 8.1 This specimen, prepared by slicing the heart in "four-chamber" projection, shows the essence of the double inlet atrioventricular connection. Note that the cavity of only one ventricle is visible. There is a second ventricle, albeit incomplete and rudimentary, but it is positioned anterosuperiorly, and so is not sectioned in this cut.

connected to the same ventricle, either through two valves (Fig. 8.3) or a common valve. It is these atrioventricular connections that determine the surgical options since, whenever hearts are found with double inlet connection as thus defined, the heart itself must perforce be functionally univentricular. Only very rarely will there be a solitary ventricle present. More frequently, in those hearts with two ventricles, one of them must be incomplete and rudimentary, lacking at least its inlet component.

Although the surgical options are the same for all patients with double inlet atrioventricular connection, the hearts themselves can show marked anatomic variation. They can exist with any arrangement of the atrial chambers, with one of three ventricular morphologies, with the variations in valvar morphology discussed above, with any ventriculo–

arterial connection, and with varied associated malformations[6]. From the surgical viewpoint, the most important differentiating feature is the morphology of the dominant ventricle in the ventricular mass. Three subsets can be distinguished. The first includes all those with the atrial chambers connected to a dominant left ventricle in the presence of a rudimentary and incomplete right ventricle. The second group comprises those with a dominant right and an incomplete and rudimentary left ventricle. The final small set is made up of those with a solitary ventricle of indeterminate morphology. These three variants must then be distinguished from other hearts that, in essence, have huge ventricular septal defects.

An obvious way of correcting surgically these hearts with double inlet is to septate the dominant or solitary ventricle[7]. The

overall morphologic arrangement, however, usually conspires to defeat this option. The most frequent surgical tactic, therefore, is to use the Fontan procedure or one of its modifications[8-10]. In this section, we will concentrate on those features influencing the Fontan procedure, although we will discuss those morphologies that lend themselves to, or compromise, septation.

The most frequent variant of double inlet ventricle is seen when both atrioventricular junctions are connected to a dominant left ventricle (Fig. 8.4). Often termed 'single ventricle with outlet chamber', the outlet chamber is, in reality, an incomplete and rudimentary right ventricle. It lacks its inlet component, either completely when the atrial chambers are exclusively connected to the dominant left ventricle, or for the greater part when there is overriding of

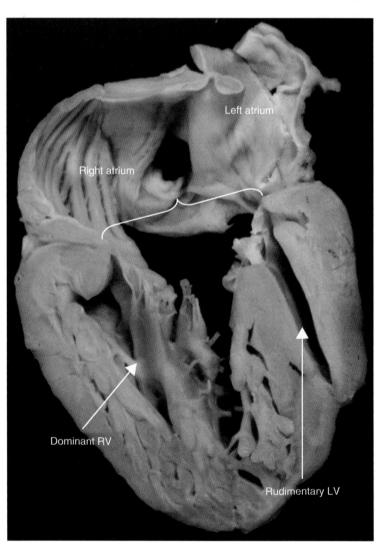

Fig. 8.2 This specimen is also prepared by making a section in "four chamber" plane. It shows double inlet to a dominant right ventricle (RV) through a common atrioventricular valve (bracket). In this example, however, because the incomplete and rudimentary left ventricle (LV) is positioned posteroinferiorly, it is included within the cut. Compare with Fig. 8.1.

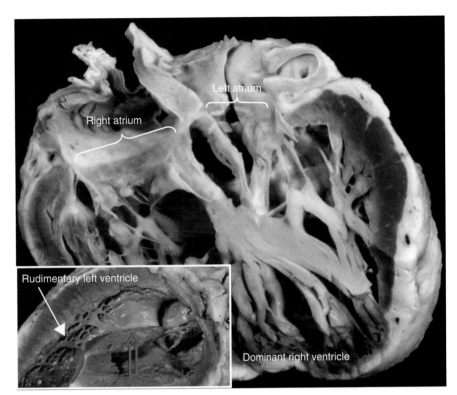

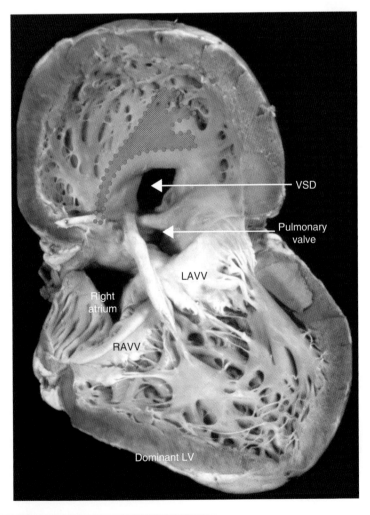

Fig. 8.3 This specimen, windowed and viewed in anatomic orientation, also has double inlet to a dominant right ventricle, but through two separate atrioventricular valves. The inset, photographed from behind, shows that one papillary muscle of the left atrioventricular valve (arrowed) retains its position within the incomplete and rudimentary left ventricle.

Fig. 8.4 This heart is an example of the commonest form of double inlet left ventricle. The dominant left ventricle (LV) has been opened in clam-like fashion, and the specimen is shown in anatomic orientation. The abnormal course of the conduction axis has been superimposed on the picture as the green cross-hatched area. LAVV – left atrioventricular valve. VSD – ventricular septal defect. RAVV – right atrioventricular valve.

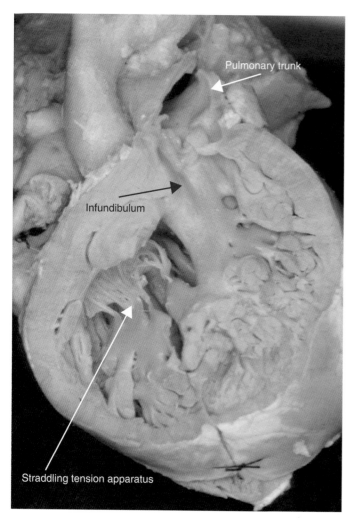

Fig. 8.5 In this specimen with double inlet left ventricle, the rudimentary right ventricle is photographed from the front with the heart positioned anatomically. The ventriculo-arterial connections are concordant, with the pulmonary trunk seen supported by an infundibulum and arising from the right ventricle. The right atrioventricular valve straddles and overrides, but its greater part remains connected within the dominant left ventricle, so the connection remains one of double inlet.

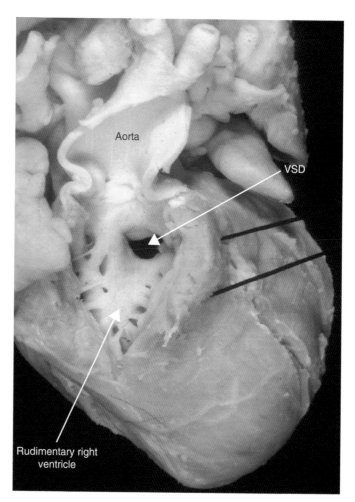

Fig. 8.6 In this specimen with double inlet left ventricle and discordant ventriculo-arterial connections, viewed anatomically, the rudimentary right ventricle, supporting the aorta, is right-sided. VSD – ventricular septal defect.

one (Fig. 8.5), or rarely both, atrioventricular junctions. The relationship of the incomplete ventricle can vary, in that it may be to the right (Fig. 8.6) or left (Fig. 8.7) of the dominant ventricle. Always, however, it is located in an anterosuperior position. The morphology of the incomplete ventricle is markedly different when it supports the pulmonary trunk (Figs. 8.5, 8.8) as opposed to the aorta (Figs. 8.6, 8.7). It is these differences which, in the past, served as the focus of whether or not the incomplete chamber should be accorded ventricular status. Irrespective of the semantic arguments, the salient anatomic point is that, in all instances, the chambers possess an apical component of morphologically right ventricular pattern. They are separated from the dominant ventricle by an apical muscular septum (Fig. 8.9) which carries the conduction system, and which is nourished by septal perforating arteries[11].

It is the precise ventriculo-arterial connections which dictate the surgical options. Usually, the ventriculo-arterial connections are discordant (Figs. 8.6, 8.7), the aorta arising from the rudimentary and incomplete right ventricle, and the pulmonary trunk connected to the dominant ventricle. The crucial feature is then the dimensions of the ventricular septal defect, since this must be of adequate size to support the systemic circulation irrespective of the surgical tactics to be adopted. Often it is restrictive, and may then need to be surgically enlarged or by-passed. The major anatomic feature of concern is the course of the axis of atrioventricular conduction tissue[12]. Although originating from an anomalously located atrioventricular node (see below), when viewed from the rudimentary right

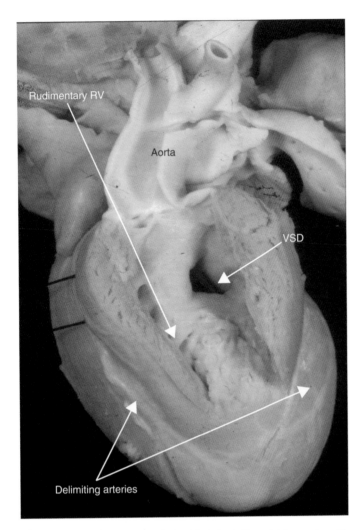

Fig. 8.7 In this specimen with double inlet left ventricle, again with discordant ventriculo-arterial connections, and viewed anatomically, the rudimentary right ventricle, supporting the aorta, is left-sided. VSD – ventricular septal defect.

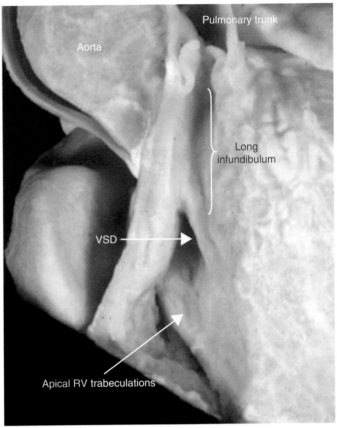

Fig. 8.8 In this specimen, again with double inlet left ventricle, but now with concordant ventriculo-arterial connections, as with the heart shown in Fig. 8.5, the right-sided rudimentary right ventricle supports the pulmonary trunk, with the aorta arising from the dominant left ventricle. This is the so-called "Holmes Heart". Note the length of the infundibulum of the rudimentary ventricle (RV) when it supports the pulmonary trunk, compared to those supporting the aorta (Figs. 8.6, 8.7). VSD – ventricular septal defect.

ventricle, irrespective of the location of the rudimentary right ventricle, the axis is always seen posteroinferior to the defect, being carried on the left ventricular aspect of the septal crest (Fig. 8.4). When the ventriculo-arterial connections are discordant, the rudimentary ventricle usually has a very short outlet portion, and a more extensive apical trabecular component (Figs. 8.6, 8.7). The safest way to enlarge the defect surgically, therefore, is to remove a wedge of the muscular septum closest to the obtuse margin of the heart, the latter being marked by the left-sided delimiting coronary artery[12] (Fig. 8.10).

Less frequently in hearts with double inlet left ventricle, the ventriculo-arterial connections may be concordant, or there

can be double outlet from the dominant or rudimentary ventricle. The variant with concordant connections is of most interest. Often described as the 'Holmes Heart'[13], the rudimentary right ventricle in this setting is markedly different from the variant with discordant ventriculo-arterial connections. The outlet component is much longer when the pulmonary trunk arises from the incomplete right ventricle, and the chamber is virtually indistinguishable from the rudimentary right ventricle seen in hearts with tricuspid atresia (compare Figs. 8.8 & 8.11). The ventricular septal defect is typically restrictive in this form of double inlet left ventricle, and the same rules pertain should it require surgical enlargement. This is unlikely to be

performed, however, unless a septation is also attempted. The more likely approach will be to perform a Fontan procedure. The rudimentary right ventricle will then be excluded from the circulation.

Taken overall, the Fontan procedure, or one of its modifications, will be the likely operation of choice for most patients with double inlet left ventricle. It can successfully be used for all the various anatomic variants whenever the haemodynamic criterions are satisfactory[14]. Almost always, the procedure includes connecting the right atrium directly, in one way or another, to the pulmonary arteries. This is now usually achieved either by creating a conduit within the right atrium to produce a so-called total cavopulmonary

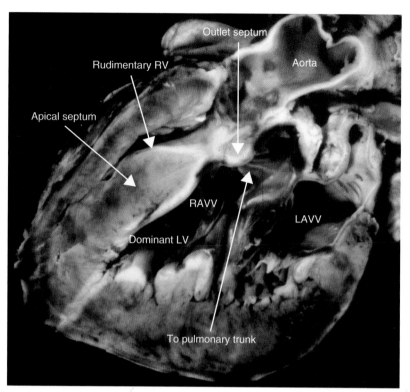

Fig. 8.9 This specimen with double inlet left ventricle and discordant ventriculo-arterial connections has been sectioned to replicate the parasternal long axis view, and is photographed in anatomical orientation. Note that the apical ventricular septum is positioned between the apical components of the dominant left (LV) and rudimentary right (RV) ventricles. This septum is the remnant of the true ventricular septum, since it carries the conduction axis, and is nourished by the septal perforating arteries. RAVV, LAVV – right and left atrioventricular valves.

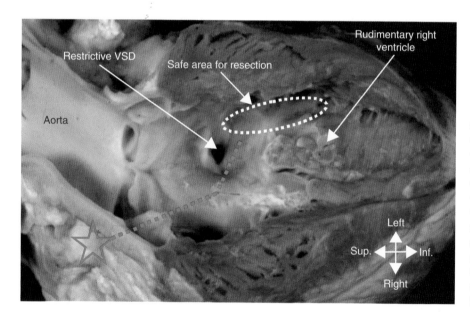

Fig. 8.10 This specimen, photographed in surgical orientation, shows the relationship of the axis of atrioventricular conduction tissue to the ventricular septal defect in double inlet left ventricle with discordant ventriculo-arterial connections when viewed from the rudimentary and incomplete right ventricle. The ventricular septal defect (VSD) is restrictive. The course of the conduction axis is superimposed in green, with the site of the anomalous atrioventricular node shown by the star, whilst the white dotted oval shows the area that can be removed without inflicting trauma to the conduction tissues.

connection[15], or else inserting an extra-conduit to connect directly the inferior caval vein to the pulmonary arteries, combining this with a Glenn procedure[16]. In the past, it was usual to anastomose directly the roof of the atrium at its junction with the appendage to the pulmonary trunk. Such an atriopulmonary connection remains an option. With juxtaposition of the atrial appendages, a not infrequent associated

malformation with double inlet left ventricle, this anastomosis becomes even simpler. If the atrium is to be connected to the pulmonary arteries, either directly or by construction of an internal conduit, the important structures to be avoided are the sinus node and its arterial supply. In this respect, the crucial area is the interatrial groove, through which courses the artery to the sinus node irrespective of its arterial origin (Fig. 8.12). Use of an internal or

external conduit obviously obviates the need to isolate surgically the systemic venous return from the right atrioventricular valve, an added manoeuvre that is essential if attempting an atriopulmonary connection. If this has to be done, there are at least two options open to the surgeon. It can be done by securing a patch across the vestibule of the valve. It can also be achieved by deviating the atrial septum to the parietal border of

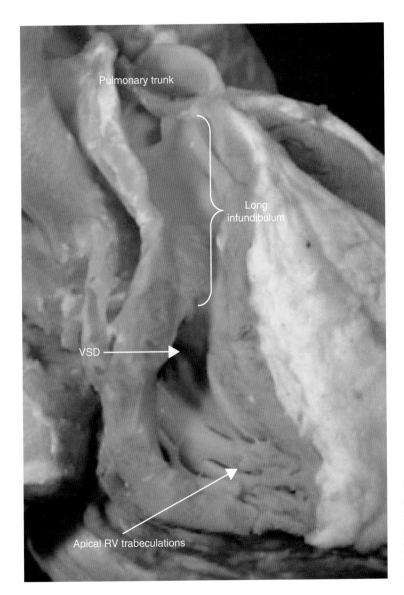

Fig. 8.11 This specimen has classical tricuspid atresia with concordant ventriculo-arterial connections, and is photographed in anatomic orientation. Note the similarity in morphology between the rudimentary right ventricle (RV) in this setting, with its long infundibulum, and that seen in the "Holmes heart" (compare with Fig. 8.8). VSD – ventricular septal defect.

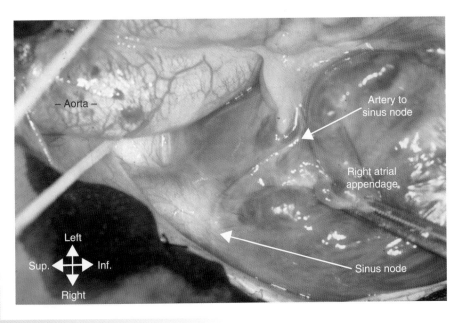

Fig. 8.12 In this heart, photographed in the operating room, the artery to the sinus node, arising from the right coronary artery, is seen coursing through the interatrial groove to cross the cavoatrial junction at the crest of the right atrial appendage. The sinus node is visible as a pale area within the terminal groove.

the right atrium, thus leaving both valves draining to the dominant ventricle. With both of these options, it is important to avoid the atrioventricular node. One distinguishing feature of hearts with double inlet left ventricle is that the node giving rise to the axis of atrioventricular conduction tissue is not located within the apex of the triangle of Koch[17]. This is because the muscular ventricular septum, carrying the ventricular conduction tissues, does not reach to the crux of the heart. Instead, it rises to the acute margin of the ventricular mass (Fig. 8.4). The atrioventricular node, therefore, is located within the quadrant of the junction related to the mouth of the right atrial appendage (Fig. 8.13). This area is the major site of danger but, irrespective of its precise location, the node can be avoided by securing the patch at least one centimetre above the attachments of the leaflets of the right atrioventricular valve (Fig. 8.13).

As we have discussed, it is now more frequent to insert an extracardiac conduit, or to construct a conduit within the right atrium, so as to direct the inferior caval venous blood to the lungs or to the superior caval vein. The superior caval vein itself is divided, and both ends are

anastomosed to the pulmonary arteries if there is an intracardiac tunnel. This produces the total cavopulmonary connection[16], said to have advantages in terms of the pattern of flow into the pulmonary arteries. When constructing an internal baffle, the major areas to be avoided are again the sinus node and its arterial supply. These problems are obviously avoided if the surgeon chooses to insert an extracardiac conduit.

As already mentioned, most centres throughout the world now favour the Fontan procedure or one of its modifications for surgical 'correction' of double inlet left ventricle. Some, nonetheless, continue to espouse septation as the most logical surgical option[7]. Only a few patients will have suitable anatomy for successful septation. Both atrioventricular valves must be competent structures, and the relationships of dominant and rudimentary ventricle must permit the construction of a patch to channel flow from the left atrioventricular valve to the ventricular septal defect. This means that the rudimentary right ventricle should be left-sided (Fig. 8.7) or, at worst, directly anterior. The dominant ventricle also needs to be of good size, which means that septation is unlikely to be attempted in

infancy. If the pulmonary circulation is not protected by naturally occurring stenosis, this must be achieved by banding the pulmonary trunk. Banding itself tends to promote hypertrophy of the ventricular myocardium, and narrowing of the ventricular septal defect. It may also be necessary, therefore, to combine enlargement of the defect (Fig. 8.10) with septation. The presence of naturally occurring subpulmonary stenosis may dictate the insertion of a conduit from the dominant ventricle to the pulmonary arteries. All these considerations suggest that relatively few patients will be suitable candidates for septation. In those that are, the overwhelming consideration during surgery will be to avoid the axis of atrioventricular conduction tissue, thus avoiding iatrogenic heart block. It is also necessary to preserve the sinus node and its arterial supply (Fig. 8.12).

As has already been discussed, the conduction axis in hearts with double inlet left ventricle takes its origin from an anomalous node located anterocephalad within the right atrioventricular junction, beneath the mouth of the appendage (Fig. 8.13). From this anterior node, the atrioventricular bundle penetrates through the lateral end of the area of fibrous

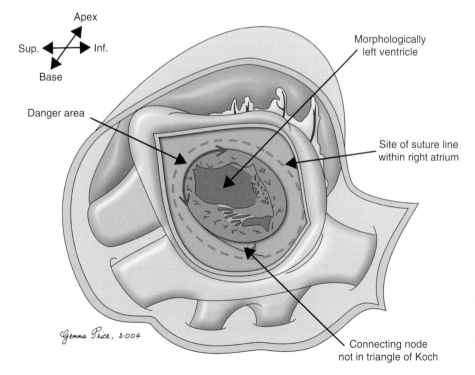

Apex

Sup. ◄──► Inf.

Base

Danger area

Morphologically left ventricle

Site of suture line within right atrium

Gemma Price, 2004

Connecting node not in triangle of Koch

Fig. 8.13 This cartoon, drawn in surgical orientation, shows the danger area of the right atrioventricular orifice (red double headed arrow) in hearts with double inlet left ventricle, and the way the conduction tissue can be avoided by suturing above the level of the atrioventricular junction (blue dotted line).

continuity between the leaflets of the pulmonary and the right atrioventricular valves. When the rudimentary right ventricle is left-sided, as it will be in most cases suitable for septation, the non-branching atrioventricular bundle then encircles the anterior quadrants of the pulmonary orifice to reach the rightward margin of the ventricular septum (Fig. 8.4). The left bundle branch then cascades down the left ventricular aspect of the septum, the axis of conduction tissue itself being located anterocephalad to the ventricular septal defect when viewed either through a fish-mouth incision in the dominant left ventricle (Fig. 8.14), or through the right atrioventricular valve (Fig. 8.15). Unless a conduit is also placed from the dominant left ventricle to the pulmonary arteries, the line of sutures used to septate the dominant ventricle must cross this course of the axis of conduction tissues (Fig. 8.14). The axis itself is relatively narrow as it emerges from the area of fibrous continuity between the pulmonary and right atrioventricular valves. If this site is known with precision, the sutures can be arranged to avoid the axis. All of these considerations, taken together, indicate

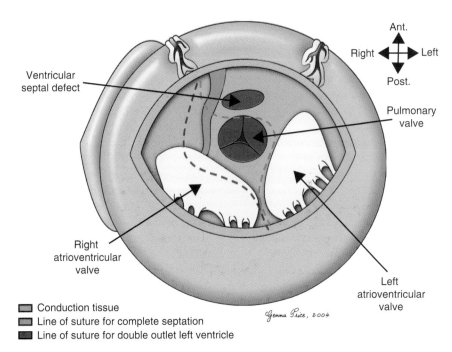

- ▢ Conduction tissue
- ▢ Line of suture for complete septation
- ▢ Line of suture for double outlet left ventricle

Gemma Price, 2004

Fig. 8.14 In this cartoon, the dominant left ventricle with double inlet is seen as through a fishmouth incision in the apex of the ventricle. The conduction axis is marked in green (see also Fig. 8.4). The potential line for complete septation, placing the pulmonary trunk in communication with the systemic venous return, (blue dotted line) crosses the conduction axis. To avoid the conduction axis (green dotted line), it is necessary to deviate the site of septation so that both outflow tracts remain in communication with the pulmonary venous return through the left atrioventricular valve.

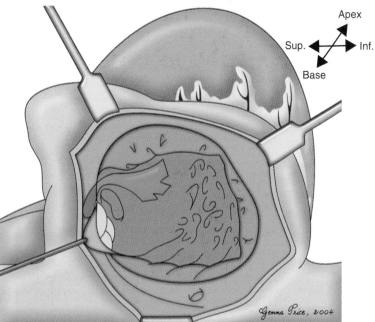

Gemma Price, 2004

Fig. 8.15 This cartoon, again drawn in surgical orientation, shows the view of the dominant left ventricle in the setting of double inlet left ventricle with discordant ventriculo-arterial connections, and the course of the conduction axis, in green, as it would be seen by the surgeon working through the right atrioventricular valve. The leaflets of the pulmonary valve are coloured yellow.

that septation is a formidable surgical procedure if the pathways through the dominant ventricle are to be separated without insertion of a conduit or involuntary induction of atrioventricular dissociation. Septation is also a potentially feasible option for patients with double inlet left ventricle and concordant ventriculo-arterial connections (the 'Holmes Heart'). If attempted, the same rules hold good for the disposition of the axis of conduction tissue.

Other variants of double inlet ventricle are much rarer, and hardly ever are suitable for septation. Double inlet right ventricle (Fig. 8.16) is seen most frequently with double outlet from the dominant right ventricle, often with straddling and overriding of the left atrioventricular valve[18] (Fig. 8.3). The rudimentary and incomplete left ventricle, usually found in left-sided position, although sometimes found to the right, is then nothing more than a pouch with left ventricular apical trabeculations (Fig. 8.17). The Fontan procedure is the most likely therapeutic surgical option, in which case the landmarks within the atrial chambers, together with the surgical caveats, are as discussed for double inlet left ventricle. Sometimes, double inlet right ventricle can be found with concordant ventriculo-arterial connections (Fig. 8.18), usually with a common valve guarding the atrioventricular junctions (Figs. 8.3, 8.19). The axis of atrioventricular conduction in this setting descends from a node located within its usual position in the triangle of Koch. The exception is when the rudimentary left ventricle is right-sided, the conduction axis then arising from an anomalous node[19], as in congenitally corrected transposition (see below).

Those rare hearts with double inlet to a solitary and indeterminate ventricle usually co-exist with isomerism of the atrial appendages, when the multiple associated malformations, particularly the anomalous venoatrial connections, dominate the picture. Rare examples can be found with usual arrangement of the atrial chambers. In this setting, the crossing of tension apparatus from the

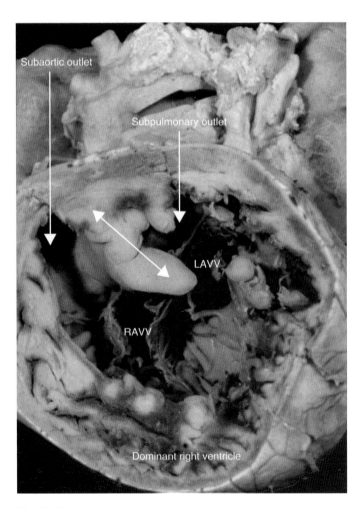

Fig. 8.16 This specimen with double inlet and double outlet right ventricle is photographed in anatomic orientation. Note that both atrioventricular valves are tethered within the dominant right ventricle, while the extensive outlet septum (white arrow) separates the origins of the two arterial trunks from the dominant right ventricle. RAVV, LAVV – right and left atrioventricular valves.

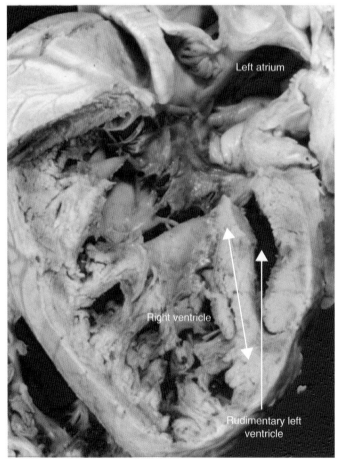

Fig. 8.17 This picture, again viewed in anatomic orientation, shows the location of the left-sided rudimentary and incomplete left ventricle in the heart shown in Fig. 8.16 with double inlet right ventricle. The rudimentary ventricle is no more than an outpouching from the dominant ventricle. The white double-headed arrow shows the apical ventricular septum between the dominant right and the rudimentary left ventricle.

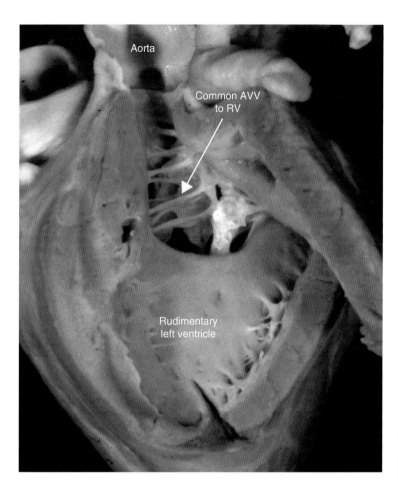

Fig. 8.18 In this picture, again in anatomic orientation, an example is seen of double inlet right ventricle in which the rudimentary left-sided left ventricle gives rise to the aorta. There is a common atrioventricular valve (AVV) joining both atriums to the dominant right ventricle (RV), shown in cross-section in Fig. 8.2.

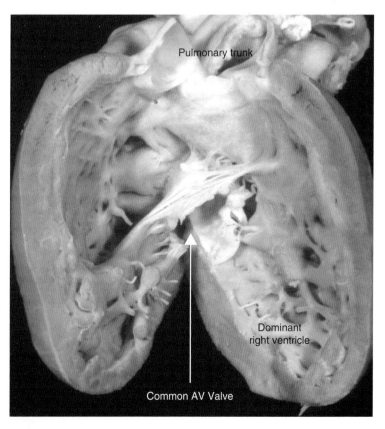

Fig. 8.19 This is another picture of the dominant right ventricle from the heart shown in Fig. 8.18. Both atriums drain to the dominant ventricle through the common atrioventricular (AV) valve. The ventriculo-arterial connections are concordant.

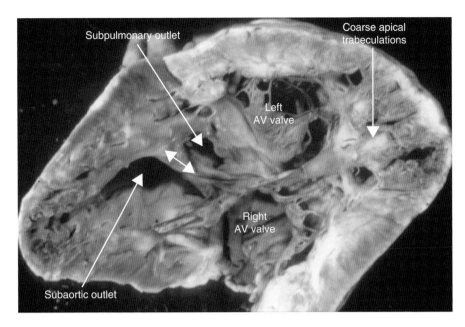

Fig. 8.20 This specimen, seen in anatomic orientation, with the ventricle opened in clam-like fashion, has double inlet to and double outlet from a solitary ventricle of indeterminate morphology, which has very coarse apical trabeculations. Note that the tension apparatus of both atrioventricular (AV) valves has a common origin, making septation exceedingly difficult, if not impossible.

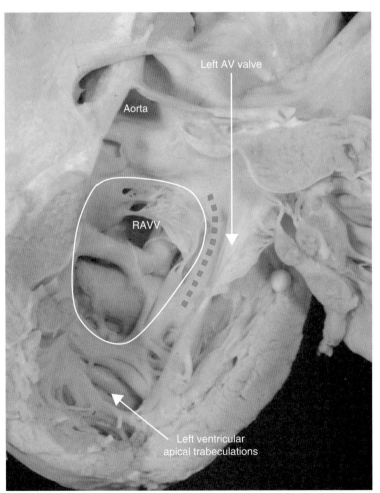

Fig. 8.21 This view, in anatomic orientation, shows the left ventricle in a heart with concordant atrioventricular connections and a huge ventricular septal defect. The site of the axis of atrioventricular conduction tissue has been marked in green dots on the left ventricular aspect of the septum. The white line shows the extent of the deficiency of the muscular septum. The right atrioventricular valve (RAVV) is connected within the right ventricle, hence the concordant nature of the atrioventricular connections.

atrioventricular valves, along with the particularly coarse indeterminate apical trabeculations, tend to conspire against septation (Fig. 8.20). Patients with solitary ventricles, therefore, are also most likely to undergo repair by means of the Fontan option, and the same rules apply as discussed above.

Hearts with huge ventricular septal defects (Fig. 8.21) can sometimes be confused with double inlet to a solitary and indeterminate ventricle. Even in those with huge septal defects, septation remains a formidable undertaking. In these rare patients, it is the persisting rim of muscular septum separating the apical trabecular components, together with the inlet septum rising to the crux, which provide the anatomic landmarks. The axis of conduction tissue descends from the regular atrioventricular node when the atrioventricular connections are concordant in this setting (Fig. 8.21).

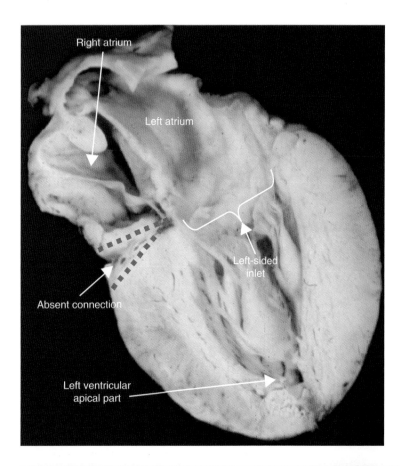

Fig. 8.22 This heart has been sectioned in "four chamber" echocardiographic equivalent, showing complete absence of the right atrioventricular connection (open red dotted triangle). This is the essence of "classical" tricuspid atresia. Note that the section passes only through the dominant left ventricle (compare with Fig. 8.1).

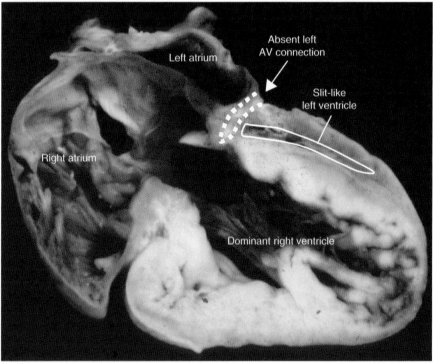

Fig. 8.23 This heart with classical mitral atresia comes from a patient with hypoplasia of the left heart. There is complete absence of the left atrioventricular (AV) connection (white dotted lines). Note that the four chamber section has transected the ventricular septum, showing the site of the rudimentary left ventricle (white oval – compare with Fig. 8.2).

TRICUSPID AND MITRAL ATRESIA

In most instances, tricuspid atresia is produced by complete absence of the right atrioventricular connection (Fig. 8.22). Many hearts with mitral atresia exist because of absence of the left atrioventricular connection (Fig. 8.23). In these hearts, the ventricular morphology is comparable to that seen with double inlet (see Fig. 8.2), with the obvious difference that only one valve enters the dominant ventricle when one connection is absent, since perforce only one atrioventricular junction will be present to make connection with the ventricular mass. The variations in terms of ventricular morphology are just as great when one atrioventricular connection is absent as for double inlet ventricle. By far the greatest number of cases encountered, however, has what can be considered to represent "classical" types of valvar atresia. It is on these "classical" variants that we will concentrate our attention.

In tricuspid atresia, it is the morphologically right atrium which is blind-ending, usually with no vestige of the tricuspid valve in its floor[20] (Fig. 8.24).

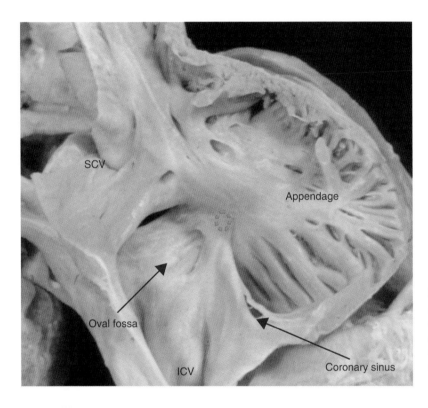

Fig. 8.24 This view, of the opened right atrium seen in anatomic orientation from a specimen with tricuspid atresia, shows the muscular floor due to complete absence of the right atrioventricular connection. The site of the atrioventricular node has been superimposed in green, and is closely related to the "dimple". ICV, SCV – inferior and superior caval veins.

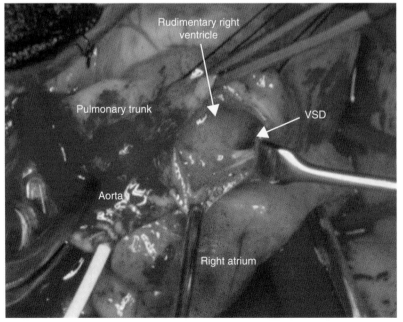

Fig. 8.25 This operative view, taken through a median sternotomy in a patient with tricuspid atresia and concordant ventriculo-arterial connections, shows the morphology of the rudimentary right ventricle, which lacks totally its inlet component, having only apical and outlet parts. VSD – ventricular septal defect.

Because of the absent connection, the right ventricle is rudimentary and incomplete (Fig. 8.25), lacking completely its inlet component[21]. The apical trabecular part of the incomplete ventricle, as with double inlet (Fig. 8.9), is separated from the left ventricle by the apical muscular ventricular septum (Fig. 8.26). Again as in double inlet left ventricle, this septum does not extend to the crux, but rather extends to the acute margin of the ventricular mass (Fig. 8.27). The surgical procedure for 'correction' is again the Fontan operation, or one of its modifications. In hearts with concordant ventriculo-arterial connections, attempts were often made during the early period of evolution of the Fontan procedure to incorporate the rudimentary right ventricle into the pulmonary circulation[22]. Presently, most surgeons have shifted to constructing total cavopulmonary connections, either using internal or external conduits. If the conduit is to be constructed within the right atrium, its muscle bundles, and the arterial supply, should be disturbed as little as possible. Preservation of the sinus node and its blood supply is particularly important, as atrial arrhythmia is a recognised life-threatening postoperative complication, particularly in the long term. The rules for avoidance of these structures are as described above for double inlet ventricle. Whenever a well-formed Eustachian valve is encountered, it should be preserved. Such a valve can be incorporated in an internal baffle. Should the option be to join the atrium directly to the pulmonary arteries, this can be done using a valved aortic homograft, but it is much more usual for the surgeon to make a direct and wide connection between the right atrium and the pulmonary arteries. The artery to the sinus node may be particularly at risk

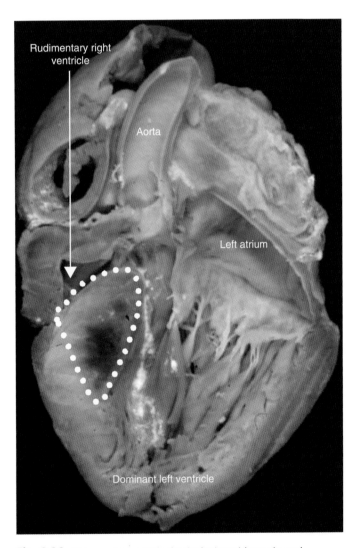

Fig. 8.26 This specimen with classical tricuspid atresia and concordant ventriculo-arterial connections has been sectioned in parasternal long axis fashion, and is photographed positioned on its apex. The apical ventricular septum (white dotted line) separates the apical parts of the dominant and rudimentary ventricles. Compare with Fig. 8.9.

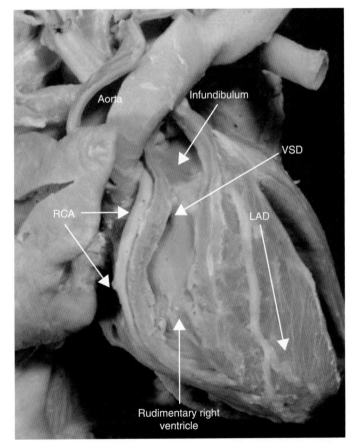

Fig. 8.27 This dissection of a specimen with tricuspid atresia, again with concordant ventriculo-arterial connections, viewed in anatomic orientation, shows that the right delimiting coronary artery descends at the acute margin of the ventricular mass from the right coronary artery (RCA), rather than the crux. The other delimiting artery (white arrow) is the left interventricular descending artery (LAD). Note the anterosuperior location of the rudimentary and incomplete right ventricle.

during this procedure as the artery traverses the interatrial groove.

When the Fontan procedure is performed in hearts with discordant ventriculo-arterial connections, it may be necessary to resect the margins of the ventricular septal defect should it be restrictive. This must be done in a way that avoids the atrioventricular conduction axis on the left ventricular aspect of the septum[12]. When seen from the right ventricle, this runs posteroinferior to the septal defect as in double inlet left ventricle, (Fig. 8.28). The rare exception is when the typical muscular ventricular

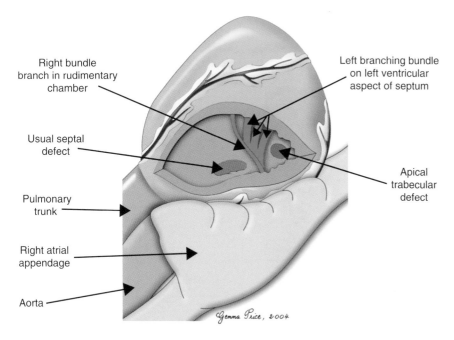

Right bundle branch in rudimentary chamber

Left branching bundle on left ventricular aspect of septum

Usual septal defect

Apical trabecular defect

Pulmonary trunk

Right atrial appendage

Aorta

Gemma Price, 2004

Fig. 8.28 This cartoon, in surgical orientation, shows the route of the axis of atrioventricular conduction tissue, shown in green, relative to the usual ventricular septal defect in tricuspid atresia, and to a defect opening between the apical trabecular component of the incomplete and rudimentary right ventricle and the dominant ventricle. In the latter situation, the axis is superior relative to the defect.

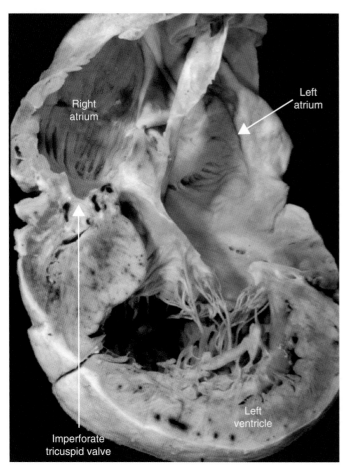

Right atrium

Left atrium

Left ventricle

Imperforate tricuspid valve

Fig. 8.29 This specimen is sectioned in four-chamber plane. There is pulmonary atresia with intact ventricular septum, but additionally the tricuspid valve is imperforate. The atrioventricular connections are concordant.

septal defect is atretic, and an apical trabecular defect provides the interventricular communication (Fig. 8.28).

In very rare cases, tricuspid atresia may be produced because an imperforate valvar membrane is interposed between the right atrium and ventricle. This is typically seen as part of pulmonary atresia with intact ventricular septum (Fig. 8.29). More rarely, the imperforate valve is found together with a ventricular septal defect (Fig. 8.30), or as part of Ebstein's malformation[23] (Fig. 8.31). We are unaware of any patient in whom the imperforate junction has been of sufficient size to permit its resection and replacement with a valvar prosthesis.

Operative treatment of mitral atresia is complicated because of its usual association with aortic atresia. This, of course, is the one of the typical combinations producing hypoplasia of the left heart[24]. Direct surgical correction involves reconstruction of the arterial pathways as an initial procedure, following the Norwood protocol[25], or one of its modifications. This is followed by a subsequent modified Fontan procedure. The options in these procedures are dictated by the anatomy of the aortic

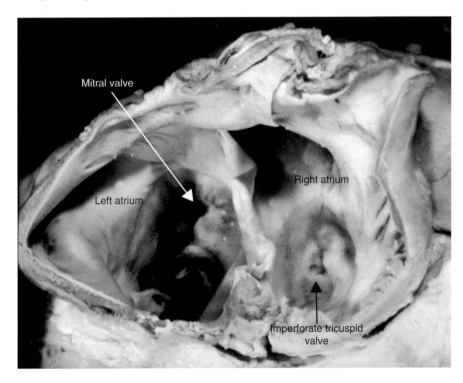

Fig. 8.30 This specimen is viewed from above and behind, in anatomic orientation, to show the right atrial aspect of an imperforate tricuspid valve. In this heart, the atrioventricular connections were again concordant, and there was a ventricular septal defect.

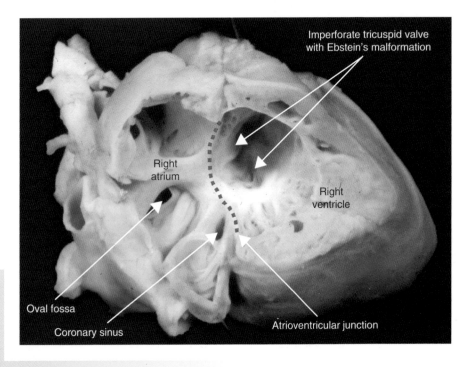

Fig. 8.31 In this heart, once again with an imperforate tricuspid valve and concordant atrioventricular connections, the tricuspid valve itself is deformed by Ebstein's malformation.

pathways rather than the ventricular morphology, with the key features being the relations of the arterial duct (Figs. 8.32, 8.33), and the size of the aortic root (Figs. 8.34, 8.35). In some patients having atresia of the left atrioventricular valve, however, the aortic outflow tract is patent. "Mitral atresia" may not be the best term for description of all these patients. This is because, in many, the morphology suggests that, had the left atrioventricular connection been formed, it would have been guarded by a morphologically tricuspid valve. The right atrium is this setting is connected to a morphologically

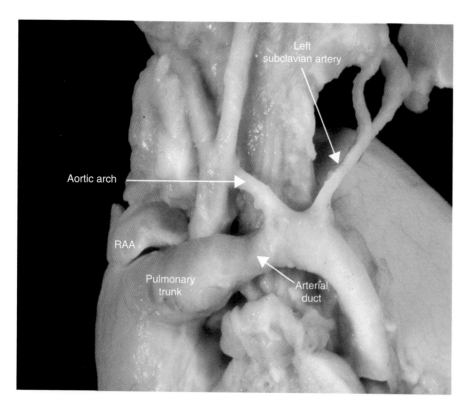

Fig. 8.32 This specimen, viewed from the left side in anatomic orientation, shows the typical arrangement of the arterial trunks in hypoplastic left heart syndrome due to combined aortic and mitral atresia, but with the subclavian artery arising distally to the arterial duct.

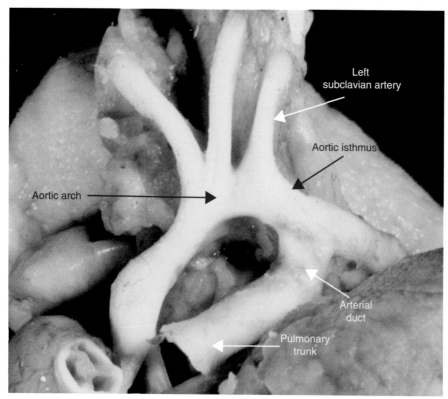

Fig. 8.33 This specimen, again viewed from the left side in anatomic orientation, shows the typical arrangement of the arterial trunks in hypoplastic left heart syndrome due to combined aortic and mitral atresia, but this time with the subclavian artery arising in its normal position proximal to the arterial duct. Compare with Fig. 8.32.

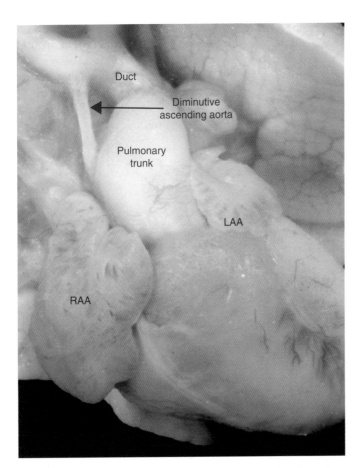

Fig. 8.34 This specimen, viewed in anatomic orientation from the front, again shows the typical arrangement of the arterial trunks in hypoplastic left heart syndrome due to combined aortic and mitral atresia, here with a diminutive ascending aorta. RAA, LAA – right and left atrial appendages.

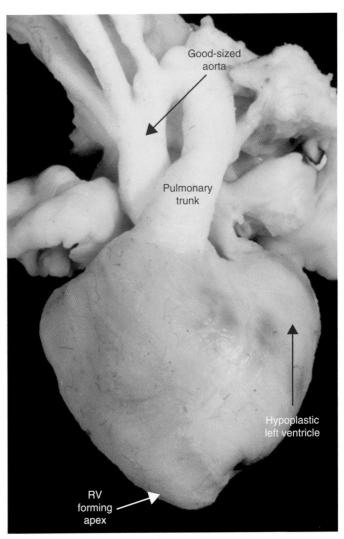

Fig. 8.35 This specimen, again viewed in anatomic orientation from the front, shows the hypoplastic left heart syndrome with combined aortic and mitral atresia, but in this heart, the aorta is of good size, despite the left ventricle being grossly hypoplastic, with the right ventricle (RV) forming the ventricular apex.

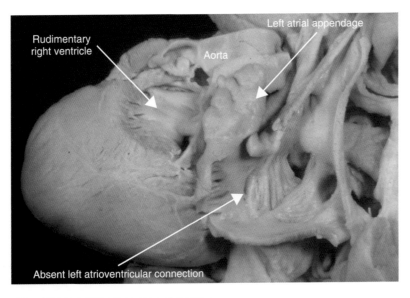

Fig. 8.36 As shown by this specimen, shown in anatomic orientation viewed from the left, "mitral atresia" is not always part of hypoplasia of the left heart. In this example, there is absence of the left atrioventricular connection, but the right atrium is connected to a dominant ventricle with left ventricular trabeculations (not seen). The rudimentary right ventricle, supporting the aorta, is left-sided and anterior. Had the left atrioventricular valve been formed, it would almost certainly of been of tricuspid morphology, but it does not help to consider this heart as showing "tricuspid atresia".

left ventricle, with the rudimentary and incomplete right ventricle being anterior and left-sided, usually with discordant ventriculo-arterial connections (Fig. 8.36). In this setting, the pulmonary venous return has no direct route to the dominant left ventricle, but must cross an atrial septal defect and traverse the right-sided atrioventricular valve. Initial survival in these cases, therefore, depends on the state of the atrial septum. Should the septum be restrictive, it will need to be enlarged. Some sort of modified Fontan procedure will then be the final option, usually a cavopulmonary connection.

As with tricuspid atresia, left-sided atresia can be produced by an imperforate atrioventricular valve rather than being due to absence of the left atrioventricular connection. The imperforate valve can be found with biventricular (Fig. 8.37) or double inlet (Fig. 8.38) atrioventricular connections. Irrespective of the specific

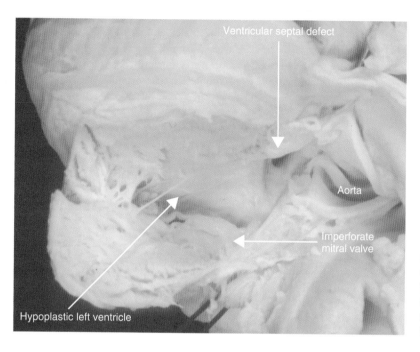

Fig. 8.37 In this specimen, again seen in anatomic orientation and photographed from the left side, there is an imperforate mitral valve in the setting of concordant atrioventricular connections. Note that the aorta arises from the hypoplastic left ventricle, and there is a ventricular septal defect.

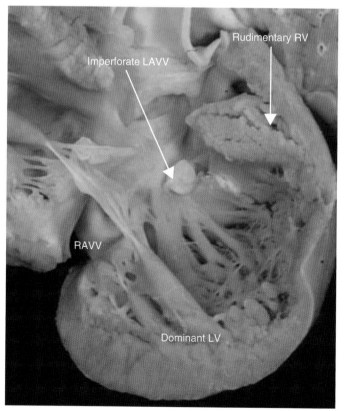

Fig. 8.38 In this specimen, seen in anatomic orientation having opened the dominant left ventricle (LV) from the front, there is double inlet to the dominant ventricle, with the rudimentary right ventricle (RV) in left-sided position, but with an imperforate left atrioventricular valve (LAVV). The right atrioventricular valve (RAVV) is patent.

morphology, the only surgical option will be to create a functionally univentricular connection, the Fontan circulation being constructed following one of the options discussed above.

TRANSPOSITION

This malformation is found when the atrial chambers are connected to their appropriate ventricles, but with discordant ventriculo-arterial connections. Most refer to this combination simply as "transposition". This usage, although

widespread, is less than precise. In the past, disagreements were frequent as to whether "transposition" should be used only to describe hearts with discordant ventriculo-arterial connections[26], or for description of any heart with an anterior aorta[27]. More significantly, when used to describe discordant ventriculo-arterial connections, "transposition" is not restricted to this arrangement at the ventriculo-arterial junctions in the setting of concordant atrioventricular connections. "Transposition", if defined simply on the basis of discordant

ventriculo-arterial connections, can coexist with discordant atrioventricular connections, with double inlet ventricle, with absence of one atrioventricular connection, or with isomerism and biventricular atrioventricular connections. It is these latter anomalies that then become the dominant features. There is, therefore, a need for a term that describes only the combinations of concordant atrioventricular and discordant ventriculo-arterial connections (Fig. 8.39). Previously, our preferred term had been "complete transposition". We now

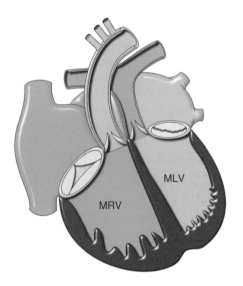
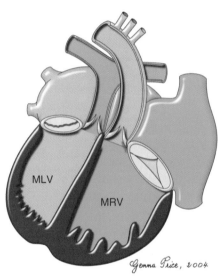

Usual arrangement

Mirror-image arrangement

Gemma Price, 2004

Fig. 8.39 The cartoon shows the segmental combinations of concordant atrioventricular and discordant ventriculo-arterial connections that produce the lesion usually described simply as "transposition". Note that the arrangement can exist in usual and mirror-imaged variants.

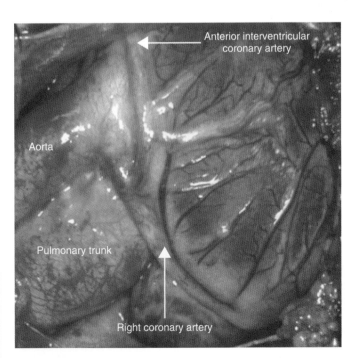

Fig. 8.40 This surgical view, taken through a median sternotomy, shows a patient with transposition (concordant atrioventricular and discordant ventriculo-arterial connections) in which the aorta is anterior and leftward relative to the pulmonary trunk.

recognise that this term itself is less than perfect. The adjective "complete" was first used to indicate that both arterial trunks were transposed across the ventricular septum, thus distinguishing the arrangement from "partial" transposition, in which only the aorta was transposed across the septum. The latter anomaly, of course, is now universally described as double outlet right ventricle. This does not alter the fact that, in the strictest sense, all examples of discordant ventriculo-arterial connections represent "complete" transposition[28]. We suggest, therefore, that the combination of discordant ventriculo-arterial with concordant atrioventricular connections

be considered the default option for "transposition". If discordant ventriculo-arterial connections are found in other settings, we describe them as congenitally corrected transposition, or tricuspid atresia with transposition, and so on. It should be remembered, however, that the often-popular term "d-transposition" cannot be used as the same default option. This latter term does not accurately describe all those cases with the usual atrial arrangement, concordant atrioventricular connections, discordant ventriculo-arterial connections, and a left-sided aorta (Fig. 8.40). Nor does "d-transposition" accurately describe that majority of patients with the combinations

of segmental arrangements producing transposition with mirror-imaged atrial arrangement (Fig. 8.41). It should also be noted that transposition, defined according to our preference, refers only to patients with usual and mirror-imaged atrial arrangements. When discordant ventriculo-arterial connections occur in the setting of isomerism of the atrial appendages, it is the anomalies at the venoatrial and atrioventricular junctions that usually dominate the anatomical and clinical considerations. These cases are, therefore, excluded from the category of transposition described here.

From the surgical standpoint, the two major subgroups of hearts with

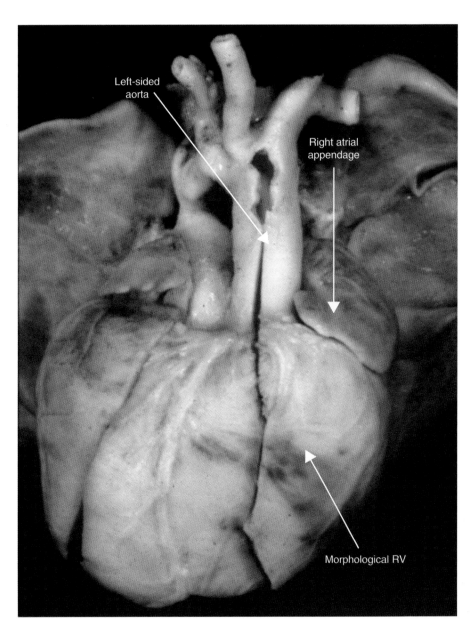

Left-sided aorta

Right atrial appendage

Morphological RV

Fig. 8.41 In this heart, with concordant atrioventricular and discordant ventriculo-arterial connections, shown in anatomical orientation from the front, the aorta is again left-sided relative to the pulmonary trunk. In this case, the heart is in the right chest, with the apex pointing to the right, in the setting of mirror-imaged atrial arrangement.

transposition are those without any major additional complicating lesions, usually described as simple transposition, and those with additional malformations sufficiently severe to complicate the

clinical picture. The morphological aspects of the complicating lesions will be dealt with in turn, but the atrial anatomy is comparable within the whole group.

Nowadays, corrective surgical procedures are almost always performed at the arterial level. Operations designed to redirect venous blood at the atrial level should not be forgotten, however,

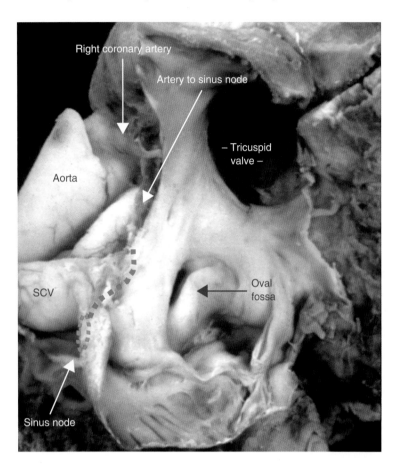

Fig. 8.42 This dissection of a specimen of transposition seen in surgical orientation from the right side shows the relationship of the artery to the sinus node (red dotted line) to the superior rim of the oval fossa. The location of the node itself is shown by the green dotted oval.

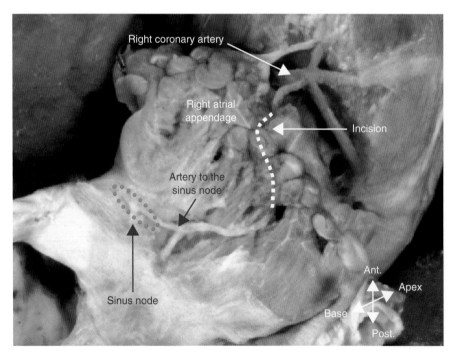

Fig. 8.43 This anatomic specimen with transposition is photographed in surgical orientation from the right side to show how an artery to the sinus node, with the site of the node shown by the green dotted oval, arising laterally from the right coronary artery (white dotted line), has been transacted by a standard incision in the right atrial appendage.

particularly since these manoeuvres are an integral part of double switch procedures. When planning these operations, known as the Mustard and Senning options, it is the disposition of the cardiac nodes and their blood supply that is probably the most important factor. The presence of discordant ventriculo–arterial connections does not in any way affect the position of the sinus node, so the rules enunciated in Chapter 2 for avoidance of this node, and discussed above in the setting of the Fontan procedure, are equally applicable in the setting of transposition. The entire terminal groove should be avoided, as the sinus node may occupy a 'horseshoe' position over the crest of the junction of the superior caval vein with the right atrium, although it is usually in a lateral position. The nodal artery may enter the groove across the crest of the appendage or after it has taken a retrocaval course. Of more importance is the course taken by the nodal artery as is ascends the interatrial groove. The artery frequently burrows into the atrial musculature, running within the superior border of the oval fossa (Fig. 8.42). It is at risk in this position when incising the septum for either a Senning or Mustard procedure, or during a Blalock-Hanlon septostomy. A lateral course across the atrial appendage is also significant (Fig. 8.43).

Other considerations remain significant when carrying out a venous switch procedure. Cannulation of the superior caval vein should be performed a good distance from the cavoatrial junction, incising the right atrium well clear of the terminal groove. Traction, suction, or suturing should be avoided in the area of the superior border of the groove. If an incision is required across the groove to widen the newly constructed pulmonary venous atrium in Mustard's operation, it can be made between the right pulmonary veins without fear of damaging the sinus node or its artery.

This discussion is also pertinent to the genesis of arrhythmias after Mustard's operation or the Senning procedure. It had been suggested that the arrhythmias are due to damage to the so–called 'specialised internodal pathways'[29]. As explained in Chapter 2, there are no such insulated pathways to be found within the atrial myocardium. Instead, the atrioventricular impulse is conducted from the sinus node through the thicker muscles of the right atrial wall and septum, with the anisotropic arrangement of the fibres favouring preferential conduction (Fig. 8.44). It is advantageous, therefore, to preserve at least one of these routes. If the terminal crest is to be divided to enlarge the new pulmonary

venous atrium, this is a further reason to preserve the superior border of the oval fossa. These procedures, together with scrupulous avoidance of the sinus node and its blood supply, mean that arrhythmias can be considerably reduced, if not totally avoided, after atrial redirection procedures.

It is always important to avoid the atrioventricular node. The landmarks to this vital structure are the same as in the normal heart. Providing all surgery is performed outside the triangle of Koch, injury to the node will be avoided. The technique of cutting back the coronary sinus should be carefully considered. It is possible to perform this procedure without damaging the node and its zones of transitional cells, but the incision will undoubtedly cross one of the preferential routes of conduction. For this reason, it is safer to place the inferior suture line so as to avoid completely the triangle of Koch.

It is also important to place the interatrial baffles so as to minimise the risk of subsequent venous obstruction, either in the pulmonary or venous pathways. Although it was suggested that venous obstruction was less likely to complicate the Senning procedure, those who became skilled in the Mustard procedure were able to achieve excellent results with a minimal incidence of late

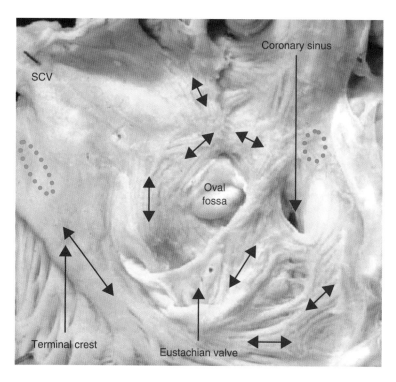

Fig. 8.44 This dissection is made in a normal heart, orientated anatomically, by removing the endocardium from the inner surface of the right atrium. It shows the non-uniform anisotropic arrangement of the muscle fibres. There is preferential conduction along the major axis of the muscle bundles (blue arrows), but no insulated and "specialised" tracts within the atrial musculature. The sites of the sinus and atrioventricular nodes are shown by the green dotted areas. SCV – superior caval vein.

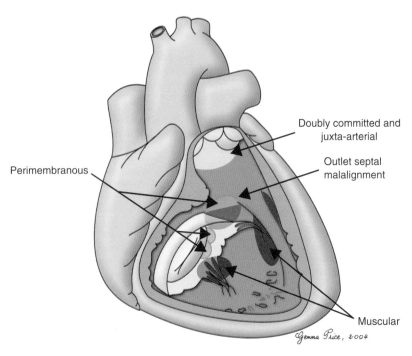

Doubly committed and
juxta-arterial

Outlet septal
malalignment

Perimembranous

Muscular

Gemma Price, 2004

Fig. 8.45 The cartoon shows how the ventricular septal defect in hearts with transposition, as in the normal heart, can be perimembranous, muscular, or doubly committed and juxta-arterial. The cartoon emphasises, however, the potential for malalignment of the muscular outlet septum, a particular feature of the ventricular septal defect in the setting of transposition.

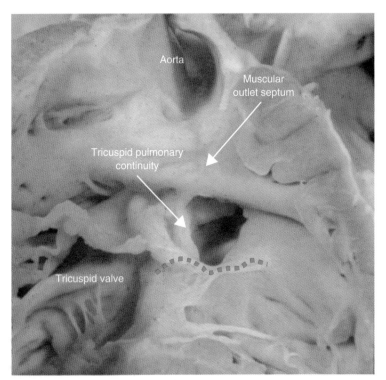

Aorta

Muscular
outlet septum

Tricuspid pulmonary
continuity

Tricuspid valve

Fig. 8.46 This view of a specimen with transposition, seen in anatomic orientation from the right ventricle, shows the right ventricular aspect of a perimembranous defect opening to the subaortic outlet with malalignment of the outlet septum and overriding of the leaflets of the pulmonary valve. The conduction axis is shown by the green dots.

venous obstruction[30]. Almost certainly, therefore, it is the surgical technique which determines the likelihood of postoperative venous obstruction.

The major complicating lesion in transposition is the presence of a ventricular septal defect, with or without obstruction of the left ventricular outflow tract. Any other lesion can coexist if anatomically possible, and the anatomy will then be as described for the lesion in isolation.

Ventricular septal defects in hearts with discordant ventriculo–arterial connections can be as variable as when found in isolation (Fig. 8.45). The majority of defects open between the outlet components of the ventricular mass, and have their own peculiar characteristics. In such setting, with malalignment of the outlet septum, they can either be perimembranous (Fig. 8.46), or have a muscular posteroinferior rim (Fig. 8.47). The distinguishing feature, as in tetralogy

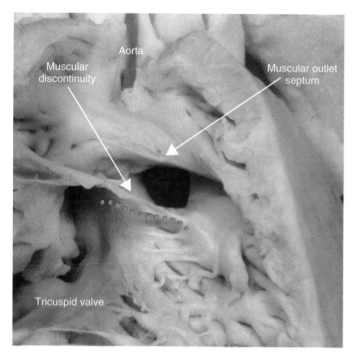

Fig. 8.47 This specimen, again seen in anatomic orientation from the right side, has a ventricular septal defect opening to the outlet of the right ventricle as in Fig. 8.46, but this time with a muscular posteroinferior rim. Note the malalignment of the outlet septum. The muscular rim protects the conduction axis, shown by the green dotted line.

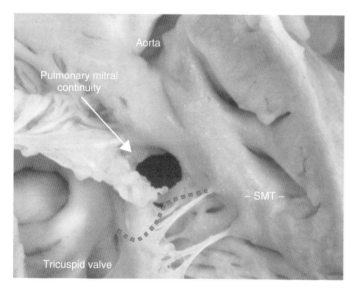

Fig. 8.48 In this heart with transposition, seen in anatomic orientation from the right side, a perimembranous defect opens to the inlet of the right ventricle. The conduction axis, shown by the green dots, is deviated posteroinferiorly, but still relates directly to the rim of the defect.

of Fallot, is whether or not the posterior limb of the septomarginal trabeculation fuses with the ventriculoinfundibular fold. If there is fusion (Fig. 8.47), the resultant muscle bar will buttress the conduction axis, and there will be discontinuity between the leaflets of the tricuspid and pulmonary valves. If there is no fusion of the muscular bundles, the defect will be perimembranous, and there will be fibrous continuity between the valvar leaflets. The penetrating bundle will be at risk in this area of fibrous continuity (Fig. 8.46).

These defects have other features of surgical significance. The tension apparatus of the tricuspid valve tends to course over the defect, attaching itself to the outlet septum or to the ventriculoinfundibular fold. This makes closure of the defect difficult without producing damage to the tricuspid valve, albeit that this is of less significance when the tricuspid valve is in the pulmonary circuit after an arterial switch. Of more significance is the divergence of the margins of the parietal and anterior heart walls. In hearts with concordant

ventriculo–arterial connections, the anterior margin of a ventricular septal defect is usually well-circumscribed. In the setting of transposition, the muscular outlet septum frequently becomes malaligned relative to the rest of the muscular ventricular septum as it inserts into the anterior wall of the right ventricular outflow tract. The defect, therefore, is more difficult to close at this anterior margin (Figs. 8.46, 8.47).

Defects can open to the inlet of the right ventricle, and again be perimembranous (Fig. 8.48) or muscular

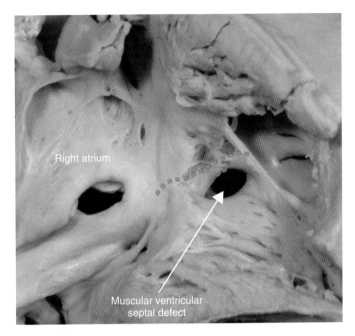

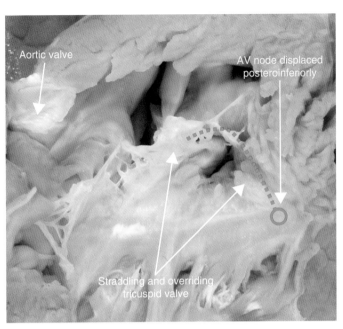

Fig. 8.49 This heart, again with transposition, and photographed through the right atrioventricular junction, has a muscular defect opening to the inlet of the right ventricle. In this setting, the conduction axis, shown by the green dots, courses anterosuperior relative to the defect.

Fig. 8.50 In this heart with transposition, this time shown in surgical orientation, there is straddling and overriding of the tricuspid valve. Because of the malalignment between the atrial and ventricular septums, the atrioventricular node (green circle) is no longer at the apex of the triangle of Koch, being deviated posteroinferiorly, as shown by the superimposed course of the conduction axis (green dotted line).

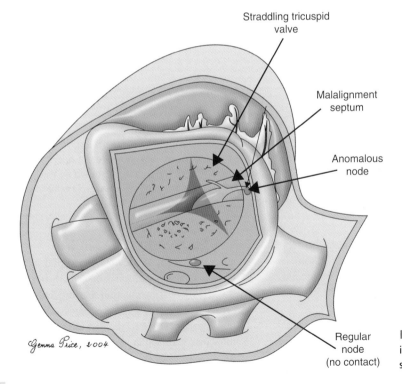

Fig. 8.51 The cartoon, shown in surgical orientation, illustrates the location of the conduction axis in a heart with straddling and overriding of the tricuspid valve.

(Fig. 8.49). Some muscular defects open centrally, while others open apically, often being multiple. Defects opening to the ventricular inlet which are also perimembranous are the harbingers of straddling and overriding of the tricuspid valve. This should always be suspected when the right ventricle is hypoplastic (Fig. 8.50). A straddling valve increases markedly the risks of surgery, not least because of the abnormal disposition of the conduction tissues (Fig. 8.51). Doubly

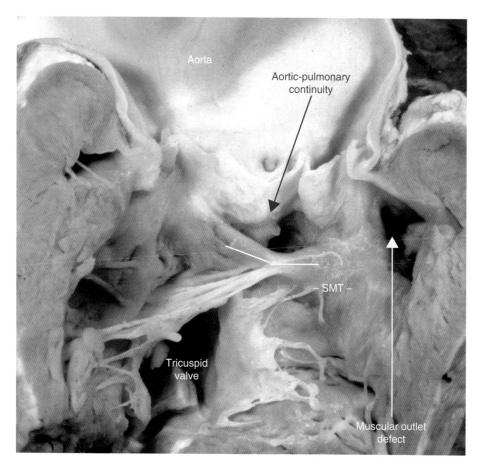

Aorta

Aortic-pulmonary
continuity

SMT –

Tricuspid
valve

Muscular outlet
defect

Fig. 8.52 In this heart with transposition, seen in anatomic orientation from the front, the major defect is doubly committed and juxta-arterial, with fibrous continuity between the leaflets of the aortic and pulmonary valves. There is a muscular posteroinferior rim to the defect (white line) that protects the conduction axis. Note the additional muscular outlet defect in front of the septomarginal trabeculation (SMT).

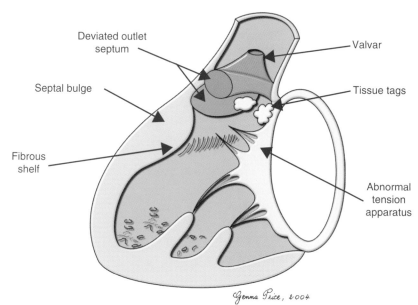

Deviated outlet
septum

Valvar

Septal bulge

Tissue tags

Fibrous
shelf

Abnormal
tension
apparatus

Gemma Price, 2004

Fig. 8.53 The cartoon shows the lesions that can produce subpulmonary obstruction in the setting of transposition. Exactly the same lesions will produce subaortic obstruction in hearts with concordant ventriculo-arterial connections.

committed and juxta-arterial defects can also be found, but are the rarest variant (Fig. 8.52).

Subpulmonary obstruction in transposition (Fig. 8.53) can be produced by any lesion which, in the normal heart, would produce subaortic obstruction (see Figs. 7.110–7.117). Valvar stenosis often accompanies the subvalvar abnormalities. Rarer lesions, such as anomalous insertion of the tension apparatus of the atrioventricular valve, are probably beyond surgical repair. Aneurysm of the membranous septum, or similar fibrous tissue "tags" (Fig. 8.54) should be readily amenable to removal, although a subpulmonary fibrous diaphragm poses more problems as it directly overlies the left bundle branch (Fig. 8.55). The difficulties are compounded when the fibrous obstruction is more extensive,

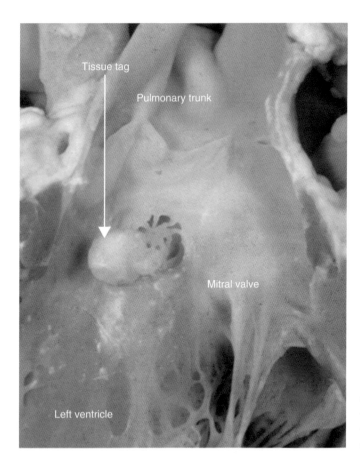

Fig. 8.54 This view of the left ventricle from a specimen with transposition, seen in anatomic orientation from the left, shows a tissue tag from the septal leaflet of the tricuspid valve herniating through a perimembranous ventricular septal defect and producing subpulmonary obstruction.

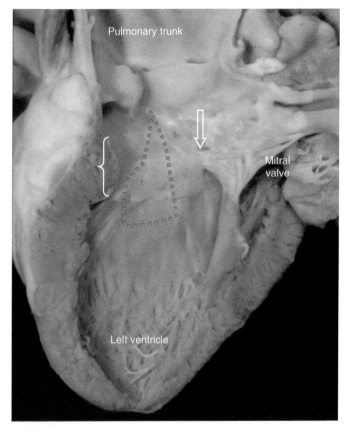

Fig. 8.55 In this view of the left ventricular outflow tract of a specimen with transposition, seen in anatomic orientation, there is obstruction due to an extensive fibrous diaphragm (bracket) that extends onto the leaflet of the mitral valve (arrow). The course of the left bundle branch is shown by the green dotted area.

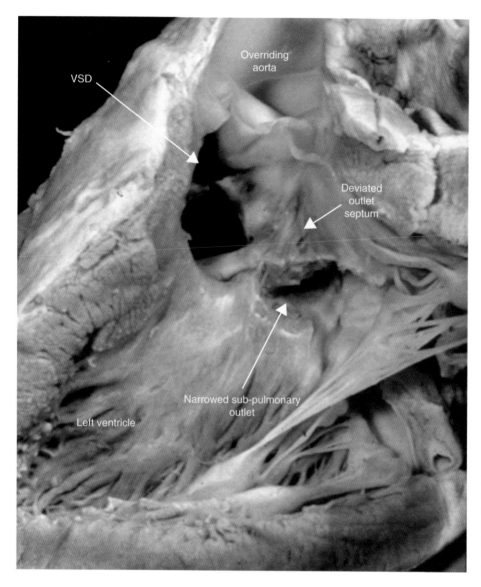

Overriding aorta

VSD

Deviated outlet septum

Narrowed sub-pulmonary outlet

Left ventricle

Fig. 8.56 This specimen of transposition, seen from the left ventricle in anatomic orientation, has the type of defect with posterior deviation of the outlet septum through the ventricular septal defect (VSD) that is most suitable for the Rastelli procedure.

because then it can form a subvalvar tunnel. The other quadrants of the outflow tract are also vulnerable because of their proximity to the left coronary artery, or because they are formed by leaflets of the mitral valve. The safest area for resection is beneath the remnant of the left margin of the ventriculoinfundibular fold. When subpulmonary obstruction coexists with a ventricular septal defect, there is almost always posterior deviation and insertion of the outlet septum into the left ventricle. This usually means that the aortic valve overrides the septum. When the septal defect is substantial this combination sets the scene for a Rastelli procedure (Fig. 8.56). Should the defect be restrictive, and a Rastelli operation is

still desirable, it is possible to resect safely the outlet septum, which never harbours conduction tissue. Should the defect be situated other than between the ventricular outlets, the chances of successfully accomplishing a Rastelli procedure are considerably reduced.

Thus far, we have devoted attention exclusively to the segmental anatomy of transposition. There is, of course, further variation in terms of both arterial relationships and infundibular anatomy. These variations do not alter the intracardiac anatomy, and are of relatively minor surgical significance. For example, the aorta is usually anterior and to the right in complete transposition (Fig. 8.57) but, in some cases, as already illustrated,

the aorta may be anterior and to the left (Figs. 8.40, 8.41). In even rarer cases, it may be posterior and to the right of the pulmonary trunk (Fig. 8.58). These different relationships do not alter the basic anatomy. They do show why it is inadvisable to use the term "d-transposition" as a unifying terminology, since it makes little sense to use this term for description of the patient in whom the aorta is left-sided.

There are some clues to associated lesions to be drawn from these unexpected arterial relationships. With a left-sided aorta (Fig. 8.59), there is a high incidence of septal defects which are doubly committed and juxta-arterial (Fig. 8.52). This arrangement is convenient for direct

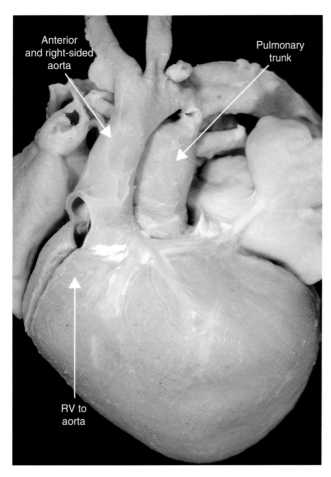

Anterior and right-sided aorta

Pulmonary trunk

RV to aorta

Fig. 8.57 This heart is shown in anatomic orientation, demonstrating the usual relationship of the aorta in the setting of transposition, anterior and to the right of the pulmonary trunk. The arrow shows the cut from the right ventricle (RV) to the aorta.

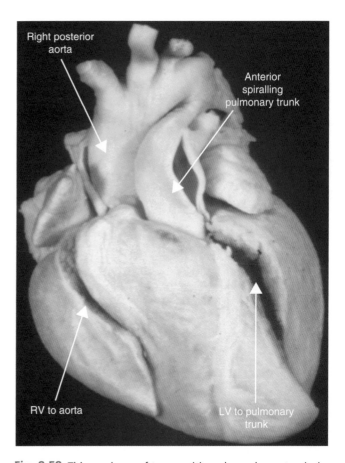

Right posterior aorta

Anterior spiralling pulmonary trunk

RV to aorta

LV to pulmonary trunk

Fig. 8.58 This specimen of transposition, shown in anatomical orientation from the front, has the aorta in posterior and rightward position relative to the pulmonary trunk, with spiralling of the arterial trunks, so-called "normal relations", but still with discordant ventriculo-arterial connections. The cuts show that the right ventricle (RV) supports the aorta, while the left ventricle (LV) gives rise to the pulmonary trunk.

connection of the aorta to the left ventricle and Rastelli's procedure. When the aorta is posterior, there is usually a subpulmonary infundibulum, with the aortic valve in fibrous continuity with the mitral valve through the roof of a perimembranous septal defect. This unusual anatomy can create difficulty both at initial diagnosis and at subsequent surgery. Variations in infundibular morphology in themselves are unlikely to give problems. The expected subaortic muscular infundibulum in the right ventricle is most frequently encountered along with fibrous continuity between the leaflets of the pulmonary and mitral valves in the left ventricle. Rarely, there may be a complete muscular infundibulum in both ventricles (Fig. 8.60). Even more rarely, as

described above, there may be a subpulmonary infundibulum with continuity between the leaflets of the aortic and mitral valve, particularly when the discordantly connected aorta is in posterior position.

The feature currently of greatest surgical importance in patients with transposition is now the morphology of the coronary arteries. This is because of the universal acceptance of the arterial switch procedure as the surgical treatment of choice. This operation involves transecting the ascending aorta and pulmonary trunk, and reconnecting them to their morphologically appropriate ventricles. The significant morphological feature is that, thus far without reported exception, the coronary arteries arise from

those aortic sinuses that are adjacent to the pulmonary trunk (Fig. 8.61). When performing the arterial switch, therefore, the surgeon is required to transfer the origins of the coronary arteries across a relatively short distance (Fig. 8.62). This holds true irrespective of the relationship of the aorta to the pulmonary trunk.

The variable relationships between the aorta and the pulmonary trunk, however, produces problems in naming the aortic sinuses and, hence, the origin of the coronary arteries. Truly formidable conventions are created if attempts are made to catalogue each and every pattern[31], while use of simple alphabetic codes[32] is self-evidently procrustean. As suggested by the group from Leiden[33], it

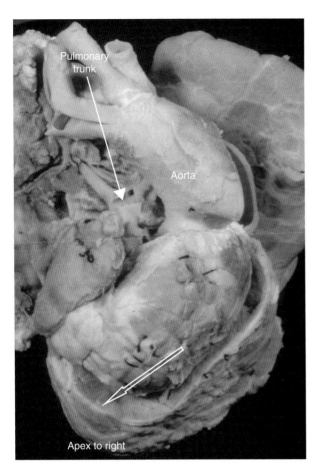

Fig. 8.59 This specimen with transposition, seen in anatomical orientation from the front, is the heart with the doubly committed and juxta-arterial defect shown in Fig. 8.52. When seen from the exterior, the aorta is anterior and to the left of the pulmonary trunk, and the apex is pointing to the right (white arrow). These findings should raise the suspicion of a doubly committed defect.

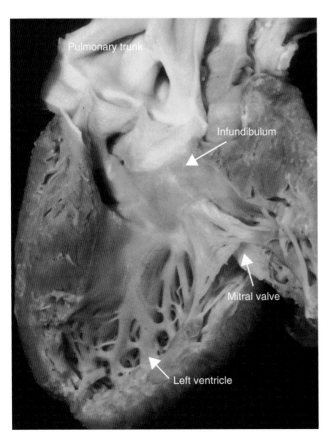

Fig. 8.60 This heart, photographed through the left ventricle in anatomic orientation, shows a large subpulmonary infundibulum separating the leaflets of the pulmonary and mitral valves.

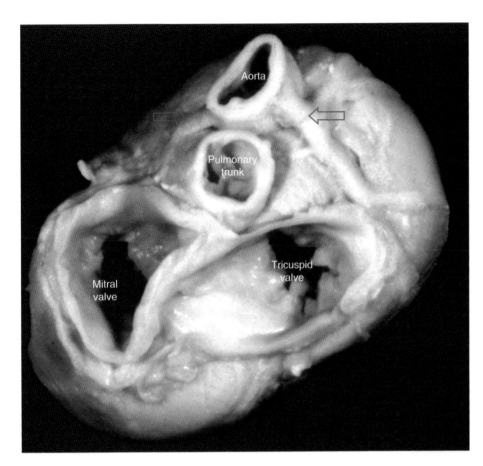

Fig. 8.61 In this heart, the short axis is viewed from above in anatomic orientation having removed the atrial myocardium and the arterial trunks. The ventriculo-arterial connections are discordant. The dissection shows how the coronary arteries (red arrows) arise from the two aortic sinuses adjacent to the pulmonary trunk.

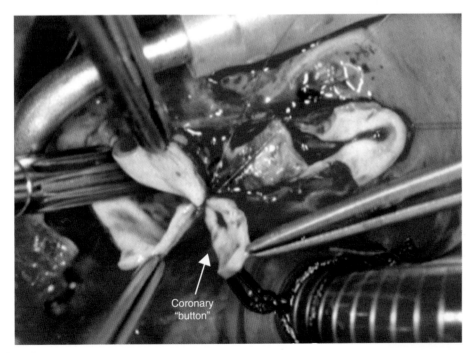

Fig. 8.62 These operative views demonstrate how a button supporting one of the coronary arteries, having been liberated from the aorta, may be transferred to the pulmonary trunk during the arterial switch procedure. The relatively short distance allows an anastomosis free of tension.

is best to name the aortic sinuses as viewed from the stance of the observer standing in the non-adjacent sinus of the aorta and looking towards the pulmonary trunk (Fig. 8.63). One sinus is then always to the observer's right hand. This is designated as sinus #1. The other sinus is to the left hand, and is called sinus #2. The three major coronary arteries can arise from either of these sinuses, giving only eight possible patterns of sinusal origin. Transfer of the arteries during the switch

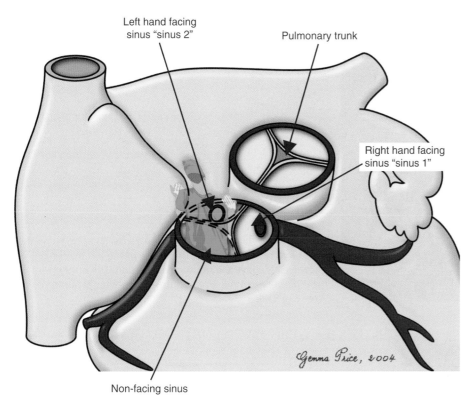

Fig. 8.63 The cartoon shows how the two aortic sinuses that face the pulmonary trunk can always be described accurately as being to the surgeon's left hand or right hand, when standing in the non-facing sinus of the aorta and looking towards the pulmonary trunk, irrespective of the relationships of the arterial trunks. Conventionally, the sinus to the right hand is described as '#1', while that to the left hand is '#2'.

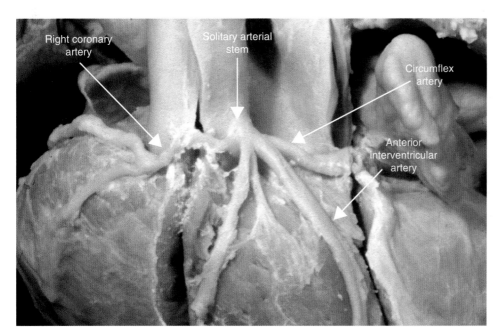

Fig. 8.64 In this heart, photographed in anatomic orientation from the front, the right and the left coronary arteries arise from a solitary vessel, with the right coronary artery and the circumflex artery then passing in front of the arterial pedicle.

procedure can be compromised by anomalous course of the coronary arteries themselves in relation to the vascular pedicle (Fig. 8.64), albeit that such variations can be suitably accommodated by appropriate surgical technique. An intramural course of the origin of the coronary artery across a valvar commissure[34,35] (Figs. 8.65, 8.66) creates greater problems, but these can also be solved. The origin of the artery to the sinus node can be very close to the origin of one coronary artery from an aortic sinus, or the sinus nodal artery can originate separately from the sinus. Also of note is mismatch between the commissures of the aortic and pulmonary valves[35] (Fig. 8.67). Despite all these anatomic variations, surgeons now find it possible to perform the arterial switch procedure with remarkable success.

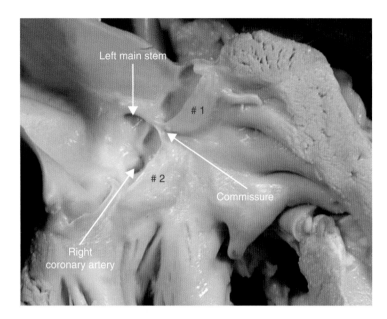

Fig. 8.65 In this heart, both coronary arteries arise within the left hand facing sinus (#2). The orifice of the left main stem, however, is above the sinutubular junction. This artery courses between the arterial trunks in intramural fashion (see Fig. 8.66).

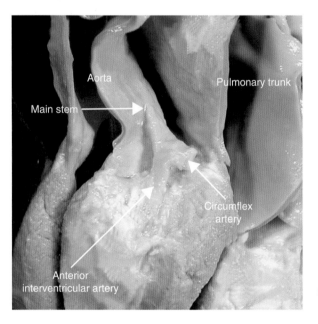

Fig. 8.66 This is the same heart as shown in Fig. 8.65. The left main stem is embedded within the wall of the aorta as it runs towards the anterior surface of the heart, dividing into circumflex and anterior interventricular branches.

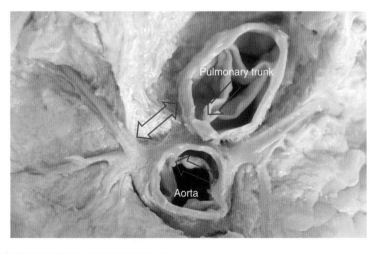

Fig. 8.67 In this heart, in which the atrial myocardium and the arterial trunks have been removed, the heart being photographed from the atrial aspect, there is gross mismatch between the zones of apposition of the leaflets of the aortic and pulmonary valves (double headed red arrow). Because of this, the distance for transfer of the left coronary artery is increased (red single headed arrows).

CONGENITALLY CORRECTED TRANSPOSITION

We use the term 'congenitally corrected transposition' to describe the combination of discordant atrioventricular and ventriculo-arterial connections. As thus defined, congenitally corrected transposition can exist with the atrial chambers in their usual arrangement, or in mirror-imaged position (Fig. 8.68). It cannot, by definition, be found when there is isomerism of the atrial appendages.

The complexities of congenitally corrected transposition reflect the fact that, with usual atrial arrangement, there is malalignment between the inlet part of the muscular ventricular septum and the atrial septum[36]. These two septal structures are in line at the crux but, when traced forwards, they diverge markedly. This produces a gap into which is wedged the subpulmonary outflow tract from the morphologically left ventricle (Fig. 8.69). This abnormal feature accounts for the most important surgical aspect of congenitally corrected transposition, namely the unusual disposition of the atrioventricular conduction tissues. Because of the septal malalignment, it is not possible for the normal atrioventricular node, positioned at the apex of the triangle of Koch, to penetrate through the fibrous atrioventricular junction and make contact with the ventricular conduction tissues. Instead, an anomalous atrioventricular node, found in an anterolateral position (Fig. 8.70), as in double inlet left ventricle, gives rise to the penetrating atrioventricular bundle. This bundle penetrates the insulating plane of the atrioventricular junction lateral to the area of fibrous continuity between the leaflets of the pulmonary and mitral valves. A long non-branching bundle then runs round the anterior quadrants of the subpulmonary outflow tract, crossing the characteristic anterior recess of the morphologically left ventricle, before descending onto the muscular ventricular septum (Fig. 8.71). Having branched, the fan-like left branch is distributed in the right-sided morphologically left ventricle, while the cord-like right branch of the bundle penetrates the septum to reach the left-sided morphologically right ventricle[36]. The discordantly connected aorta arises from this morphologically right ventricle, typically above a complete muscular infundibulum, and usually in a left-sided position (Fig. 8.72).

When congenitally corrected transposition exists without any other anomaly, the circulation of the blood is normal. This situation is very much the exception. Usually, one or more of three associated lesions are found. These are a ventricular septal defect, pulmonary stenosis, or anomalies of the left-sided atrioventricular valve[37]. It is these associated lesions that require surgical treatment.

A ventricular septal defect is present in up to three-quarters of patients. As in the patient with concordant atrioventricular connections, it may be perimembranous, muscular, or doubly committed and juxta-arterial (Fig. 8.73). Usually it is of the perimembranous type, and opens between the ventricular inlets. Then, because of the wedge position of the pulmonary valve, the pulmonary trunk tends to override the defect (Fig. 8.74). When seen from the right atrium, it is shielded by the superior end of the zone of apposition between the leaflets of the right-sided morphologically mitral valve (Fig. 8.75). The abnormal position of the atrioventricular node and the non-branching atrioventricular bundle must be borne in mind when closing the defect. The atrioventricular bundle arises from the anomalous anterolateral node, penetrates the area of pulmonary-mitral valvar continuity, and then runs round the subpulmonary outflow tract to descend on the anterosuperior margin of the defect (Fig. 8.71).

The safest way of closing the defect without damaging the conduction system[38] is to place sutures from the left-sided morphologically right ventricular aspect (Fig. 8.76). Although the defect opens mostly between the ventricular inlets, it can extend to become doubly committed and juxta-arterial. It is then

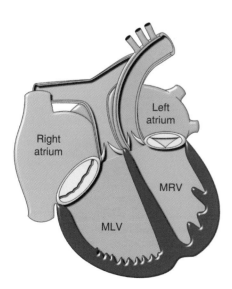

Usual arrangement

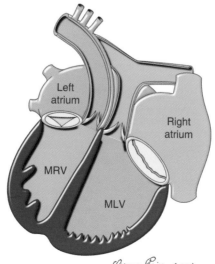

Genna Price, 2004

Mirror-imaged arrangement

Fig. 8.68 The cartoon shows the segmental combinations of discordant atrioventricular and ventriculo-arterial connections that produce the lesion best described as congenitally corrected transposition. As shown, the arrangement can be found in usual and mirror-imaged variants. MRV, MLV – morphologically right and left ventricles.

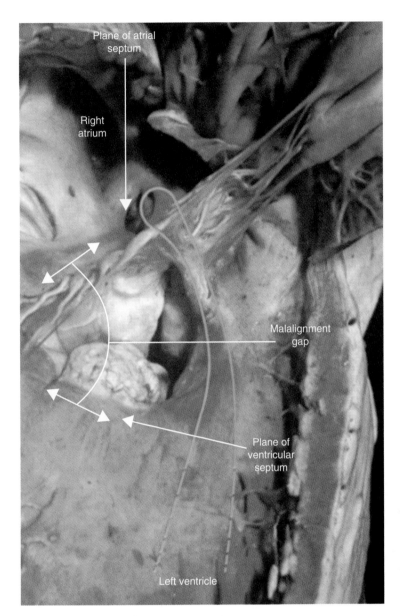

Plane of atrial
septum

Right
atrium

Malalignment
gap

Plane of
ventricular
septum

Left ventricle

Fig. 8.69 This specimen with congenitally corrected transposition, viewed in anatomical orientation from the morphologically left ventricle, shows the malalignment between the atrial and ventricular septal structures, with the subpulmonary outflow tract wedged into this gap. The site of the atrioventricular conduction axis has been superimposed in green. Reproduced by kind permission of Prof. Anton Becker, University of Amsterdam.

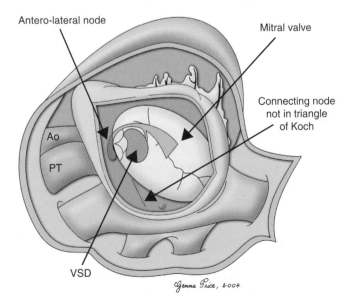

Antero-lateral node

Mitral valve

Connecting node
not in triangle
of Koch

Ao

PT

VSD

Gemma Price, 2004

Fig. 8.70 The cartoon shows the view of the morphologically mitral valve in congenitally corrected transposition as seen by the surgeon working through a right atriotomy. The location of the atrioventricular node and the conduction axis has been marked in green, with the leaflets of the pulmonary valve highlighted in yellow. There is a perimembranous ventricular septal defect (VSD). Ao – aorta; PT – pulmonary trunk.

Morphologically left ventricle

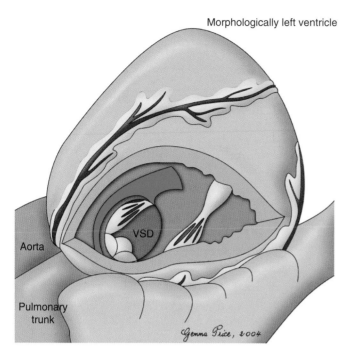

Fig. 8.71 In this cartoon, we show the view of the ventricular septal defect (VSD) in congenitally corrected transposition as would be seen by the surgeon working through a generous incision in the right-sided morphologically left ventricle. The course of the conduction axis has been marked in green.

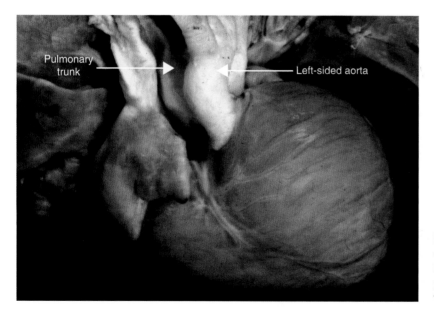

Fig. 8.72 This specimen is photographed in anatomic orientation from the front, showing the usual left-sided location of the aorta relative to the pulmonary trunk in congenitally corrected transposition.

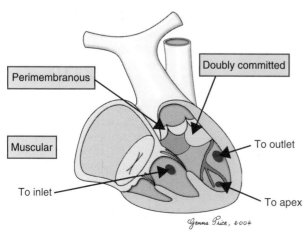

Fig. 8.73 The cartoon shows that, in congenitally corrected transposition as in the otherwise normal heart, the ventricular septal defect can be perimembranous, muscular, or doubly committed and juxta-arterial. In congenitally corrected transposition, however, the conduction axis, shown in green, takes a grossly abnormal course relative to the defects.

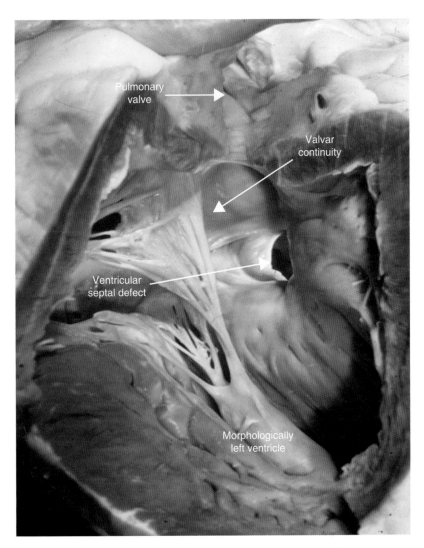

Fig. 8.74 This view of a specimen with congenitally corrected transposition, shown in anatomic orientation from the front, illustrates the relationships of a perimembranous ventricular septal defect opening to the inlet of the morphologically left ventricle. Reproduced by kind permission of Prof. Anton Becker, University of Amsterdam.

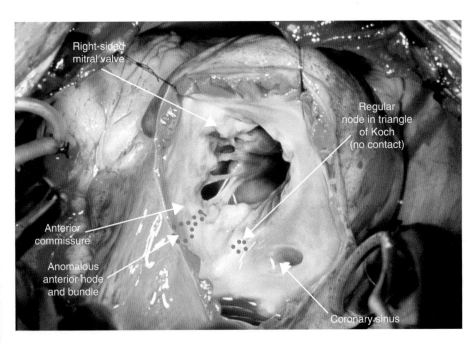

Fig. 8.75 This surgical view of a perimembranous inlet ventricular septal defect in congenitally corrected transposition, seen through the right-sided morphologically mitral valve, shows how the defect and the subpulmonary outflow tract are shielded behind the anteroseptal commissure of the valve. The green dotted areas show the connecting and non-connecting atrioventricular nodes. Reproduced by kind permission of Dr. Jan Quaegebeur, Columbia University, New York.

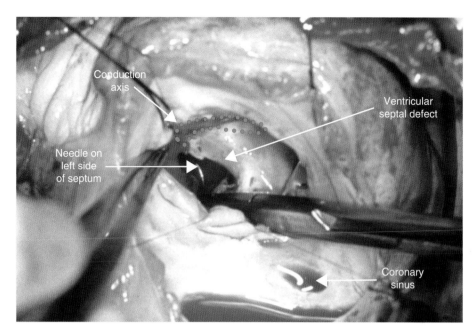

Conduction axis

Ventricular septal defect

Needle on left side of septum

Coronary sinus

Fig. 8.76 This further view of the patient shown in Fig. 8.75 illustrates how the axis of conduction tissue (shown in green) can be avoided by placing sutures through the defect on its morphologically right ventricular aspect (left-sided). Reproduced by kind permission of Dr. Jan Quaegebeur, Columbia University, New York.

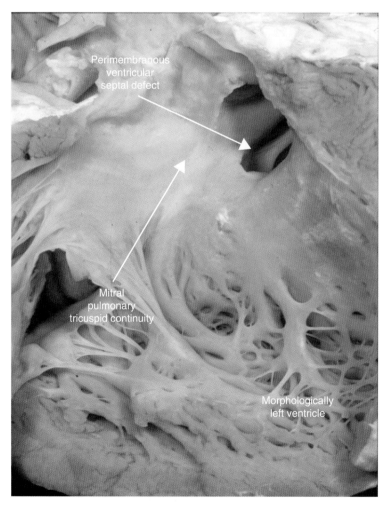

Perimembranous ventricular septal defect

Mitral pulmonary tricuspid continuity

Morphologically left ventricle

Fig. 8.77 In this specimen, viewed in anatomic orientation, the perimembranous ventricular septal defect extends to become doubly committed and juxta-arterial, being roofed by fibrous continuity between the leaflets of the aortic and pulmonary valves.

roofed by the conjoined leaflets of the aortic and pulmonary valves (Fig. 8.77). When it is perimembranous and juxta-arterial, the conduction tissue remains in anterior position. In some patients, however, there can be a muscular inferior rim between the leaflets of the pulmonary and mitral valves. It is still likely that the conduction tissue remains in anterosuperior position relative to the defect. A comparable case has been seen with both a perimembranous and a

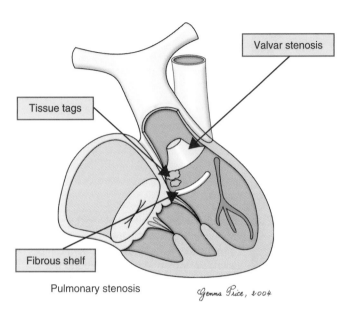

Valvar stenosis

Tissue tags

Fibrous shelf

Pulmonary stenosis

Gemma Price, 2004

Fig. 8.78 The cartoon shows the lesions that can produce subpulmonary obstruction in the setting of congenitally corrected transposition. Note the anterior position of the conduction axis, shown in green. As with transposition, the same lesions produce subaortic obstruction in the setting of concordant ventriculo-arterial connections.

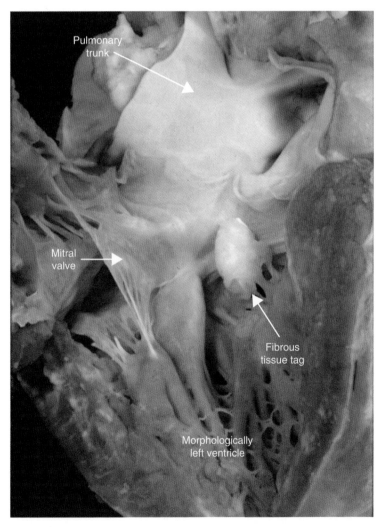

Pulmonary trunk

Mitral valve

Fibrous tissue tag

Morphologically left ventricle

Fig. 8.79 In this specimen, viewed in anatomic orientation through the morphologically left ventricle, a fibrous tissue tag derived from the septal leaflet of the left-sided morphologically tricuspid valve herniates into the subpulmonary outflow tract.

muscular outlet defect. The conduction axis descended the muscle bar between them.

As with transposition, any of the lesions that produces obstruction of the left ventricular outflow tract will produce pulmonary stenosis when the transposition is congenitally corrected (Fig. 8.78). Valvar stenosis in isolation is rare, but frequently coexists with subvalvar obstructive lesions. Particularly significant in this respect are fibrous tissue tags (Fig. 8.79). Fibrous diaphragmatic

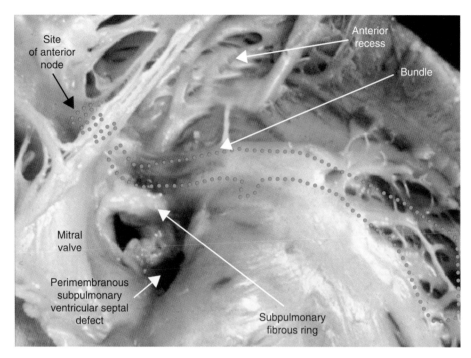

Site of anterior node

Anterior recess

Bundle

Mitral valve

Perimembranous subpulmonary ventricular septal defect

Subpulmonary fibrous ring

Fig. 8.80 In this specimen, seen in anatomic orientation through the morphologically left ventricle, a fibrous shelf produces subpulmonary obstruction in presence of a perimembranous ventricular septal defect. The site of the axis of atrioventricular conduction tissue has been superimposed in green.

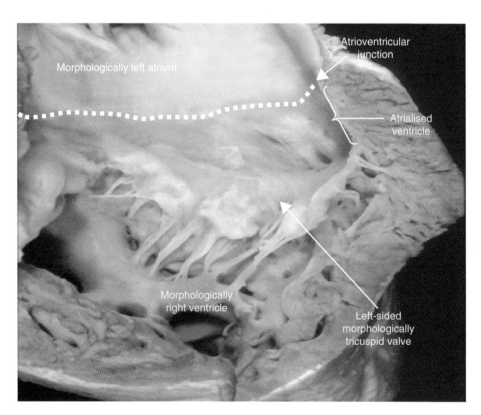

Morphologically left atrium

Atrioventricular junction

Atrialised ventricle

Morphologically right ventricle

Left-sided morphologically tricuspid valve

Fig. 8.81 This specimen with congenitally corrected transposition, seen in anatomical orientation from the left side, shows Ebstein's malformation of the left-sided morphologically tricuspid valve. There is no thinning of the musculature of the inlet component of the morphologically right ventricle.

lesions (Fig. 8.80), or muscular obstruction, are also encountered[39]. The overwhelming consideration in all of these types of stenosis is the presence of the non-branching bundle running round the anterior quadrants of the outflow tract. Apart from tissue tags, this relationship makes it very difficult to resect these various lesions. Placement of a conduit is the safest means of avoiding postoperative heart block.

Ebstein's malformation is the lesion which most frequently afflicts the left-sided morphologically tricuspid valve, involving downward displacement of the septal and mural leaflets (Fig. 8.81). Only rarely is the inlet part of the ventricle

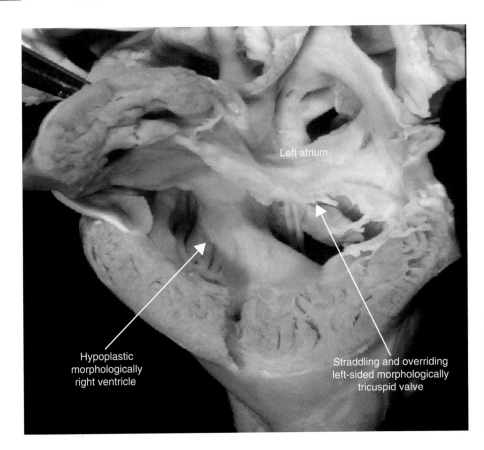

Fig. 8.82 In this heart with congenitally corrected transposition, viewed in anatomic orientation from the left-sided morphologically right ventricle, there is straddling and overriding of the left-sided morphologically tricuspid valve. Note the hypoplastic nature of the morphologically right ventricle.

dilated and thinned, as occurs so frequently in Ebstein's malformation with concordant atrioventricular connections. Should replacement of the valve become necessary, the location of the conduction tissues in the right-sided atrioventricular junction takes them out of the area of danger.

The other anomaly that affects the left valve, and that can also affect the right valve[40], is straddling of its tension apparatus and overriding of the valvar orifice (Fig. 8.82). These anomalies do not alter the origin of the conduction tissues from an anterolateral node, but will markedly increase the risks of surgery. Indeed, in the presence of straddling atrioventricular valves, some may opt for functionally univentricular rather than biventricular surgical correction. Those who use biventricular correction have observed disappointing results subsequent to simple correction of the associated lesions, because these manoeuvres leave the morphologically right ventricle supporting the systemic circulation. Because of this, the trend is now to correct the patients using the so-called double

switch procedure, combining atrial redirection with either an arterial switch[41] or use of an interventricular tunnel to the aorta, placing a conduit from the morphologically right ventricle to the pulmonary atrium[42]. This also makes it possible to correct patients with co-existing pulmonary atresia.

DOUBLE OUTLET VENTRICLE

When describing the ventriculo-arterial connections in the setting of overriding arterial valves, we have found it useful to apply the '50 percent rule'. On this basis, we define double outlet ventricle whenever more than half of the circumference of both arterial valves take their origin from the same ventricle[43]. In many patients, this problem does not arise, since both arterial trunks arise unequivocally from the one ventricle. Even when overriding, there is usually little question as to the anatomical assignment of the abnormal valve, since rarely does it appear to be equally committed to both chambers. Even then, if the decision is made according to the

connection of the leaflets as seen in short axis[44], there is little problem (Fig. 8.83). Making such designations on the basis of long axis views by means of angiography or echocardiography, however, can be misleading. Variations either in the angle of view, or streaming of the angiographic material, can make the appropriate assignment difficult. Nonetheless, if the '50 percent rule' is accepted as a pragmatic convention for decision-making, the subject of double outlet ventricle becomes straightforward, if not even simple.

Double outlet ventriculo-arterial connection can exist with such a wide variety of cardiac configurations that the possible combinations seem almost limitless. The cases which we will illustrate are those with both arteries arising from the right ventricle in the setting of concordant atrioventricular connections. The principles to be established are equally applicable in the setting of the other atrioventricular connections. Almost always, there is a co-existing ventricular septal defect[45]. It is then the anatomic relationship between

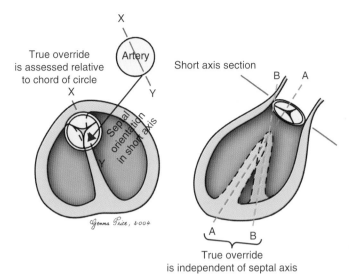

True override
is assessed relative
to chord of circle

Artery

Short axis section

Septal orientation in short axis

Gemma Price, 2004

True override
is independent of septal axis

Fig. 8.83 The cartoon shows how overriding arterial valves are assigned to one or other ventricle on the basis of their connection as judged in the short axis, left hand panel, in which it is possible to assess the tangent drawn by the ventricular septum (X-Y) relative to the short axis of the overriding arterial trunk, rather than the long axis of the ventricular septum (A-B in right hand panel), which can change depending on the motion of the heart.

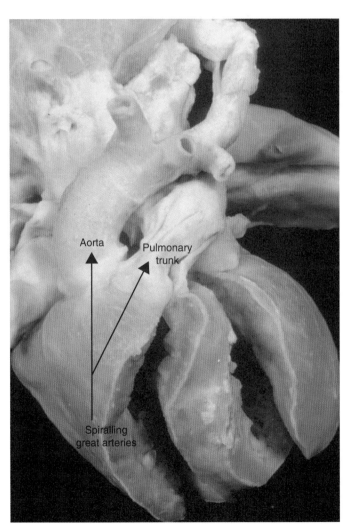

Aorta

Pulmonary trunk

Spiralling great arteries

Fig. 8.84 This specimen, shown in anatomic orientation from the front, has double outlet from the right ventricle with the interventricular communication in subaortic position. The great arterial trunks spiral in normal relationships as they leave the base of the heart.

the great arteries and the defect that is important to the surgeon. Also of significance is the presence of other associated anomalies.

In the majority of cases, the aorta and the pulmonary trunk are related more or less normally. The aortic valve, therefore, is posterior and to the right of the pulmonary valve, and the pulmonary trunk spirals round the aorta as it extends towards its bifurcation (Fig. 8.84). In the remainder, the arterial trunks arise from

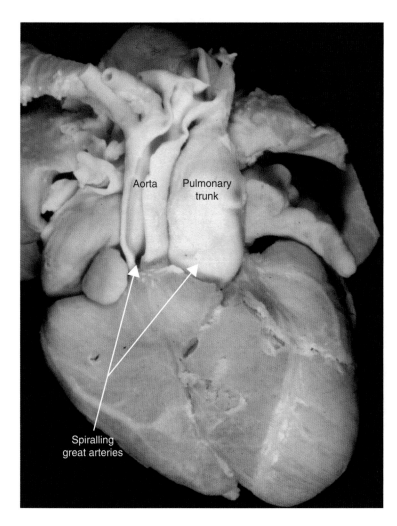

Aorta

Pulmonary trunk

Spiralling great arteries

Fig. 8.85 In this specimen, also seen in anatomical orientation from the front, and also with double outlet from the right ventricle, the interventricular communication was in subpulmonary position. The arterial trunks rise in parallel fashion as they exit from the base of the heart (compare with Fig. 8.84).

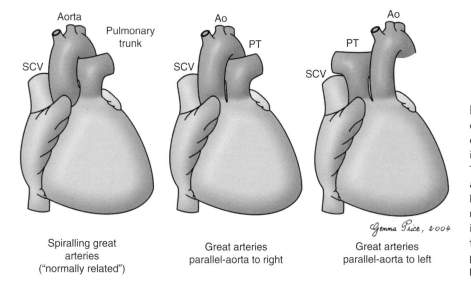

Aorta

Pulmonary trunk

SCV

Ao

PT

SCV

Ao

PT

SCV

Spiralling great arteries ("normally related")

Great arteries parallel-aorta to right

Great arteries parallel-aorta to left

Gemma Price, 2004

Fig. 8.86 The cartoon, drawn in anatomical orientation, shows the three typical orientations of the arterial trunks to be found in hearts with double outlet right ventricle. The arrangements with spiralling and parallel arterial trunks with the aorta to the right have been shown in Figs. 8.84 and 8.85. The rarest variant, shown in the right hand panel, is for the arterial trunks to rise in parallel fashion, but with the aorta in left-sided position. SCV – superior caval vein; Ao – aorta; PT – pulmonary trunk.

the base of the heart in parallel fashion, as anticipated when the ventriculo-arterial connections are discordant. For a good proportion of these, the arterial valves are side-by-side (Fig. 8.85), otherwise, the aortic valve is anterior. In a few cases, the aorta is posteriorly located because the pulmonary trunk is enlarged. Almost always the aorta is to the right but, in a small number of cases, the aorta can be left-sided relative to the pulmonary trunk (Fig. 8.86).

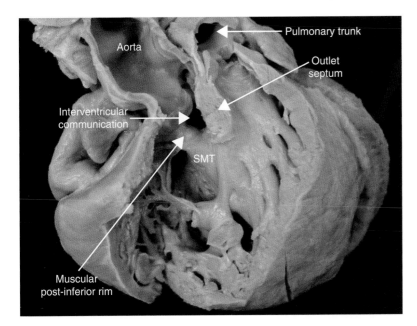

Fig. 8.87 In this specimen, shown in anatomic orientation from the front, the interventricular communication is cradled within the limbs of the septomarginal trabeculation (SMT). Note that the posterior limb of the trabeculation fuses with the ventriculo-infundibular fold, the muscular buttress thus formed protecting the atrioventricular conduction axis. The interventricular communication is directly adjacent to the aortic valve.

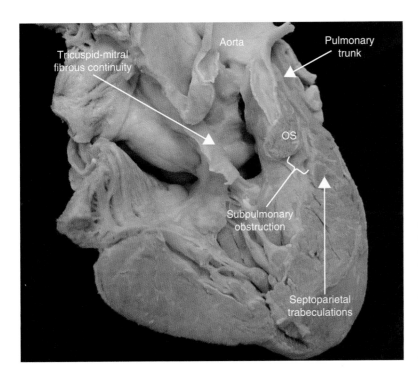

Fig. 8.88 In this specimen, shown in anatomic orientation, the outlet septum (OS) is attached to the anterior limb of the septomarginal trabeculation and the defect is subaortic. There is also extensive fibrous continuity between the leaflets of the mitral and tricuspid valves, making the defect perimembranous, despite the presence of bilateral infundibulums. Note that the subpulmonary infundibulum is obstructed, giving the morphology of tetralogy of Fallot, but with double outlet ventriculo-arterial connection and a subaortic infundibulum.

The most important associated anomaly is the interventricular communication, also described as the ventricular septal defect. Its anatomy should be considered in two ways. The first feature of significance is its proximity to the great arteries[45]. The second feature concerns its own intrinsic morphology[44]. When combining these two approaches, it must be remembered that, when there is double outlet from the right ventricle, the muscular ventricular septum itself separates only the inlet and apical trabecular components of the ventricles. The outlet septum, if present as muscular tissue, is found between the two outlets from the right ventricle. It is, therefore, exclusively a right ventricular structure, and does not form the roof of the interventricular communication[44].

Except when non-committed, the defect is to be found cradled between the limbs of the septomarginal trabeculation.

Its other borders vary depending on several features[44]. The first is whether the septomarginal trabeculation fuses with the ventriculoinfundibular fold. If it does, there is a muscular inferior rim to the defect. This then protects the conduction tissue axis as in tetralogy or transposition (Fig. 8.87). If it does not, there is continuity between the leaflets of the atrioventricular valves, and the defect is perimembranous (Fig. 8.88). The second

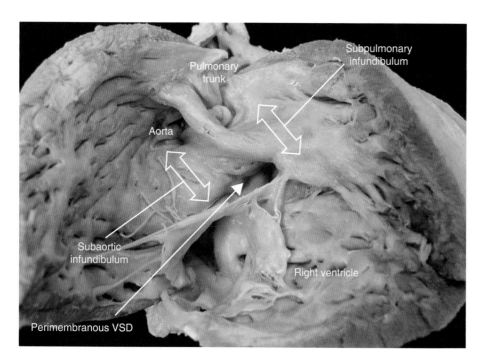

Fig. 8.89 In this specimen with double outlet right ventricle, seen in anatomic orientation, there is an extensive subaortic infundibulum, along with a long subpulmonary infundibulum (double headed arrows), but the defect is perimembranous, with fibrous continuity between the leaflets of the tricuspid and mitral valves.

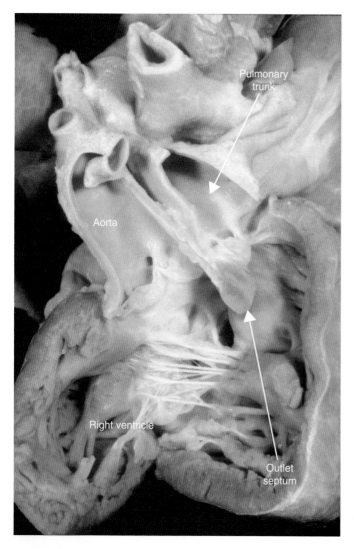

Fig. 8.90 In this specimen, seen in anatomic orientation, there is unequivocal double outlet from the right ventricle, but with fibrous continuity between the leaflets of the aortic, tricuspid, and mitral valves.

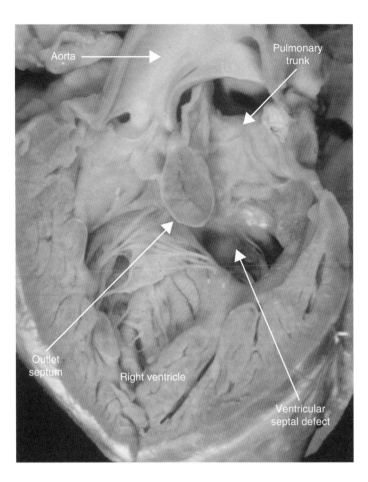

Aorta

Pulmonary trunk

Outlet septum

Right ventricle

Ventricular septal defect

Fig. 8.91 In this specimen, shown in anatomical orientation, the interventricular communication is positioned in subpulmonary location. This is the so-called "Taussig-Bing malformation". Note the attachment of the muscular outlet septum to the midpoint of the ventriculo-infundibular fold, along with bilateral infundibulums.

feature is the extent of the ventriculoinfundibular fold. When there is a well-formed fold, there are muscular infundibulums bilaterally, and the arterial valves are some distance away from the margins of the defect (Fig. 8.89). The defect can still be perimembranous in the setting of bilateral infundibulums, nonetheless, because of continuity between the leaflets of the mitral and tricuspid valves (Figs. 8.88, 8.89). When the ventriculo-infundibular fold is attenuated, the leaflets of one of the arterial valves are able to achieve fibrous continuity with an atrioventricular valve (Fig. 8.90).

The final feature is the relationship of the muscular outlet septum to the other structures. When attached to the anterior limb of the septomarginal trabeculation, the defect is subaortic (Figs. 8.87 –8.90). When, in contrast, the outlet septum is attached to the ventriculo-infundibular fold, or to the posterior limb of the septomarginal trabeculation, the defect is

placed beneath the left-sided great artery, which is almost always the pulmonary trunk (Fig. 8.91). When the outlet septum is absent, the defect is doubly committed and juxta-arterial (Fig. 8.92).

From this potential for variation, two "typical" groups of patients can be collected from those having double outlet from the right ventricle. The most frequent configuration is when the aortic valve is posterior and to the right of the pulmonary trunk (Fig. 8.84), usually with the perimembranous interventricular communication in subaortic position (Figs. 8.87–8.90). This arterial relationship can also be found with a doubly committed and juxta-arterial defect (Fig. 8.92). The second group comprise hearts in which the aorta ascends parallel to the pulmonary trunk (Fig. 8.85), usually with its valve either in anterior or side-by-side position, and to the right relative to the pulmonary valve, and with the septal defect in perimembranous or muscular

but subpulmonary position (Fig. 8.91). This is the so-called 'Taussig-Bing' variant[46].

The surgeon should be particularly wary when the interventricular communication is non-committed[47]. Almost always when it is subaortic, subpulmonary, or doubly committed, it is possible to place a patch within the right ventricle so as to connect the interventricular communication to one or other outflow tract, thus achieving biventricular connections. This may not be possible if the defect is anatomically non-committed, or else if the interventricular communication is adjacent to an outflow tract, but the potentially corrective pathways are blocked by structures such as valvar tension apparatus. Anatomical non-commitment is most usually found when the interventricular communication is between the ventricular inlets (Fig. 8.93), or is the ventricular component of an atrioventricular septal defect in patients with common atrioventricular junction.

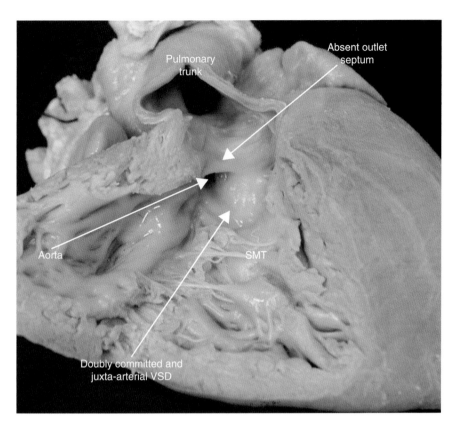

Fig. 8.92 In this specimen, shown in anatomical orientation, the interventricular communication (VSD) is double committed and juxta-arterial due to failure of formation of the subpulmonary muscular infundibulum. There is fibrous continuity between the leaflets of the aortic and pulmonary valves, and fibrous continuity also between the arterial valves and the mitral valve. SMT – septomarginal trabeculation.

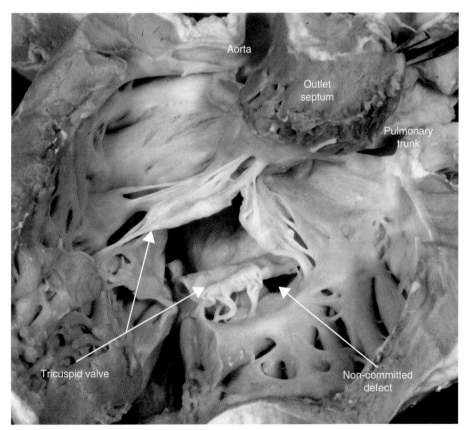

Fig. 8.93 In this specimen, shown in anatomic orientation, the interventricular communication opens between the ventricular inlets, and is shielded by the septal leaflet of the tricuspid valve. This feature, coupled with the distance from the outflow tracts, makes the defect non-committed. There is also an additional muscular inlet defect that is non-committed.

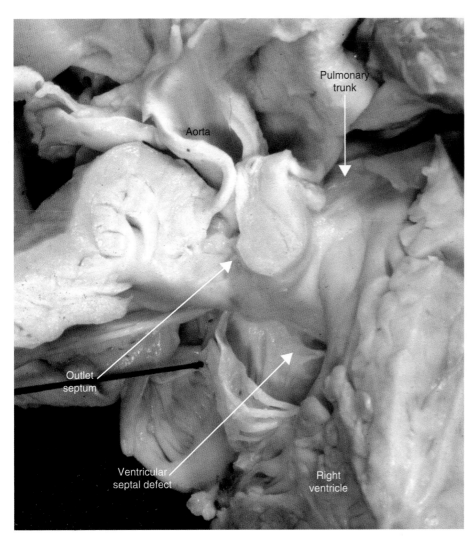

Fig. 8.94 In this specimen, also seen in anatomic orientation, the interventricular communication is again between the ventricular inlets (compare with Fig. 8.93). In this instance, however, it could be argued that, despite the relationship to the tricuspid valve, the defect could be committed surgically to the subpulmonary outlet. It is moot, therefore, as to whether the defect should be considered anatomically subpulmonary, or non-committed.

The surgeon may be able to overcome these impediments and still achieve biventricular repair[48]. In this situation, however, there may be arguments as to whether the defect is truly non-committed (Fig. 8.94). There is no question but that the defect is non-committed both anatomically and surgically when it is encased within the muscular septum and opens to the inlet of the right ventricle (Fig. 8.95).

It is also important for the surgeon to identify any other abnormalities in the extremely heterogeneous group of malformations linked together because of a double outlet ventriculo-arterial connection. By far the most common set of anomalies relates to obstruction of the arterial outlets, such as infundibular stenosis, valvar stenosis, coarctation or interruption of the aortic arch. The presence of subpulmonary infundibular stenosis is a particularly frequent finding when the septal defect is subaortic, often producing the morphology of tetralogy of Fallot, even in the setting of bilateral infundibulums (Fig. 8.88). Coarctation and interrupted arch, together with straddling of the mitral valve, are frequent accompaniments of the 'Taussig-Bing' variant[46]. Common atrioventricular valves also occur in a significant number of cases. Unusual coronary arterial anatomy, including the intramural arrangement, is found most frequently when the aorta is in anterior or side-by-side position. In this situation, special consideration is needed when performing either a right ventriculotomy or an arterial switch procedure[35].

Surgical and anatomical considerations for the potential corrective procedures relate to the particular combination of defects. It is possible, nonetheless, to establish some basic rules[49] (Fig. 8.96). The outlet septum, almost always present, serves as a guide to the arterial valves and their relationships to each other, and to the ventricular septal defect. As described above, in cases with subaortic defects the septum usually inserts into the anterior limb of the septomarginal trabeculation. With subpulmonary defects, it usually inserts into the ventriculo-infundibular fold, or into the posterior part of the ventricular septum. The outlet septum is always devoid of any vital structure, so it can be resected or used as a secure site for anchorage of sutures. In contrast, the ventriculo-infundibular fold is not a solid bar of muscle. Therefore, care must be taken to avoid extensive dissection or resection of this structure, since the right coronary artery lies within its fold.

Knowledge of the type of ventricular septal defect will, as in isolated defects, give accurate guidance to the disposition of the conduction tissue. Obstruction of the subpulmonary outflow tract requires the same attention to detail as when dealing with tetralogy of Fallot. Other cardiac anomalies will have to be dealt with in the context of the particular cardiac configuration present.

It may not have passed unnoticed that the group of hearts unified because of their double outlet ventriculo–arterial connections has been discussed thus far with little reference to the so-called "bilateral conus". This is because we do not take this feature as an integral feature of the group. To us, the term "double outlet" logically pictures a specific ventriculo-arterial connection, and that is what we have described. The presence or absence of a "bilateral conus" depends simply on whether the ventriculo-infundibular fold separates the atrioventricular and arterial valves

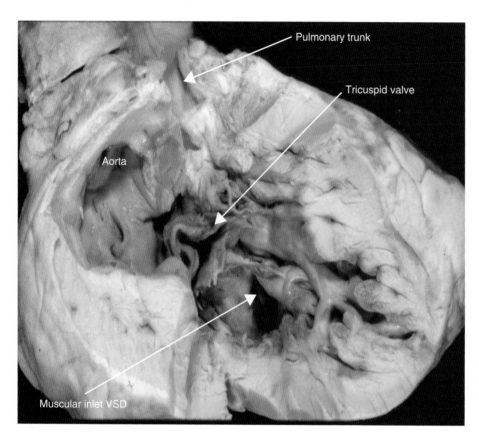

Fig. 8.95 In this specimen, again shown in anatomic orientation, the defect is within the muscular septum and opens to the right ventricular inlet. This defect is unequivocally non-committed.

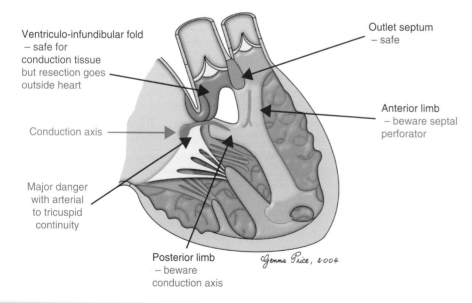

Fig. 8.96 The cartoon shows the major components of the outflow tracts, and illustrates the salient surgical features relating to each individual muscular component. The conduction axis is shown in green, and the first septal perforating artery as the red forked tongue. The ventriculo-infundibular fold is shown in red, the outlet septum in blue, and the septomarginal trabeculation in yellow.

completely, or else is attenuated at some point to permit fibrous continuity between their leaflets. Either arrangement can exist when the ventriculo–arterial connection is one of double outlet. Double outlet left ventricle can present with similar variations in the position of the arterial trunks, and their relationship to the interventricular communication, as we have described for double outlet right ventricle. As with double outlet right ventricle, double outlet left ventricle can be found with any atrioventricular connections. The rules for the disposition of the conduction tissue will then change accordingly.

COMMON ARTERIAL TRUNK

A common arterial trunk is one that supplies directly the systemic, pulmonary, and coronary arteries[50] (Fig. 8.97). In this way, the anomaly is distinguished from the other types of ventriculo–arterial connection producing single outlet from the heart, namely a solitary aortic trunk with pulmonary atresia, a solitary pulmonary trunk with aortic atresia, or a solitary arterial trunk.

We consider an arterial trunk to be solitary rather than common when it is not possible to find any evidence of intrapericardial pulmonary arteries[51]. Description in this fashion resolves the controversy as to whether the pulmonary arteries, had they been present, would have arisen from the arterial trunk or from the heart (Fig. 8.98). In patients with a solitary trunk as thus defined, it is the

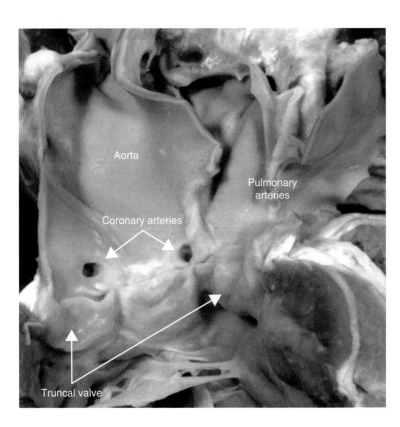

Aorta

Pulmonary arteries

Coronary arteries

Truncal valve

Fig. 8.97 The specimen, shown in anatomic orientation, illustrates the essence of a common arterial trunk. A solitary trunk leaves the base of the heart through a solitary arterial valve and supplies directly the systemic, pulmonary, and coronary arteries.

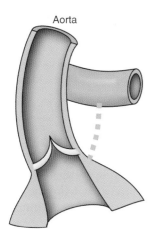

Aorta

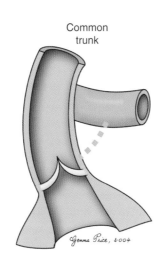

Common trunk

Gemma Price, 2004

Fig. 8.98 The cartoon illustrates the dilemma in defining the nature of an arterial trunk in the absence of any atretic intrapericardial pulmonary arteries (dotted channels). There is no way of knowing whether, had they existed, the pulmonary arteries would have originated directly from the heart (left hand panel) or from the arterial trunk itself (right hand panel). Had they originated from the heart, the patent arterial trunk would obviously have been an aorta. Had the trunk itself given rise initially to atretic pulmonary arteries, however, it would have initially have been a common trunk. In this situation, therefore, it is better to describe the arterial trunk simply as a solitary structure.

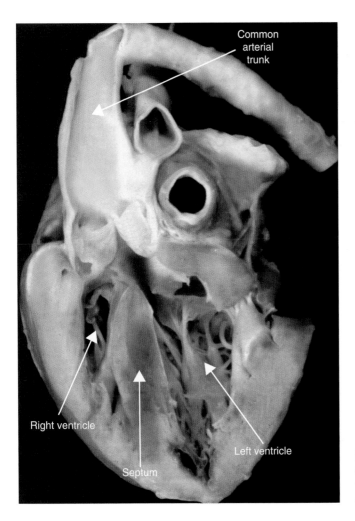

Common arterial trunk

Right ventricle

Septum

Left ventricle

Fig. 8.99 The heart has been sectioned along its long axis, and is shown in anatomical orientation, illustrating that the common arterial trunk overrides a juxta-arterial ventricular septal defect, being equally committed to both ventricles.

arterial supply to the pulmonary circulation that is the key to surgical treatment. Such patients are best considered along with tetralogy with pulmonary atresia (see page 205, Fig. 7.151).

The anatomical features that determine the success of surgical treatment for a common arterial trunk are its connection to the ventricular mass, the state of the truncal valve, the morphology of the ventricular septal defect, the presence of associated anomalies, and the arrangement of the great arteries arising from the common trunk. A common trunk can exist with any atrioventricular connection, but it is very rare to find other than concordant ones. The trunk usually overrides the ventricular septum, being more or less equally committed to the right and left ventricles (Fig. 8.99). The septal defect exists because of the complete lack of the muscular outlet septum, together with the septal

components of the sleeves of infundibular muscle. In consequence, the defect is directly juxta-arterial. It is usually cradled between the limbs of the septomarginal trabeculation, and in most patients the posterior limb fuses with the ventriculoinfundibular fold (Fig. 8.100). As with other defects of this type, the muscular structure thus formed serves to buttress the axis of atrioventricular conduction tissue from potential surgical damage. More rarely, there can be fibrous continuity between the truncal and tricuspid valves. The defect is then perimembranous, and the conduction axis is much more at risk during closure when connecting the common trunk to the left ventricle (Fig. 8.101). In the rare instance that the defect is restrictive, it is usually because the common trunk is connected exclusively or predominantly to the right ventricle (Fig. 8.102), often with a subtruncal infundibulum. If necessary, the

defect may be enlarged along its anterosuperior margins. Sometimes, a second muscular defect co-exists with the juxta-arterial defect. If present, such defects must be identified and closed. After surgical repair of a common trunk following the Rastelli technique, the truncal valve effectively becomes the aortic valve. Valvar incompetence or stenosis, if present, is therefore of considerable significance.

Variation in the arrangement of the great arteries is found in both the pulmonary and aortic pathways. Following the classical studies of Collett and Edwards[52], it has been usual to classify patients according to the mode of origin of the pulmonary arteries. The possibilities initially described were for the arteries to arise from a short confluent channel (Fig. 8.103), to arise separately and directly from the left posterior aspect of the trunk (Figs. 8.104, 8.105), or to arise separately

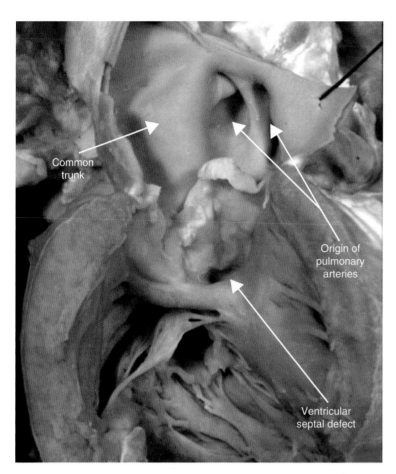

Fig. 8.100 This heart, shown in anatomic orientation as seen from the right ventricle, has a common arterial trunk overriding a ventricular septal defect with a muscular posteroinferior rim. The muscular rim protects the atrioventricular conduction axis.

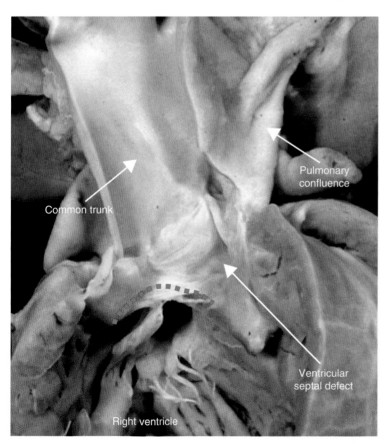

Fig. 8.101 This heart with a common arterial trunk, again viewed in anatomic orientation, has a ventricular septal defect that is perimembranous, with fibrous continuity between the leaflets of the truncal and tricuspid valves. The conduction axis, shown by the green dotted line, is at risk in the posteroinferior rim of the defect.

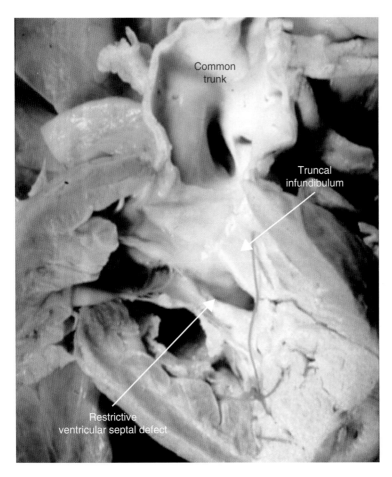

Fig. 8.102 In this heart with common arterial trunk, seen in anatomic orientation, the trunk arises exclusively from the right ventricle. The ventricular septal defect is restrictive.

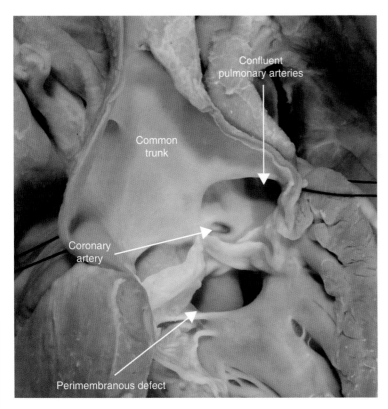

Fig. 8.103 In this heart, the common arterial trunk has been opened from the front, and is shown in anatomical orientation. The pulmonary arteries arise from the left side of the trunk via a confluent channel. The ventricular septal defect is perimembranous. Note the location of the coronary artery adjacent to a zone of apposition between two leaflets of the truncal valve.

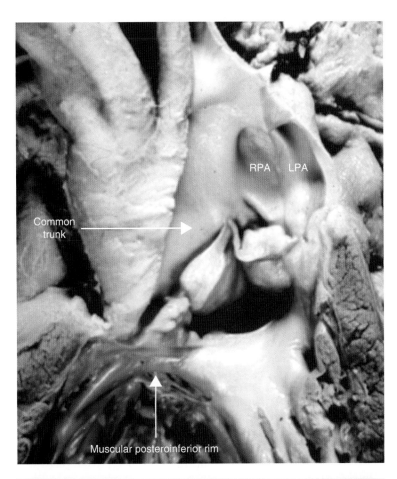

Fig. 8.104 In this heart, opened in comparable fashion to the heart shown in Fig. 103, and also photographed in anatomic orientation, the pulmonary arteries (RPA, LPA) arise by separate opening from the left posterior aspect of the common arterial trunk. In this instance, there is a muscular posteroinferior rim to the defect that protects the atrioventricular conduction axis. The truncal valve has four leaflets.

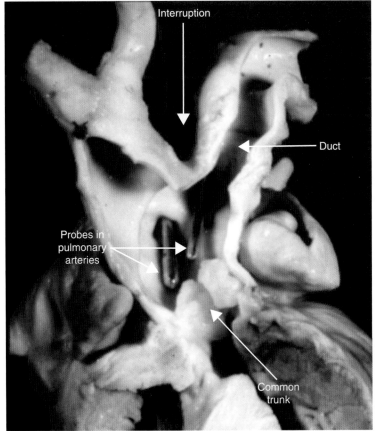

Fig. 8.105 This specimen, shown in anatomic orientation, has a common arterial trunk with interruption of the aortic arch between the left common carotid and subclavian arteries. The descending aorta is fed through the arterial duct. The probes are placed in the right and left pulmonary arteries, which arise separately from the back of the common trunk.

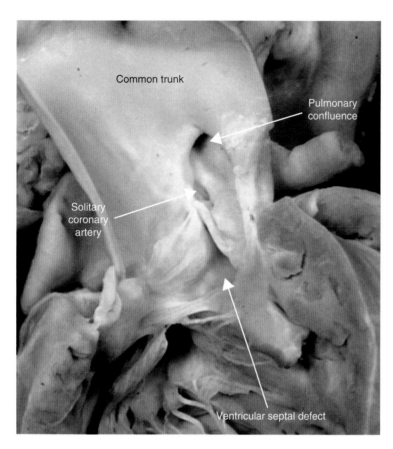

Common trunk

Pulmonary confluence

Solitary coronary artery

Ventricular septal defect

Fig. 8.106 This specimen is again opened anteriorly through a common arterial trunk, and photographed in anatomic orientation. Note the location of the solitary coronary artery, very close to the peripheral attachment of the zone of apposition between two of the leaflets of the trifoliate common truncal valve, and directly adjacent to the mouth of a confluent pulmonary channel (compare with Fig. 8.103).

from either side of the trunk. Rarer patterns also exist, such as origin of the pulmonary arteries within a truncal valvar sinus. Either of the first two patterns facilitates connection to a right ventricular conduit during complete repair. The much rarer variant, in which each pulmonary artery arises from the side of the trunk, makes complete repair more difficult, though not impossible. The so-called 'type IV' of Collett and Edwards[52], where there is no evidence of intrapericardial pulmonary arteries, is best considered to represent a solitary arterial trunk (see above).

Although it is the patterns of the pulmonary arteries which are traditionally used to categorise common trunk, the pattern of the aortic arch is of much more surgical significance. Usually the aorta arises in its anticipated position or, more rarely, anteriorly, but its branches continue to supply the branchiocephalic arteries, and it continues as the descending aorta. Not infrequently, however, the aortic arch is interrupted. This pattern will create problems for the surgeon. In this arrangement, the ascending aorta supplies all or only part of the arterial supply to the head, neck and arms. The interruption is usually at the isthmus, but it can occur proximal to the origin of the left subclavian artery. In either case, the descending aorta is supplied by the arterial duct (Fig. 8.105). If surgical repair is contemplated, it is imperative to recognise this arrangement, and to make appropriate modifications to the surgical procedure. Other variations in arterial pattern rarely occur in association with common trunks, such as crossed pulmonary arteries[53].

The surgeon should also take care to identify the origins of the coronary arteries[54]. Frequently, they arise above the sinutubular junction, often adjacent to the pulmonary arteries (Fig. 8.106). In this setting, they are at risk if unrecognised when the surgeon separates the pulmonary arteries from the common trunk.

References

1. Anderson RH, Macartney FJ, Tynan M, Becker AE, Freedom RM, Godman MJ, Hunter S, Quero Jimenez M, Rigby ML, Shinebourne EA, Sutherland G, Smallhorn JF, Soto B, Thiene G, Wilkinson JL, Wilcox BR, Zuberbuhler JR. Univentricular atrioventricular connection: the single ventricle trap unsprung. *Pediatr Cardiol* 1983; **4**: 273–280.

2. Anderson RH, Becker AE, Tynan M, Macartney FJ, Rigby ML, Wilkinson JL. The univentricular atrioventricular connection: getting to the root of a thorny problem. *Am J Cardiol* 1984; **54**: 822–828.

3. Anderson RH, Ho SY. What is a ventricle? *Ann Thorac Surg* 1998; **66**: 616–620.

4. Anderson RH, Becker AE, Macartney FJ, Shinebourne EA, Wilkinson JL, Tynan MJ. Is "tricuspid atresia" a univentricular heart? *Pediatr Cardiol* 1979; **1**: 51–56.

5. Bharati S, Lev M. Tricuspid atresia and univentricular heart. (Letter). *Pediatr Cardiol* 1980; **1**: 165–166.

6. Anderson RH, Baker EJ, Redington AN. Can we describe structure as well as function when accounting for the arrangement of the ventricular mass? *Cardiol Young* 2000; **10**: 247–260.

7. Kurosawa H, Imai Y, Fukuchi S, Sawatari K Koy Y, Nakazawa M, Takao A. Septation and Fontan repair of univentricular

atrioventricular connection. *J Thorac Cardiovas Surg* 1990; **99**: 314–319.

8. Gale AW, Danielson GK, McGoon DC, Wallace RB, Mair DD. Fontan procedure for tricuspid atresia. *Circulation* 1980; **62**: 91–96.

9. Laks H, Williams WG, Hillenbrand WE, Freedom RM, Talner NS, Rowe RD, Trusler GA. Results of right atrial to right ventricular and right atrial to pulmonary artery conduits for complex congenital heart disease. *Ann Surg* 1980; **192**: 382–389.

10. Fontan F, Kirklin JW, Fernandez G, Costa F, Naftel DC, Tritto F, Blackstone EH. Outcome after a "perfect" Fontan operation. *Circulation* 1990; **81**: 1520–1536.

11. Hosseinpour AR, Anderson RH, Ho SY. The anatomy of the septal perforating arteries in normal and congenitally malformed hearts. *J Thorac Cardiovasc Surg* 2001; **121**: 1046–1052.

12. Cheung HC, Lincoln C, Anderson RH, Ho SY, Shinebourne EA, Pallides S, Rigby ML. Options for surgical repair in hearts with univentricular atrioventricular connection and subaortic stenosis. *J Thorac Cardiovasc Surg* 1990; **100**: 672–681.

13. Abbott ME. *Unique case of congenital malformation of the heart.* Museum Notes. McGill University 1992; pp. 522–525.

14. Stefanelli G, Kirklin JW, Naftel DC, Blackstone EH, Pacifico AD, Kirklin JK, Soto B, Bargeron IM. Early and intermediate-term (10 year) results of surgery for univentricular atrioventricular connection ("single ventricle"). *Am J Cardiol* 1984; **54**: 811–821.

15. de Leval MR, Kilner P, Gewillig M, Bull C. Total cavopulmonary connection: a logical alternative to atriopulmonary connection for complex Fontan operations. *J Thorac Cardiovasc Surg* 1988; **96**: 682–695.

16. Marcelletti C, Corno A, Giannico S, Marino B. Inferior vena cava-pulmonary artery extracardiac conduit: a new form of right heart bypass. *J Thorac Cardiovasc Surg* 1990; **100**: 228–232.

17. Anderson RH, Arnold R, Thaper MK, Jones RS, Hamilton DI. Cardiac specialized tissues in hearts with an apparently single ventricular chamber (Double inlet left ventricle). *Am J Cardiol* 1974; **33**: 95–106.

18. Keeton BR, Macartney FJ, Hunter S, Mortera C, Rees P, Shinebourne EA, Tynan MJ, Wilkinson JL, Anderson RH. Univentricular heart of right ventricular type with double or common inlet. *Circulation* 1979; **59**: 403–411.

19. Essed CE, Ho SY, Hunter S, Anderson RH. Atrioventricular conduction system in univentricular heart of right ventricular type with right-sided rudimentary chamber. *Thorax* 1980; **35**: 123–127.

20. Anderson RH, Wilkinson JL, Gerlis LM, Smith A, Becker AE. Atresia of the right atrioventricular orifice. *Br Heart J* 1977; **39**: 414–428.

21. Orie JD, Anderson C, Ettedgui J, Zuberbuhler JR, Anderson RH. Echocardiographic-morphologic correlations in tricuspid atresia. *J Am Coll Cardiol* 1995; **26**: 750–758.

22. Bull C, de Leval M, Stark J, Macartney F. Use of a subpulmonary ventricular chamber in the Fontan circulation. *J Thorac Cardiovasc Surg* 1983; **85**: 21–31.

23. Rao PS, Jue KL, Isabel-Jones J, Ruttenberg HD. Ebstein's malformation of the tricuspid valve with atresia. *Am J Cardiol* 1973; **32**: 1004–1009.

24. Noonan JA, Nadas AS. The hypoplastic left heart syndrome. An analysis of 101 cases. *Pediatr Clin North Am* 1958; **5**: 1029–1056.

25. Norwood WI, Lang P, Hansen DD. Physiologic repair of the aortic atresia-hypoplastic left heart syndrome. *New Eng J Med* 1983; **308**: 23–26.

26. Van Praagh R. Transposition of the Great Arteries II. Transposition clarified. *Am J Cardiol* 1971; **28**: 739–741.

27. Van Mierop LHS. Transposition of the great arteries. Clarification or further confusion? Editorial. *Am J Cardiol* 1971; **28**: 735–738.

28. Jaggers JJ, Cameron DE, Herlong JR, Ungerleider RM. Congenital Heart Surgery Nomenclature and Database Project: transposition of the great arteries. *Ann Thorac Surg* 2000; **69 (Suppl 4)**: S205–S235.

29. Isaacson R, Titus JL, Merideth J, Feldt RH, McGoon DC. Apparent interruption of atrial conduction pathways after surgical repair of transposition of the great arteries. *Am J Cardiol* 1972; **30**: 533–535.

30. Ullal RR, Anderson RH, Lincoln C. Mustard's operation modified to avoid dysrhythmias and pulmonary and systemic venous obstruction. *J Thorac Cardiovasc Surg* 1979; **78**: 431–439.

31. Shaher RM, Puddu GC. Coronary arterial anatomy in complete transposition of the great arteries. *Am J Cardiol* 1966; **17**: 355–361.

32. Yacoub MH, Radley-Smith R. Anatomy of the coronary arteries in transposition of the great arteries and methods for their transfer in anatomical correction. *Thorax* 1978; **33**: 418–424.

33. Gittenberger-de-Groot AC, Sauer U, Oppenheimer-Dekker A, Quaegebeur J. Coronary arterial anatomy in transposition of the great arteries: a morphologic study. *Pediatr Cardiol* 1983; **4**: 15–24.

34. Gittenberger-de-Groot AC, Sauer U, Quaegebeur J. Aortic intramural coronary artery in three hearts with transposition of the great arteries. *J Thorac Cardiovasc Surg* 1986; **91**: 566–571.

35. Massoudy P, Baltalarli A, de Leval MR, Cook A, Neudorf U, Derrick G, McCarthy KP, Anderson RH. Anatomic variability in coronary arterial distribution with regard to the arterial switch procedure. *Circulation* 2002; **106**: 1980–1984.

36. Anderson RH, Becker AE, Arnold R, Wilkinson JL. The conducting tissues in congenitally corrected transposition. *Circulation* 1974; **50**: 911–923.

37. Van Praagh R. What is congenitally corrected transposition? *N Eng J Med* 1970; **282**: 1097–1098.

38. de Leval M, Bastos P, Stark J, Taylor JFN, Macartney FJ, Anderson RH. Surgical technique to reduce the risks of heart block following closure of ventricular septal defect in atrioventricular discordance. *J Thorac Cardiovasc Surg* 1979; **78**: 515–526.

39. Anderson RH, Becker AE, Gerlis LM. The pulmonary outflow tract in classically corrected transposition. *J Thorac Cardiovasc Surg* 1975; **69**: 747–757.

40. Becker AE, Ho SY, Caruso G, Milo S, Anderson RH. Straddling right atrioventricular valves in atrioventricular discordance. *Circulation* 1980; **61**: 1133–1141.

41. Ilbawi MN, DeLeon SY, Backer CL, Duffy LE, Muster AJ, Vales VR, Paul MH. An alternative approach to the surgical management for physiologically corrected transposition with ventricular septal defect and pulmonary stenosis or atresia. *J Thorac Cardiovasc Surg* 1990; **100**: 410–415.

42. Imai Y, Sawatori K, Hoshino S, Ishihara K, Nakazawa M, Momma K. Ventricular function after anatomic repair in patients with atrioventricular discordance. *J Thorac Cardiovasc Surg* 1994; **107**: 1272–1283.

43. Wilcox BR, Ho SY, Macartney FJ, Becker AE, Gerlis IM, Anderson RH. Surgical anatomy of double-outlet right

ventricle with situs solitus and atrioventricular concordance. *J Thorac Cardiovasc Surg* 1981; **82**: 405–417.

44. Anderson RH, McCarthy K, Cook AC. Double outlet right ventricle. *Cardiol Young* 2001; **11**: 329–344.

45. Lev M, Bharati S, Meng CCL, Liberthson RR, Paul MH, Idriss F. A concept of double-outlet right ventricle. *J Thorac Cardiovasc Surg* 1972; **64**: 271–281.

46. Stellin G, Zuberbuhler JR, Anderson, RH, Siewers RD. The surgical anatomy of the Taussig-Bing malformation. *J Thorac Cardiovasc Surg* 1987; **93**: 560–569.

47. Stellin G, Ho SY, Anderson RH, Zuberbuhler JR, Siewers RD. The surgical anatomy of double-outlet right ventricle with concordant atrioventricular connection and non-committed ventricular septal defect. *J Thorac Cardiovasc Surg* 1991; **102**: 849–855.

48. Lacour-Gayet F, Haun C, Ntalakoura K, Belli E, Houyel L, Marcsek P, Wagner F, Weil J. Biventricular repair of double outlet right ventricle with non-committed ventricular septal defect (VSD) by VSD rerouting to the pulmonary artery and arterial switch. *Eur J Cardiothorac Surg* 2002; **21**: 1042–1048.

49. Capuani A, Uemura H, Ho SY, Anderson RH. Anatomic spectrum of abnormal ventriculoarterial connections: surgical implications. *Ann Thorac Surg* 1995; **59**: 352–360.

50. Crupi G, Macartney FJ, Anderson RH. Persistent truncus arteriosus. A study of 66 autopsy cases with special reference to definition and morphogenesis. *Am J Cardiol* 1977; **40**: 569–578.

51. Anderson RH, Thiene G Editorial. Categorization and description of hearts with a common arterial trunk. *Eur J Cardiothorac Surg* 1989; **3**: 481–487.

52. Collett RW Edwards JE. Persistent truncus arteriosus. A classification according to anatomic types. *Surg Clin North Am* 1949; **29**: 1245–1270.

53. Jue KL, Lockman LA, Edwards JE. Anomalous origins of pulmonary arteries from pulmonary trunk ("crossed pulmonary arteries"). Observations in a case with 18 trisomy syndrome. *Am Heart J* 1966; **71**: 807–812.

54. Suzuki A, Ho SY, Anderson RH, Deanfield JE. Coronary arterial and sinusal anatomy in hearts with a common arterial trunk. *Ann Thorac Surg* 1989; **48**: 792–797.

9

Abnormalities of the great vessels

ANOMALOUS SYSTEMIC VENOUS DRAINAGE

Abnormal systemic venous connections are usually of little surgical significance, since their clinical consequences are limited. The anomalies are apt to be encountered as the surgeon pursues a more complex associated intracardiac anomaly, and are of most significance in the setting of isomeric atrial appendages (visceral heterotaxy). They may be grouped into the following categories: absence or abnormal drainage of the right caval vein(s); persistence or abnormal drainage of the left caval vein(s); and abnormal hepatic venous connections. Abnormalities of the coronary sinus usually fall into one of these groups, except the so-called 'unroofed' coronary sinus, which has been already discussed in Chapter 7.

Abnormalities of the right superior caval vein

These are extremely rare. The vein may be diminished in size. Alternatively, it may be completely absent when the venous return from the head, neck and arms passes through a persistent left superior caval vein to the right atrium by way of the coronary sinus (Fig. 9.1) or, rarely, directly into the left atrium. Only this last situation requires surgical intervention. The other conditions, if encountered during an open-heart operation, would require some adjustment from the usual technique used for cannulation. Though there is no definite evidence to this effect, we would not expect these abnormalities to affect the location of the sinus node.

Abnormalities of the inferior caval vein

The inferior caval vein has been described to connect directly to the morphologically left atrium[1], producing right-to-left shunting, albeit that we have never seen such a lesion. When the inferior caval vein does drain to the left atrium, this is usually because a persistent Eustachian valve directs flow from the right atrium through the oval fossa (Fig. 9.2). Such right-to-left shunting can also be an iatrogenic phenomenon, occasionally observed when low-lying atrial septal defects are improperly closed (see Chapter 7). The more frequent anomaly afflicting the inferior caval vein is interruption of its terminal segment, with return of the venous blood from the lower body through the azygos or hemiazygos venous systems[2]. This malformation is seen most frequently with isomerism of the left atrial appendages[3] (Fig. 9.3). The hepatic veins then usually drain independently into the right-sided or left-sided atrium, although there can be a confluent suprahepatic channel. Interruption of the inferior caval vein with azygos continuation can also occur in individuals with lateralised atrial chambers. The hepatic veins then always connect to the right atrium through a suprahepatic segment of the inferior caval vein (Fig. 9.4).

Persistence of the left superior caval vein

The commonest malformation involving the caval veins is persistence of the left superior caval vein (Fig. 9.1). In this setting, the persisting left vein is joined to the right superior caval vein by a brachiocephalic vein in about three-fifth of reported cases[4]. When arranged in this fashion, the left caval vein can simply be clamped or ligated, so as to avoid flooding the field when the heart is opened. If connections with the right vein are not apparent, a trial period of occlusion will usually indicate whether venous hypertension will give problems. A left superior caval vein is found not infrequently in patients with cyanotic heart disease, being reported in up to one-fifth of patients with tetralogy of Fallot, and one-twelfth of patients with Eisenmenger's syndrome[5]. This venous

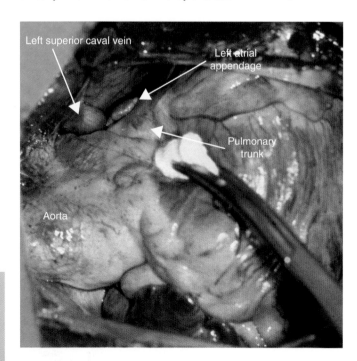

Fig. 9.1 This operative view through a median sternotomy shows a left superior caval vein entering the pericardial cavity between the left atrial appendage and the pulmonary trunk.

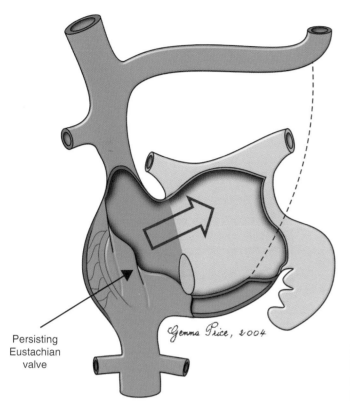

Persisting
Eustachian
valve

Gemma Price, 2004

Fig. 9.2 The cartoon shows the most frequent mechanism by which the venous return through the inferior caval vein drains to the left atrium. It is deflected across a defect within the oval fossa (red arrow) due to persistence of the Eustachian valve.

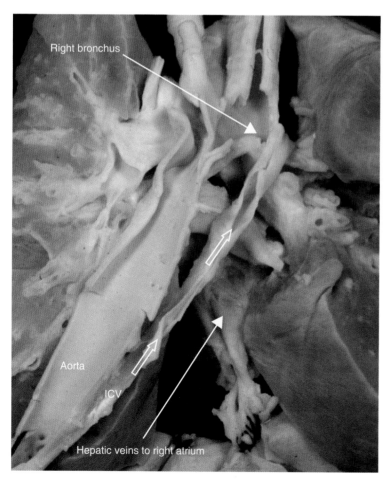

Right bronchus

Aorta

ICV

Hepatic veins to right atrium

Fig. 9.3 The heart is photographed from the right side, showing interruption of the abdominal course of the inferior caval vein, with the venous return from the abdomen returned to the heart through the azygos system of veins (arrows). There was associated isomerism of the left atrial appendages.

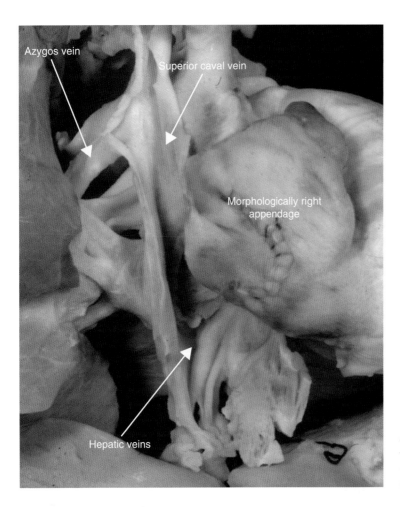

Fig. 9.4 This heart, again photographed from the right side in anatomic orientation, also has interruption of the inferior caval vein with return of venous blood from the abdomen through the azygos system of veins. In this instance, there is usual atrial arrangement. Note the structure of the morphologically right appendage.

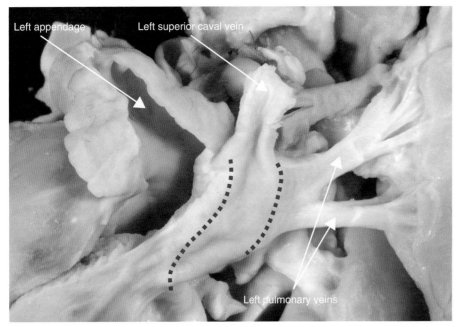

Fig. 9.5 The heart is photographed from behind in anatomic orientation. A persistent left superior caval vein enters the left atrioventricular groove between the left appendage and the left pulmonary veins, with its course through the groove marked by the red dotted lines. The opening in the right atrium through the enlarged coronary sinus is shown in Fig. 9.6.

channel can be the route of partially or totally anomalous pulmonary venous connection. It can also empty directly into the left atrium, so-called 'unroofing of the coronary sinus'. Much more frequently, it is encountered as an isolated lesion that usually receives the hemiazygos vein before penetrating the pericardium and passing between the left atrial appendage and the left pulmonary veins (Fig. 9.5). It then connects with the coronary sinus behind the heart to empty into the right atrium

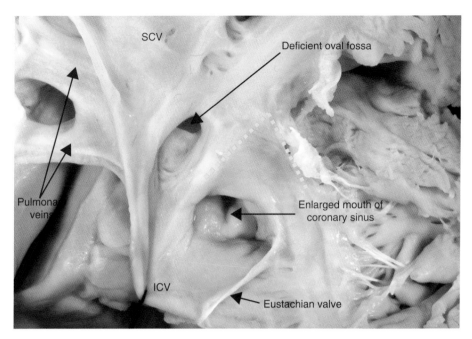

Fig. 9.6 This photograph, again in anatomical orientation, shows the enlarged orifice of the coronary sinus within the right atrium of the heart shown in Fig. 9.5. Note the location of the triangle of Koch (yellow dotted lines). SCV – right superior caval vein; ICV – inferior caval vein.

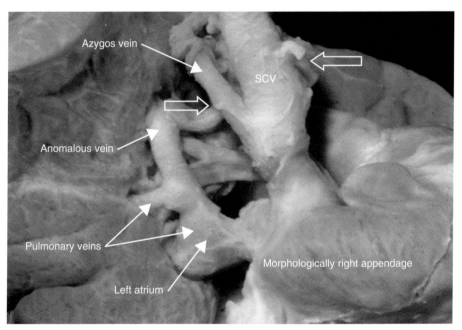

Fig. 9.7 This specimen, from a patient with hypoplasia of the left heart, photographed in anatomic orientation, shows the course of the so-called levoatrial cardinal vein. The pulmonary veins connect in normal fashion to the left atrium, but the anomalous vein drains the atrial contents to the superior caval vein. Thus, there are normal venous connections, but anomalous drainage.

through a larger than normal orifice (Fig. 9.6). In such hearts, the Thebesian valve is often attenuated or absent.

Levoatrial cardinal vein

Another anomaly that, although rare, warrants consideration is the levoatrial cardinal vein[6,7]. This channel connects the left atrium to the systemic venous system. It is found with associated lesions such as mitral atresia, where it functions as the only route for pulmonary venous return (Fig. 9.7). Then, although the pulmonary

veins are normally connected to the morphologically left atrium, the pattern of venous return is comparable to the 'snowman' types of anomalous pulmonary venous connection (see below).

ANOMALOUS PULMONARY VENOUS CONNECTION

Very rarely, the pulmonary veins may be obstructed or totally atretic at their atrial junction[8]. This is unlikely to be a surgically remedial situation. Much more commonly, the pulmonary venous system,

either totally or in part, has an anomalous connection. There is a plethora of possibilities for abnormal pulmonary venous connections[9–11]. The arrangements should be described as specifically and as unambiguously as possible (Fig. 9.8). The pulmonary veins connect anomalously when they are not joined to the morphologically left atrium. Consequently, if all the veins from one lung connect to a site other than the left atrium, the arrangement can be described as unilateral totally anomalous pulmonary venous connection. If all the veins from

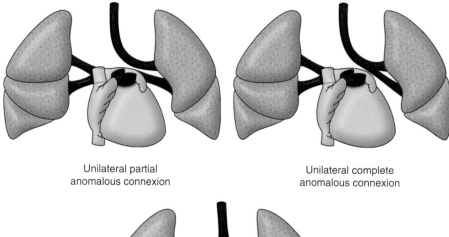

Unilateral partial
anomalous connexion

Unilateral complete
anomalous connexion

Total anomalous connexion
(bilateral and complete)

Fig. 9.8 This cartoon, in anatomic orientation, shows how anomalous connection of the pulmonary veins can be well accounted for by describing the connection of the veins from each lung as separate entities, and then describing partially as opposed to totally anomalous drainage on each side. The site of drainage needs to be specified separately (see Fig. 9.9).

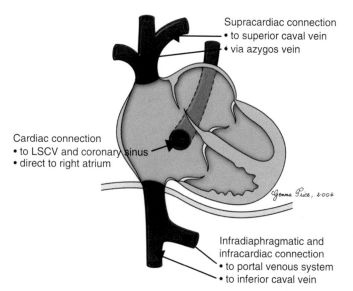

Supracardiac connection
• to superior caval vein
• via azygos vein

Cardiac connection
• to LSCV and coronary sinus
• direct to right atrium

Infradiaphragmatic and
infracardiac connection
• to portal venous system
• to inferior caval vein

Fig. 9.9 This cartoon, in anatomic orientation, shows the potential sites for anomalous connection of the pulmonary veins. (LSCV – left superior caval vein).

both lungs connect to sites other than the morphologically left atrium, there is totally anomalous pulmonary venous connection. This, of necessity, implies bilateral totally anomalous connection.

Any combination can readily be described by treating each lung as an entity. The unifying feature in all of these combinations is the connection of one or more pulmonary veins to the systemic venous system or to the right atrium. It is equally important, therefore, that the site of drainage be identified. Historically, this has been described as supradiaphragmatic or infradiaphragmatic (Fig. 9.9). The supradiaphragmatic group can be subdivided into supracardiac and cardiac groups. Supracardiac connection may be to a right or left superior caval vein, the brachiocephalic (innominate) vein, or even the azygos vein. Connection to the brachiocephalic vein is most frequent. The combination of drainage via a vertical vein and thence via the brachiocephalic vein to the superior caval vein (Fig. 9.10) produces the typical 'snowman' configuration as seen on chest radiography. Drainage directly to the right atrium is typically through the coronary sinus (Fig. 9.11). In our

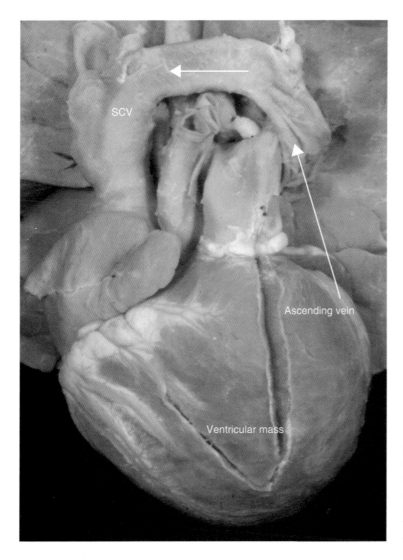

SCV

Ascending vein

Ventricular mass

Fig. 9.10 This heart, photographed from the front in anatomic orientation, has totally anomalous pulmonary venous connection to the superior caval vein (SCV). With this arrangement, the heart forms the body of the "snowman" seen in the chest radiograph, with the anomalous vein forming the head of the snowman as it courses to drain in the caval vein (arrow).

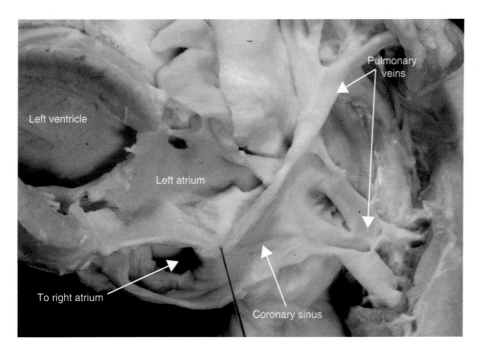

Pulmonary veins

Left ventricle

Left atrium

To right atrium

Coronary sinus

Fig. 9.11 This specimen, viewed from behind in anatomic orientation, has anomalous connection of all four pulmonary veins to the coronary sinus.

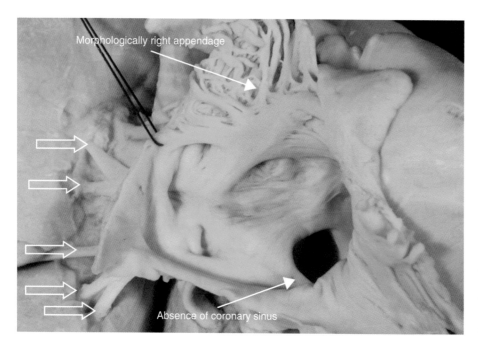

Fig. 9.12 In this heart, all four pulmonary veins (arrows) are connected directly to the right atrium, the lowermost vein through two tributaries. There was isomerism of the right atrial appendages. Note the absence of the coronary sinus.

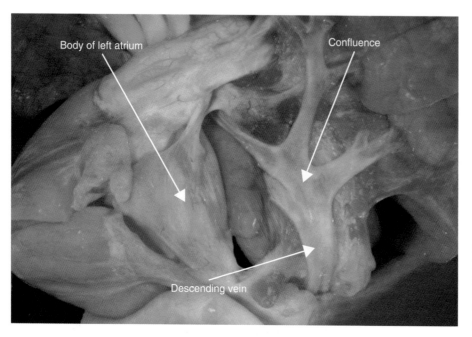

Fig. 9.13 This specimen, viewed from behind in anatomic orientation, has anomalous connection of all pulmonary veins to a descending channel that passes through the diaphragm to join the portal venous circulation.

experience, totally anomalous connection to the right atrium other than through the coronary sinus has been seen only in the setting of isomerism of the right atrial appendages (Fig. 9.12). Infradiaphragmatic connection is usually total except when there is partially right-sided connection to the inferior caval vein. This latter arrangement is the so-called 'scimitar syndrome', a name taken from its likeness to a Turkish sword when seen roentgenographically[12]. In the usual infradiaphragmatic connection, the common channel connecting both lungs lies outside the pericardium posterior to the left atrium. A vertical vein drains through the diaphragm as a single channel to enter the portal vein or the venous duct (Fig. 9.13). Occasionally, the channel breaks up into a series of branches which connect to the gastric veins (Fig. 9.14). It is very rare to find infradiaphragmatic connection directly to the inferior caval vein.

The salient anatomical features relating to surgical repair of anomalous pulmonary connections include the type of abnormal connection, for example, total, unilateral or mixed, the site of anomalous connection, and the proximity of the anomalous veins to the left atrium. As pointed out in Chapter 7, an interatrial communication in the mouth of the superior caval vein, the so-called sinus venosus defect, is always accompanied by anomalous connection of the right pulmonary veins to the superior caval vein. The need to safeguard the sinus node and its blood supply has already been emphasised.

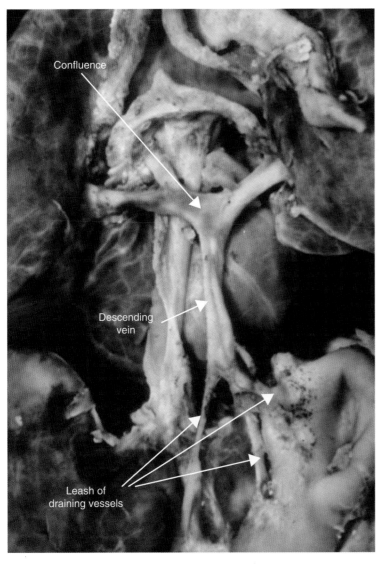

Confluence

Descending
vein

Leash of
draining vessels

Fig. 9.14 In this heart, also with totally anomalous pulmonary venous connection, the descending channel fragments into a leash of small veins that join the gastric veins. Viewed from behind in anatomic orientation.

Other sites of connection, or potential sites of anastomosis, often require construction of an extensive atrial junction to guard postoperatively against pulmonary venous obstruction. The appropriate landmarks must be borne in mind. Two types of anomalous connection pose particular problems. The first is when the anomalous venous return is by way of the coronary sinus (Fig. 9.11). We initially thought that the myocardium between the coronary sinus and the left atrium was common to both structures. We now know that the sinus has its own myocardial wall, separate from that of the left atrium[13]. It is possible, nonetheless, to incise both walls so as to unroof the sinus. At the same time, the orifice of the coronary sinus can be made confluent with the atrial septal defect, which is almost invariably within the oval fossa.

It is important to remove enough of the walls to ensure that the patch placed across the orifice of the coronary sinus and oval fossa does not produce obstruction at the site of the incised sinus septum. Ideally, the incised walls of atrium and coronary sinus should also be repaired, since the incisions create a route to the inferior atrioventricular groove. Thus far, however, we are unaware of any reports of tamponade following such procedures. The surgeon should be aware, nonetheless, that a potential opening is created to the extracardiac spaces. When incising the coronary sinus, it is also important to avoid the atrioventricular node at the apex of the triangle of Koch.

The second problematic type of connection is the infradiaphragmatic variant. The extrapericardial common pulmonary venous trunk is further from

the posterior left atrial wall than might be expected. Because of this, the anastomosis constructed between the trunk and left atrium is vulnerable to obstruction, particularly at its lateral extreme. This may become evident only when bypass is discontinued and the heart fills with blood.

ANOMALIES OF THE AORTA

The congenital anomalies of the thoracic aorta that are of interest to the surgeon include coarctation, the spectrum of partial to complete interruption of the aorta, and vascular "rings" and "slings".

Aortic coarctation

Coarctation is a congenitally-derived discrete shelf-like lesion within the aorta which causes obstruction to the flow of

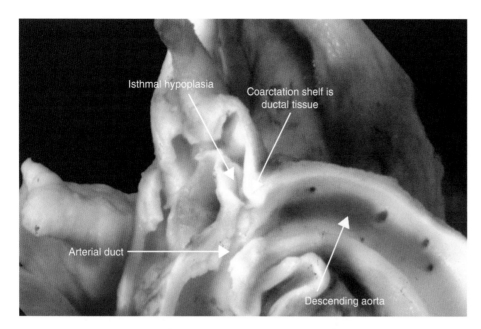

Fig. 9.15 This specimen, viewed in anatomic orientation shows the ductal tissue that forms the shelf lesion of aortic coarctation. Note the co-existing hypoplasia of the aortic isthmus.

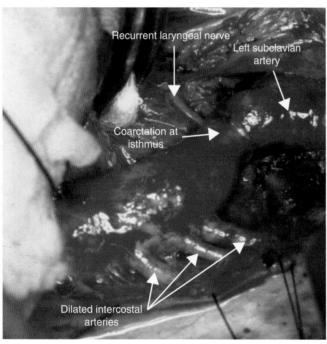

Fig. 9.16 This operative view, through a left thoracotomy, shows aortic coarctation with enlarged intercostal arteries, part of a well-developed collateral circulation.

blood. It is most often found just distal to the left subclavian artery, but can occur proximally or more distally, and even in the abdominal aorta. It is usually accompanied by some degree of tubular hypoplasia of the aorta, but is anatomically independent of the hypoplasia. It can co-exist with other lesions that diminish left-sided flow, but coarctation can, and does, occur independently. Tubular hypoplasia, when involving the isthmic segment of the aortic arch, can then be considered as part of a spectrum leading to atresia or interruption of the aortic arch.

Much has been made of the role of ductal tissue in the aetiology of coarctation. Although there was a time when some doubted its significance, the evidence supporting its inclusion in the coarctation shelf (Fig. 9.15) is now unequivocal[14–16]. Certainly the surgeon needs to be aware of the importance of removing all the ductal tissue during repair. The significance of the duct itself devolves upon its patency. If the duct is patent, typically there is an associated congenital anomaly that promotes increased flow of blood through the

pulmonary trunk, and diverts blood away from the proximal aorta. In these circumstances, the associated anomaly tends to dominate the picture, and will determine the most appropriate surgical therapy. On the other hand, coarctation with a closed duct is very likely to be an isolated lesion, except for the occasional association with a bifoliate aortic valve[17].

The chief concerns of the surgeon relate to the specific anatomy of the coarctation. The nature of the collateral circulation is of particular significance. With well-developed collateral arteries (Fig. 9.16)

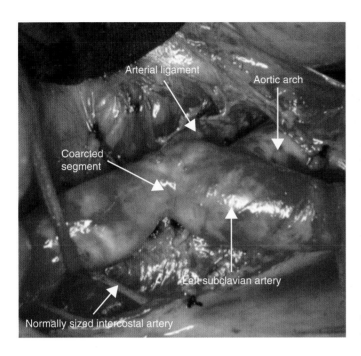

Fig. 9.17 In this operative view through a left thoracotomy, again from a patient with aortic coarctation (compare with Fig. 9.16), the collateral circulation is not well-developed.

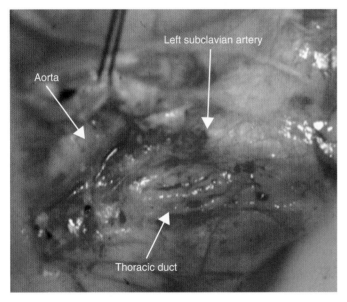

Fig. 9.18 This view through a left lateral thoracotomy shows the thoracic duct as it passes from the area of coarctation behind the left subclavian artery.

there is little danger of cross-clamping the aorta during repair. If the collaterals are less well-developed (Fig. 9.17), however, clamping the aorta may have several deleterious consequences. These include strain on the left ventricle due to proximal hypertension, which may also induce a cerebrovascular accident secondary to rupture of a 'berry' aneurysm. There may be distal aortic hypotension, at pressures of less than 50 millimeters of mercury, which endangers the splanchnic and spinal vascular beds. Irrespective of the nature of the collaterals, the spinal circulation is best preserved by interrupting none, or as few as possible, of the intercostal vessels. Temporary occlusion of the intercostal vessels adjacent to the operative field seems to be a reasonable compromise in this difficult situation.

Other noteworthy features include the position of the thoracic duct (Fig. 9.18), and the occasional presence of an anomalous artery (Fig. 9.19), sometimes referred to as 'Abbott's artery'. When present, this artery arises from the posteromedial aspect of the proximal descending aorta. Whether it is an enlarged bronchial artery, or 'persistence of the evanescent fifth arch', as suggested by Hamilton and Abbott[18], is irrelevant, albeit that the latter seems unlikely since the fifth arch has yet to be discovered during normal development. What is important is that the surgeon be aware of the existence of this anomalous vessel that, if not properly managed, can lead to substantial bleeding during the repair[19].

Interruption of the aortic arch

Discontinuity of the aorta, as opposed to coarctation, has been variously referred to as absence, atresia or interruption of the arch. Included in this group are those

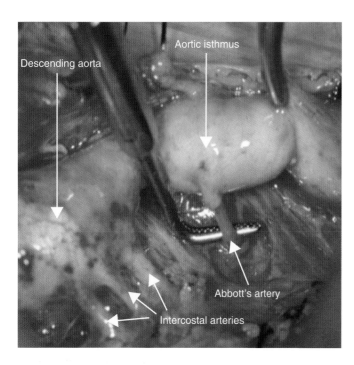

Fig. 9.19 As seen through a left thoracotomy, the proximal descending aorta and distal arch have been rotated anteriorly. The large collateral vessel referred to as 'Abbott's artery' is seen arising proximally to the area of coarctation.

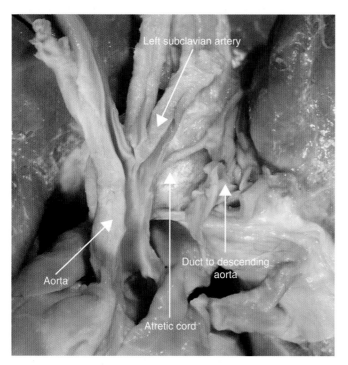

Fig. 9.20 This specimen, photographed in anatomic orientation, has atresia of the isthmus, with a thin fibrous cord running from the site of effective interruption at the left subclavian artery to the distal descending aorta, which is fed through the arterial duct.

cases with a fibrous cord or bridge of tissue (Fig. 9.20), as well as those with a gap, or absolute discontinuity, at some point in the arch (Fig. 9.21). Interruption can occur at one of three positions: at the isthmus; between the left subclavian and left common carotid arteries; and between the left common carotid and brachiocephalic arteries (Fig. 9.22). These lesions typically are found in the setting of a unilateral left aortic arch but, rarely, a right arch can be similarly affected[20]. Since patients with discontinuity of the aorta are unlikely to survive without surgical treatment, they are a particular challenge to the clinician. The associated cardiovascular malformations are of critical importance, for they affect the operative outcome as much as does interrupted arch itself.

Almost always there is a patent connection to the distal aorta through the duct (Fig. 9.21). A 'proximal' septal defect is also the rule. This is most frequently a ventricular septal defect but, occasionally, an aortopulmonary window is found. The ventricular septal defect is usually perimembranous, and is typically associated with posterior and leftward displacement of the outlet septum,

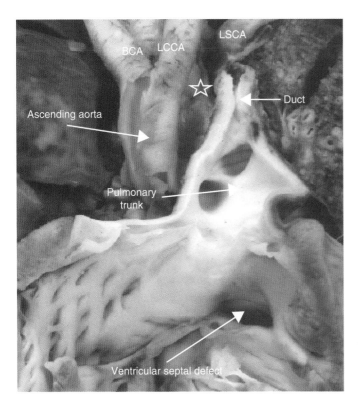

Fig. 9.21 In this specimen, shown in anatomic orientation as photographed from the front, the aortic arch is interrupted (star) between the left common carotid artery (LCCA) and the left subclavian artery (LSCA), the latter fed from the pulmonary trunk via the arterial duct. The ascending aorta is hypoplastic, and also gives rise to the brachiocephalic artery (BCA). Note the muscular ventricular septal defect, with posterior malalignment of the outlet septum (see Fig. 9.23).

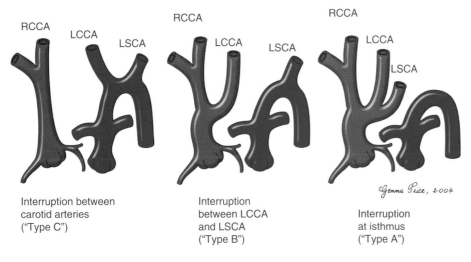

Interruption between carotid arteries ("Type C")

Interruption between LCCA and LSCA ("Type B")

Interruption at isthmus ("Type A")

Fig. 9.22 This cartoon, in anatomic orientation, shows the different sites of interruption of the aortic arch. The ascending aorta, and the vessels it feeds, are shown in red. The pulmonary trunk, and the vessels fed via the arterial duct, are shown in blue. RCCA – right common carotid artery; LCCA – left common carotid artery; LSCA – left subclavian artery. The right subclavian artery usually takes origin from the brachiocephalic trunk, but can have retro-oesophageal origin from the descending aorta (see Fig. 9.27).

resulting in subaortic stenosis (Fig. 9.23). Any type of defect, nonetheless, can be found. Abnormal ventriculo-arterial connections are not unusual, and present their own particular problems for operative reconstruction[21].

A less lethal, but fairly frequently associated, arterial abnormality is aberrant origin of a retro–oesophageal right subclavian artery from the distal aorta. Since the arch is interrupted, symptoms of a vascular ring are unlikely unless a ring is created while reconstructing the arch. Conversely, if the aberrant artery is brought forward, it can be useful in repairing the aorta. This emphasises the importance of defining clearly the nature and effect of associated abnormalities. Successful anatomical correction is as dependent on appropriate management of these accompanying lesions as it is on establishing aortic continuity.

Vascular rings

Aortic rings are malformations associated with abnormal regression of part of a 'double aortic arch'. Knowledge of the development of the aortic arches may be a genuine aid to understanding the morphology of these anomalies, although it is undesirable to use embryological hypothesis as proven fact. Initially, the arterial system is bilaterally symmetrical, with five sets of arches encircling the gut, along with an hypothetical fifth set that has yet to be found during normal development (Fig. 9.24). Of these, only the third, fourth and sixth arches remain recognizable in the postnatal heart. Remnants of the third arch supply the head, the left fourth arch becomes part of

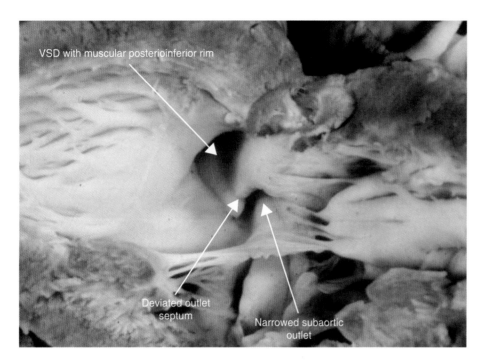

VSD with muscular posterioinferior rim

Deviated outlet septum

Narrowed subaortic outlet

Fig. 9.23 This view of the left ventricle of a specimen with interrupted aortic arch, seen in anatomic orientation, shows posterior deviation of the outlet septum into the left ventricle, with obstruction of the subaortic outflow tract.

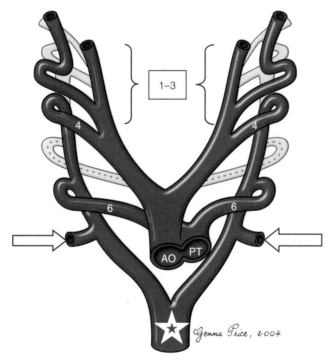

1–3

4   4

6   6

AO   PT

Gemma Price, 2004

Fig. 9.24 This cartoon, in anatomic orientation, shows the patterns of formation of the aortic arches believed to exist during embryological development. The numbers refer to the arteries supplying the pharyngeal arches of the developing embryo. It is most unlikely that there is ever a fifth aortic arch. The arrows show the seventh segmental arteries, which will becomes the subclavian arteries. Initially they are distal to the insertion of the sixth aortic arch. AO – aorta; PT – pulmonary trunk.

the definite aortic arch, and the left sixth arch becomes the duct (Fig. 9.25). The subclavian arteries, which are the seventh cervical intersegmental arteries, come to take origin from the fourth arch between the third and sixth arches when the heart migrates inferiorly[22]. Thus, normally during early development, most of the right-sided structures regress, leaving a left arch and a left-sided aorta (Fig. 9.25). Failure of this regression would leave a double arch, forming a 'ring' around the trachea and the oesophagus. The so-called hypothetical double aortic arch[23] is a concept that explains malformations encircling the tracheo-oesophageal pedicle on the basis of incomplete regression. The hypothetical pattern comprises a midline anterior aorta, continued anteriorly on each side by the fourth arches to bilateral posterior aortic segments, which join to form a midline descending aorta. Common carotid and subclavian arteries arise from each fourth arch in the hypothetical system, whilst an arterial duct connects each arch to its companion pulmonary artery (Fig. 9.26). Persistent patency of the entire double arch will obviously cause problems, while inappropriate interruption or atresia at any part of the ring can produce multiple variations of abnormal anatomy. Such a situation is illustrated in Fig. 9.27, which shows a left aortic arch

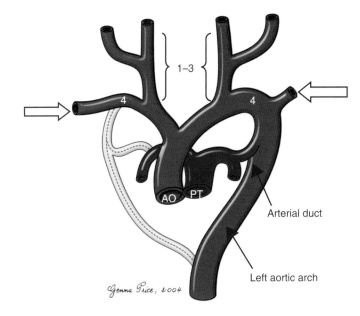

Fig. 9.25 This cartoon shows how the definitive system of aortic arches is derived from the embryologic primordiums depicted in Fig. 9.24. Note that the subclavian arteries (arrows), derived from the seventh segmental arteries, have migrated proximal to the origin of the ducts, and that the right aortic arch has atrophied (yellow and red dotted channels). The left sixth arch persists as the arterial duct.

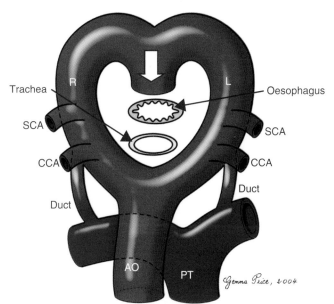

Fig. 9.26 The cartoon shows the perfect hypothetical double arch, with right (R) and left (L) components, and with a subclavian (SCA), common carotid (CCA) and arterial duct arising from each arch. The descending aorta (arrow) is in the midline, or in a "neutral" position.

with an aberrant right subclavian artery, and a ligamentous left-sided duct. Stewart and colleagues[23] provided an exhaustive list of the potential malformations, which they catalogued in complex alpha-numeric fashion. Our preference is for descriptive analysis rather than alphanumeric notation. It should be noted that, as in the latter example of focal atresia, the atretic segment may not persist as a fibrous cord, and may not necessarily cause compression of the trachea or oesophagus. Also, the size of the component parts of the ring is at least as important in producing symptoms as the particular anatomic arrangement. This accounts for the high incidence of

symptoms associated with double aortic arch. Indeed, when only a fibrous cord is found, compression is not always apparent. Figure 9.28 shows a duct taking origin from the left subclavian artery, which arises from a right arch. The considerable tracheoesophageal compression is not obvious until the duct is divided, and its ends are allowed to spring apart (Fig. 9.29). Those wishing to explore further the various combinations of aortic rings will find most explained in the atlas of Stewart and colleagues[23].

A word must be said about the right-sided aortic arch apart from its association with vascular rings. A right-sided aortic

arch is defined as one that crosses over the main stem of the right bronchus. It may connect to the descending aorta on either the right or left side of the vertebral column. Such a right-sided aortic arch is considered abnormal with the usual atrial arrangement, but is normal in patients with the mirror-imaged arrangement. In either case, it may or may not produce problems clinically. Its chief surgical significance lies in its association with about one-quarter of cases of tetralogy of Fallot, and approximately half of all patients with common arterial trunks.

When contemplating construction of a subclavian-to-pulmonary arterial shunt, it

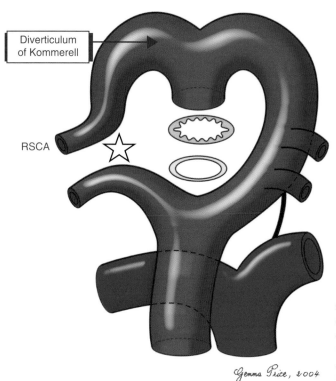

Diverticulum of Kommerell

RSCA

Gemma Price, 2004

Fig. 9.27 This cartoon shows how an aberrant origin of the right subclavian artery (RSCA) is explained on the basis of the hypothetical double arch. The proximal portion of the right arch is known as the diverticulum of Kommerell, and the initial segment of the right arch is interrupted between the right common carotid and right subclavian arteries (star). The duct, shown in left-sided position, has become ligamentous in this example.

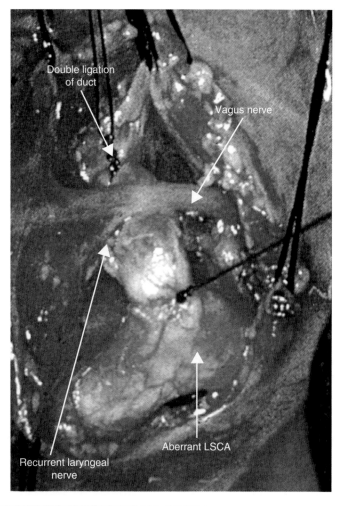

Double ligation of duct

Vagus nerve

Recurrent laryngeal nerve

Aberrant LSCA

Fig. 9.28 This operative view, taken through a left thoracotomy, shows an arterial duct that arises from an aberrant left subclavian artery (LSCA), itself coursing in retrooesophageal position from a right aortic arch. The duct has been doubly ligated prior to its division. Note the size and location of the vagus nerve and its recurrent laryngeal branch.

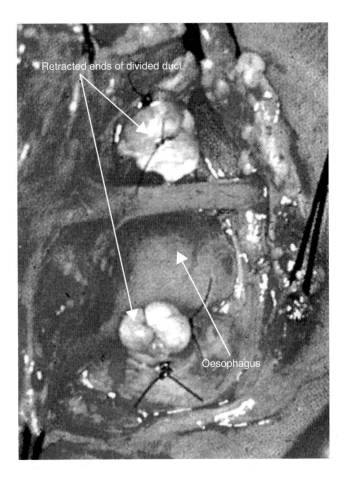

Retracted ends of divided duct

Oesophagus

Fig. 9.29 After division of the duct in the patient shown in Fig. 9.28, the ends of the arch have sprung apart to free the oesophagus.

is important to recognise that, in patients with a right aortic arch, there is usually a mirror-imaged arrangement of the brachiocephalic arteries. The first branch of the aorta beyond the coronary arteries is the brachiocephalic trunk, which gives rise to the left subclavian and common carotid arteries. Under such circumstances, the surgeon may elect to perform a left-sided anastomosis so as to avoid kinking of the right subclavian artery as it is turned down into the mediastinum. The duct, however, usually remains a left-sided structure, connecting the brachiocephalic trunk to the left pulmonary artery (Fig. 9.30). Perhaps because of this mirror-imaged arrangement, it is unusual for the subclavian artery to have an aberrant origin. Thus, under these circumstances, it is equally unusual to find a symptomatic vascular ring.

Pulmonary arterial anomalies

By far the most common malformation of the pulmonary arteries, excluding atresia or stenosis, is for either the right or left

pulmonary artery to have an aortic origin. Most frequently the anomalous artery arises via the arterial duct. Although seen in the presence of pulmonary atresia, usually with the other lung supplied by major systemic-to-pulmonary collateral arteries (Fig. 9.31), it can be found with the other pulmonary artery connected to the patent pulmonary trunk. In this arrangement, the duct will often close with time. There will then be apparent unilateral absence of that pulmonary artery that was initially fed through the duct. This is common in tetralogy of Fallot or double outlet right ventricle, but about half of the patients thus afflicted have otherwise normal hearts. In our experience, it is rare to find true absence of the hilar pulmonary artery.

Less frequently, the anomalous pulmonary artery, usually the right, can arise directly from the ascending aorta (Fig. 9.32). This is sometimes termed a 'hemitruncus', but we do not recommend use of this term, because almost always there are two normally formed arterial valves. Rarely, the right pulmonary artery

may take an unusually high origin from the right side of the ascending portion of a common arterial trunk. Even in this setting, the descriptive title of 'common trunk with anomalous origin of the right pulmonary artery' is preferable to 'hemitruncus'.

When the anomalously connected pulmonary artery arises directly from the aorta, surgical repair consists simply of detachment from the aorta and reattachment to the pulmonary trunk. This is somewhat more difficult in the presence of a common trunk, but the same basic principle is followed for repair. When the anomalous pulmonary artery is fed through a duct, or connected by a ligament, it will arise from the aortic arch or a brachiocephalic artery. Care must then be taken during surgical reconstruction to ensure that ductal tissue is not incorporated with the anastomosis, since it may subsequently constrict and produce stenosis at the site of repair. It should be remembered that, in cases with unilateral absence of a pulmonary artery, it is usual to find pulmonary hypertension and

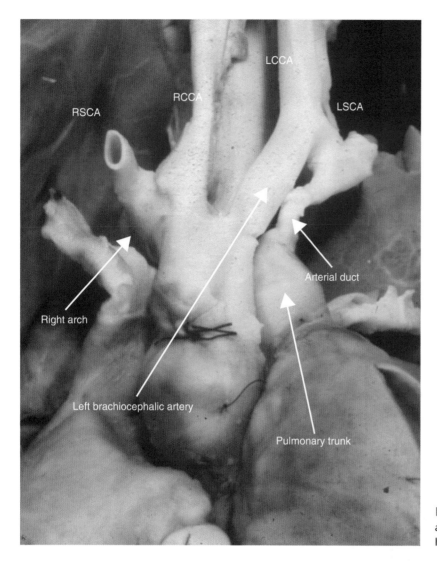

Fig. 9.30 This view of a specimen, orientated anatomically, shows a right aortic arch with a left-sided arterial duct. Abbreviations as before.

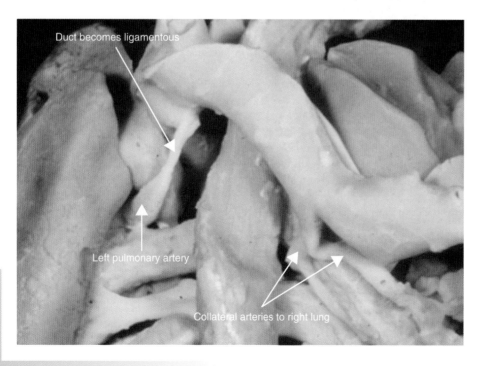

Fig. 9.31 In this specimen, photographed from behind, the left pulmonary artery was initially fed from a left-sided duct, which has become ligamentous. The right lung is fed through systemic-to-pulmonary collateral arteries.

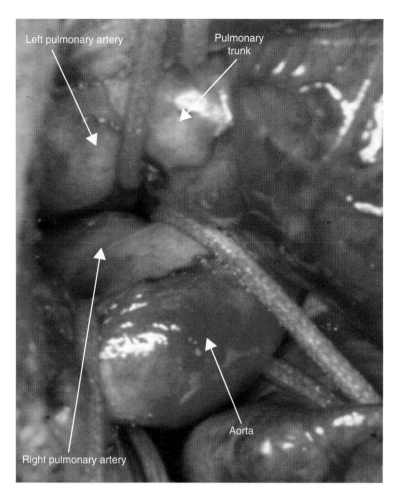

Left pulmonary artery

Pulmonary trunk

Aorta

Right pulmonary artery

Fig. 9.32 In this operative view, through a median sternotomy, the right pulmonary artery can be seen to arise directly from the aorta. This should not be described as "hemitruncus", since there are separate aortic and pulmonary pathways, albeit with the pulmonary trunk feeding only the left pulmonary artery.

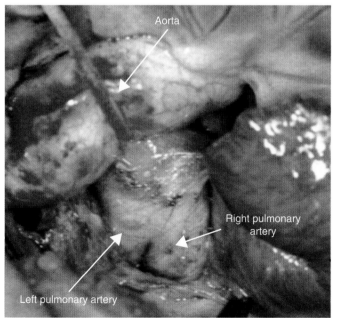

Aorta

Right pulmonary artery

Left pulmonary artery

Fig. 9.33 This operative view, through a median sternotomy, shows the left pulmonary artery arising from the right pulmonary artery. Having taken origin from the right pulmonary artery, the left artery then runs between the trachea and the oesophagus, producing the so-called pulmonary arterial sling (see Fig. 9.34).

pulmonary hypertensive vascular disease in the normally connected lung, probably because of its being disproportionately small and having to receive the entire right ventricular output[24].

A much rarer anomaly is when the left pulmonary artery arises from the right pulmonary artery. The abnormal left pulmonary artery originates within the right chest, and passes between the trachea and oesophagus to the left pulmonary hilum, creating a so-called 'vascular sling'[25] (Figs. 9.33, 9.34). This may result in repeated respiratory problems, requiring division and transplantation of the

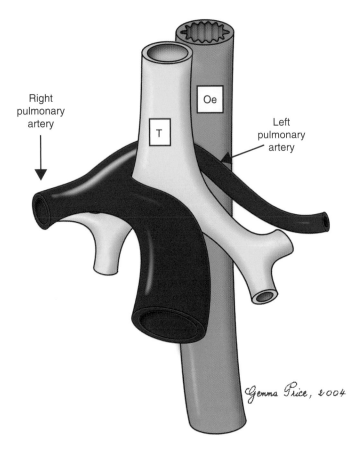

Gemma Price, 2004 **Fig. 9.34** The cartoon shows the arrangement known as the pulmonary arterial sling, illustrated in Fig. 9.33. OE – oesophagus, T – trachea.

offending artery. As discussed above, the right pulmonary artery may arise anomalously from the aorta or brachiocephalic artery, but an abnormal right pulmonary vessel arising from the left pulmonary artery has not, to our knowledge, been reported. The reason for this is not clear.

In the rare occurrence of agenesis of the right lung, displacement of the heart into the right chest may create a ring-like disposition which can obstruct the left bronchus. The displaced heart, pulling on the left pulmonary artery, draws the ligament and descending aorta across the left bronchus, compressing the bronchus against the spinal column. Division of the ligament, and grafting of the aorta, may be necessary to allow the pulmonary trunk and aorta to spring apart and 'unroof' the constricting circle[26–28].

PERSISTENCE OF THE ARTERIAL DUCT AND AORTOPULMONARY WINDOW

Persistence of the arterial duct occupies a special place in the study of cardiovascular disease, since it was the first congenital malformation to be cured by operative intervention[29]. Though the duct can now safely be closed by techniques of interventional catheterisation[30,31], its interruption remains a paradigm of the best of surgical science. The anatomy is almost always predictable, and the operative results uniformly excellent.

Because the arterial system develops with bilateral symmetry, a persistent duct may be either right- or left-sided, although the latter is overwhelmingly more common. Because the duct can persist on either side, or bilaterally, then as discussed above, it may be important as part of a vascular ring. Persistent patency may also play an important physiological role when it accompanies other complex congenital cardiovascular anomalies, such as interruption of the aortic arch, aortic or pulmonary valvar atresia, or discordant ventriculo-arterial connections. In this section, we confine our discussion to the primary congenital condition of isolated left-sided persistently patent arterial duct.

Although it is possible to approach the patent duct anteriorly, and sometimes necessary to use this route (Fig. 9.35), the normal operative approach is through a left lateral thoracotomy (Fig. 9.36). The duct arises from the posterosuperior aspect of the junction of the pulmonary trunk and left pulmonary artery. It courses posteriorly and slightly leftward to join the junction of the aortic arch and descending aorta just distal to and opposite the origin of the left subclavian artery. Its pulmonary end is covered by a fold of pericardium, and its aortic end by parietal pleura. It may be confused with the aortic isthmus, particularly in the infant, and it is possible to identify the left pulmonary artery as a patent duct. Even under the best conditions, these other structures may be mistakenly ligated in place of the duct. The caveats of this procedure have been elegantly reviewed by Pontius et al[32]. Approached laterally, the best anatomical guide to the duct is the vagus nerve and its recurrent laryngeal branch. The vagus nerve passes along the subclavian artery, crossing over the aortic arch before heading in a posterior direction to disappear behind the hilum. Just at the level of the duct, it gives off the recurrent

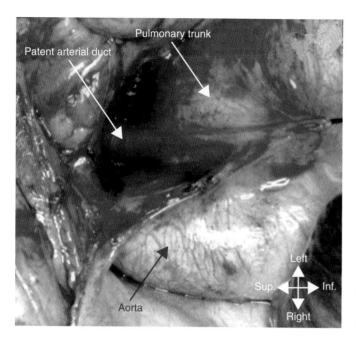

Fig. 9.35 This operative view through a median sternotomy shows the origin of a patent arterial duct from the distal extent of the pulmonary trunk.

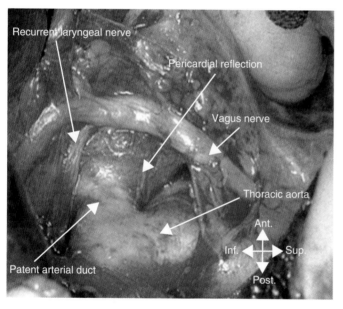

Fig. 9.36 In this operative view, a patent arterial duct is seen through a left thoracotomy (compare with Fig. 9.35). Note the location of the vagus nerve and it recurrent laryngeal branch.

nerve (Fig. 9.37), which then curves beneath the inferomedial wall of the duct before ascending along the posteromedial aspect of the aorta into the groove between the trachea and oesophagus.

Access to the duct may be achieved by incising the mediastinal parietal pleura, either between the phrenic and vagus nerves, or more posteriorly over the aorta itself. With either approach, the recurrent nerve must be visualised to guard against direct trauma or injury by traction. The fold of pericardium extending over the pulmonary end of the duct may be lifted away by sharp dissection. The

posteromedial wall of the duct is firmly attached by another more fibrous fold to the bronchus. It is this firm fibrous fold that prevents easy circumscription of the duct with a right-angle clamp. To minimise the risk of tearing the wall of the duct, this tissue must be divided by sharp dissection. This can be done through a superior approach over the aortic end of the duct, or by freeing the aorta and retracting it medially. In the latter instance, small but potentially troublesome bronchial vessels may be encountered, arising from the posterior wall of the aorta. Another anatomical note

of caution involves the thoracic duct and its tributaries in the area of the origin of the subclavian artery. Division of any of these major lymph vessels is liable to lead to chylothorax and its attendant difficulties. Should the lymphatic trunks be inadvertently divided, they must be ligated to avoid chylothorax.

The duct in an infant or small child can measure from 1 to 15 millimeters in length and diameter. Rarely, it can be aneurysmally dilated[33] (Fig. 9.38). These may be aneurysms of a truly patent duct, or may simply be a dilated ductal diverticulum with a closed pulmonary

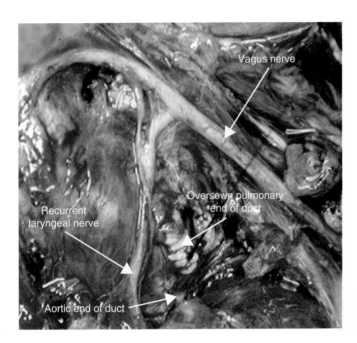

Fig. 9.37 The arterial duct shown in Fig. 9.36 has been divided and oversewn, emphasising the close relationship of the recurrent laryngeal nerve to the duct.

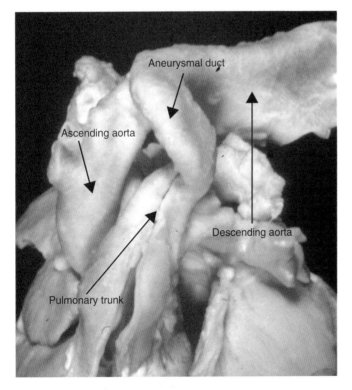

Fig. 9.38 The heart is photographed in anatomic orientation from the front. The arterial duct is patent and aneurysmal.

end. In general, the short and fat duct should be cross-clamped, divided, and oversewn to minimise the chances of incomplete ligation or tearing of the vessel wall. For the longer thin duct, a triple ligation technique has proved to be safe and effective[34].

The clinical presentation of aortopulmonary window is often similar to that of a common arterial trunk. The anatomical distinction lies in the mode of ventriculo-arterial connection. Where, in a common trunk, there is a solitary arterial valve, aortopulmonary window is always associated with separate aortic and pulmonary valves (Fig. 9.39). Though the ventricular septum is usually intact, this defect is frequently associated with additional congenital cardiovascular anomalies[35].

The defect itself is usually located in the right lateral wall of the pulmonary trunk anterior and opposite to the origin of the right pulmonary artery, which frequently overrides the window, or arises directly from the aorta (Fig. 9.39). This means that its opening into the left side of

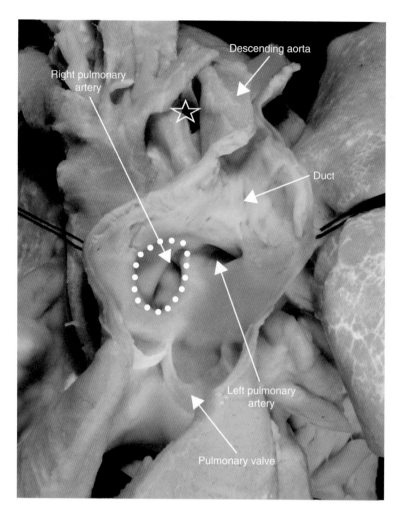

Fig. 9.39 This specimen, shown in anatomic orientation having opened the pulmonary trunk, shows an aortopulmonary window. The right pulmonary artery takes origin from the aorta, and there is interruption of the aortic arch at the isthmus (star), the descending aorta fed via the patent arterial duct.

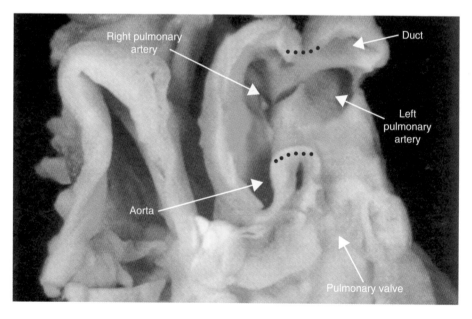

Fig. 9.40 This specimen also has an aortopulmonary window in the setting of origin of the right pulmonary artery from the aorta and interruption of the aortic arch. The heart is sectioned to replicated the left anterior oblique subcostal echocardiographic section. In this heart, the window (dotted lines) has some length.

the ascending aorta is just distal to the sinutubular junction and the orifices of the coronary arteries. It is not infrequent, however, to find one coronary artery taking anomalous origin from the pulmonary trunk. The defect may appear as a well-demarcated short tubular structure (Fig. 9.40), or it may be more like a window. Surgical repair is best accomplished through an incision in the ascending aorta using standard cardiopulmonary bypass techniques.

As a general rule, 'closed' methods are not advisable, not even for the more tubular defects. When the window supplies a vital part of the circulation, it cannot be closed without providing an alternate source of blood for the dependent segment of the circulation.

ANOMALIES OF THE CORONARY ARTERIES

Congenital malformations of the coronary arteries in otherwise normally structured hearts have, traditionally, been categorised as major or minor. This approach was rooted in the belief that the so-called major anomalies were those that produced symptomatology, whereas the minor lesions were thought to be of no clinical relevance[36]. The potential danger of such a classification became evident when it was realised that some lesions categorised as minor within this concept could be a cause of sudden cardiac death[37]. Because of this discrepancy between presumed anatomic

and revealed clinical significance, it now seems preferable to account for these malformations on a descriptive basis. Within such a descriptive categorisation, the anomalies can be grouped into those with anomalous origin of the coronary arteries from the arterial roots, those with anomalous course of the epicardial coronary arteries, those with anomalous communications between the coronary arteries and other structures within the heart, or combinations of such findings.

Anomalous origin of the coronary arteries

The coronary arteries can arise anomalously either from the pulmonary trunk or, rarely, from the right or left pulmonary artery. They can also take an anomalous origin from the aorta itself. It is anomalous origin from the pulmonary trunk that is of most clinical significance. Often described as the Bland–White–Garland syndrome, anomalous origin of

the left coronary artery from the pulmonary trunk (Figs. 9.41, 9.42) usually presents in infancy with ischaemia of the left ventricle (Fig. 9.43), although, if there is well-developed collateral circulation, presentation can be markedly delayed, some cases not presenting until childhood or even adolescence. The clinical problems are produced by the extent of ischaemia of the left ventricular myocardium, which can be extreme. It is important to reattach the artery to the aorta as soon as the diagnosis is made. In most instances, the artery arises from the right hand facing sinus of the pulmonary trunk[38], and it is relatively easy to transfer the arterial origin, together with a button of pulmonary sinus, back to the left hand facing sinus of the aorta. It is rare nowadays to create an aortopulmonary tunnel in order to reconnect the artery to the aorta[39]. Either of these procedures, nonetheless, is usually preferable to simple ligation of the coronary artery. The pattern that

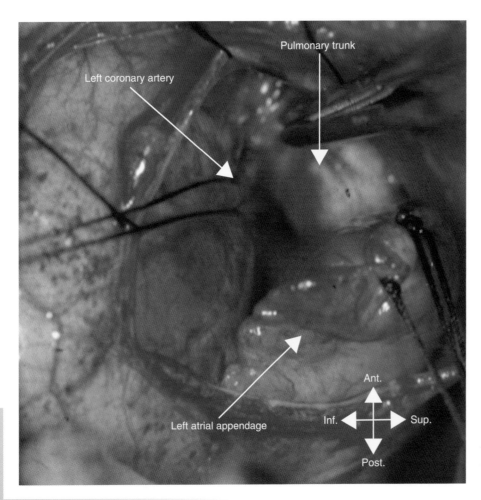

Fig. 9.41 This view through a left lateral thoracotomy shows a silk ligature encircling a left coronary artery that is arising from the pulmonary trunk.

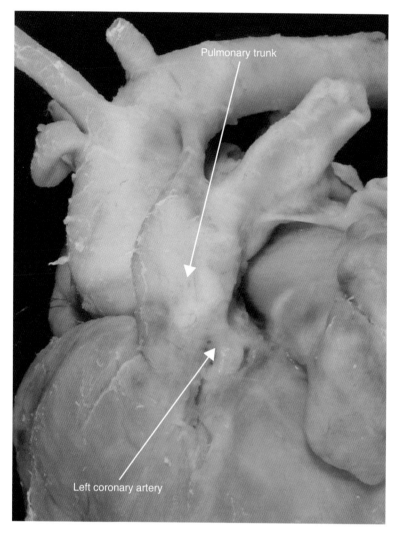

Fig. 9.42 In this specimen, photographed in anatomic orientation, the left coronary artery again takes origin from the pulmonary trunk, arising from one of the sinuses adjacent to the aorta.

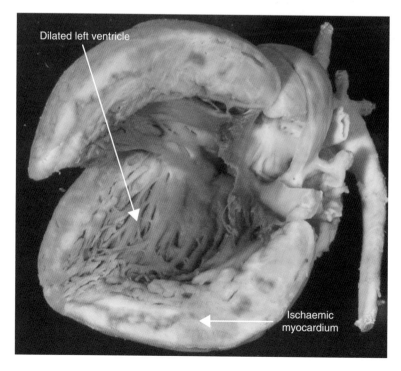

Fig. 9.43 In this anatomic specimen, photographed in anatomic orientation, the left ventricle is dilated secondary to anomalous origin of the left coronary artery from the pulmonary trunk, while the ventricular myocardium is obviously ischaemic.

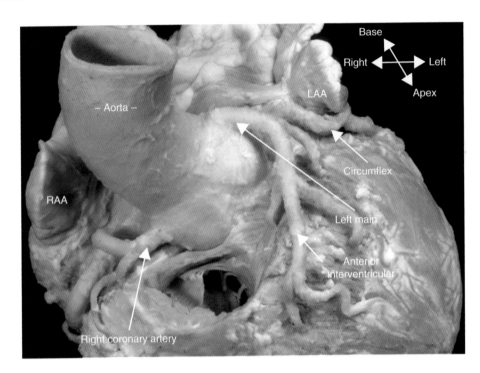

Fig. 9.44 The aortic root is photographed from the front, in anatomic orientation, to show the origin of the coronary arteries. The pulmonary valvar leaflets and subpulmonary infundibulum have been removed.

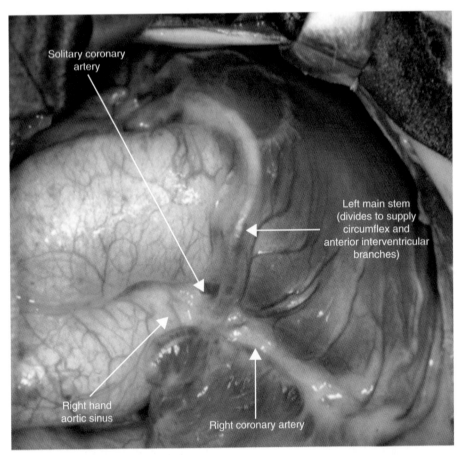

Fig. 9.45 This operative view, taken through a median sternotomy, demonstrates all the coronary arteries arising from a solitary coronary artery that takes origin from the right hand facing sinus. The main stem that divides beneath the left appendage to become the circumflex and anterior interventricular arteries crosses the origin of the pulmonary trunk from the right ventricle.

may create problems in transfer is when the artery arises from a branch of the pulmonary trunk rather than the trunk itself. Other patterns, such as anomalous origin of the right coronary artery from the pulmonary trunk, do not produce the same degree of symptomatology, and often do not come to the attention of the surgeon. If encountered, an anomalous right coronary artery can readily be transferred back to the aortic root.

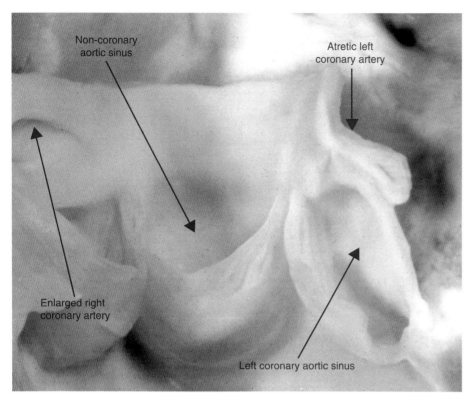

Non-coronary
aortic sinus

Atretic left
coronary artery

Enlarged right
coronary artery

Left coronary aortic sinus

Fig. 9.46 This view of the opened aortic root, photographed in anatomic orientation, shows atresia of the main stem of the left coronary artery. The specimen came from an adult who died suddenly. Note the enlarged orifice of the right coronary artery.

The significance of anomalous origin of one coronary artery from the aorta has yet to be fully established. Usually the coronary arteries arise from the two aortic sinuses that are adjacent to the pulmonary trunk. In the normal heart, the left coronary artery arises from the left hand facing sinus, while the right coronary artery arises from the right hand facing sinus (Fig. 9.44). Accessory orifices supplying either the infundibular artery, the artery to the sinus node, or an artery supplying the walls of the arterial trunks, are by no means uncommon. These accessory branches should not be interpreted as representing anomalies. The circumflex and anterior descending branches of the left coronary artery can also rarely take separate origins from the left hand facing sinus in an otherwise normal heart. Usually the arteries arise within the sinuses, but origin at the sinutubular junction, or just above it, should not be considered abnormal. High origin, however, or an oblique course of a coronary artery through the wall, particularly when crossing a commissure to give the so-called intramural course, should be considered anomalous, as should origin of the left coronary artery from the left hand facing sinus or, as

occurs very rarely, from the non-facing aortic sinus[40].

The finding of a single coronary artery also represents anomalous origin from the aortic root. This can be found in two patterns. In the first, all three coronary arteries arise from the same aortic sinus, with either one, two, or three orifices within the sinus. Usually it is the right hand sinus that gives origin to the coronary arteries. There is then an associated anomalous epicardial course of the branches of the left coronary artery as they reach the anticipated locations. This can involve the anterior interventricular branch tracking between the aorta and the pulmonary trunk, with the potential for its constriction. Alternatively, the main stem of the left coronary artery can run across the subpulmonary infundibulum, tracking towards the left atrial appendage before dividing into the circumflex and anterior interventricular arteries (Fig. 9.45). Another pattern is for the right coronary artery to take its normal origin from the right hand facing sinus, but then to continue beyond the crux as the circumflex artery, and to terminate at the obtuse margin as the anterior interventricular artery (see Fig. 4.8). This pattern probably has no clinical significance. In

addition to anomalous origin, congenital malformations can also afflict normally attached arteries, producing the effect of anomalous origin. Particularly important in this respect is congenital atresia of the main stem of the left coronary artery (Fig. 9.46). This can be another substrate for sudden death in an adolescent or young adult[41]. Unfortunately, this anomaly is unlikely to be diagnosed prior to the event, when it could readily be treated by surgical manoeuvres.

Anomalous epicardial course of the coronary arteries

Although an anomalous epicardial course can be found in otherwise normally structured hearts, it is seen more frequently in hearts that are themselves malformed, such as those with discordant ventriculo-arterial connections or common arterial trunk. The clinical significance of these anomalies has yet to be fully determined. Some are found as chance observations at autopsy, such as the origin of the circumflex coronary artery from the right coronary artery, with passage through the transverse sinus to reach the left atrioventricular groove (Fig. 9.47). Others may be of significance for sudden death,

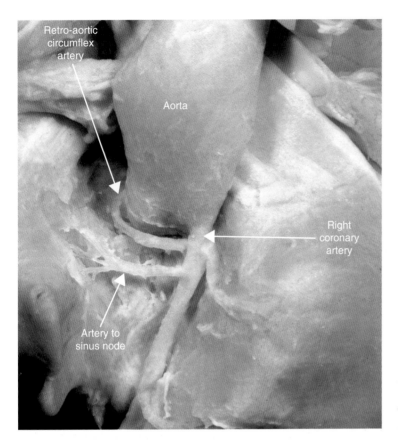

Retro-aortic circumflex artery

Aorta

Right coronary artery

Artery to sinus node

Fig. 9.47 This infant heart is photographed in anatomic orientation. The circumflex coronary artery arises from the right hand facing aortic sinus, and passes through the transverse sinus, behind the aorta, to reach the left atrioventricular groove.

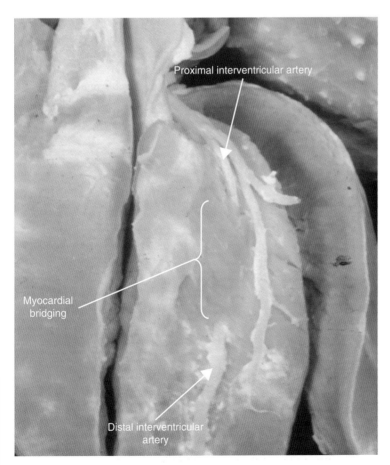

Proximal interventricular artery

Myocardial bridging

Distal interventricular artery

Fig. 9.48 In this heart, photographed from the front in anatomic orientation, there is extensive myocardial bridging across the anterior interventricular artery.

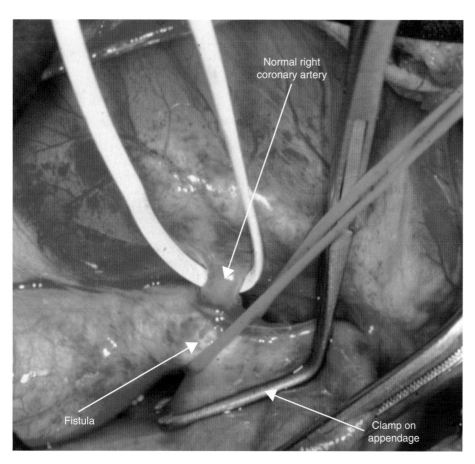

Normal right
coronary artery

Fistula

Clamp on
appendage

Fig. 9.49 This operative view through a
median sternotomy, with the right atrial
appendage retracted, shows a fistula
running from the right coronary artery to
the base of the appendage. The white loop
is placed around the normal distal segment
of the right coronary artery, while the red
loop encircles the fistula itself.

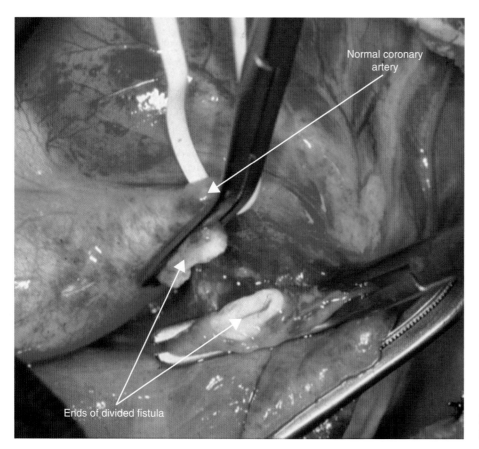

Normal coronary
artery

Ends of divided fistula

Fig. 9.50 The broad fistula shown in
Fig. 9.49 has been divided.

such as passage of the anterior interventricular artery between the aorta and the pulmonary trunk[42]. In this respect, muscular bridging of the epicardial coronary arteries (Fig. 9.48) may be of relevance, although the significance of this finding has still to be established.

Anomalous communications of the coronary arteries

Fistulous communications between the coronary arteries and the ventricles are seen most frequently when atresia of an outflow tract is seen in the setting of an intact ventricular septum, notably in pulmonary atresia with intact ventricular septum (see Chapter 7, page 208, Fig. 7.157). Such communications can also be found in otherwise normally structured hearts, and the anomalous artery can be joined to any other cardiac structure. The right coronary artery is most frequently involved, and it may connect to the right atrium (Figs. 9.49, 9.50), the superior caval vein, the coronary sinus, the right ventricle, the pulmonary trunk, a pulmonary vein, or the left ventricle. The communication itself can be a large solitary orifice (Fig. 9.50), or a complex worm-like aneurysmal cavity. When the communication is simple and large, shunting across it can be considerable and the artery itself can be markedly dilated. 'Steals' can also result, with consequent ischaemia in the area of myocardium from which the steal has occurred.

References

1. Anderson RC, Heilig W, Novick R, Jarvis C. Anomalous inferior vena cava with azygos drainage: so-called absence of the inferior vena cava. *Am Heart J* 1955; **49**: 318–322.

2. Moller JH, Nakib A, Anderson RC, Edwards JE. Congenital cardiac disease associated with polysplenia: A developmental complex of bilateral 'left-sidedness'. *Circulation* 1967; **36**: 789–799.

3. Venables AW. Isolated drainage of the inferior vena cava to the left atrium. *Br Heart J* 1963; **25**: 545–548.

4. Winter FS. Persistent left superior vena cava: survey of world literature and report of 30 additional cases. *Angiology* 1954; **5**: 90–132.

5. Bankl H. In *Congenital Malformations of the Heart and Great Vessels*. Baltimore – Munich: Urban and Schwarzenberg 1977; p 194.

6. Edwards JE, DuShane JW. Thoracic venous anomalies. 1. Vascular connection between the left atrium and the left innominate vein (levoatriocardinal vein) associated with mitral atresia and premature closure of the foramen ovale (case 1). 11. Pulmonary veins draining wholly to the ductus arteriosus (case 2). *Arch Pathol* 1950; **49**: 517–537.

7. Pinto CAM, Ho SY, Redington A, Shinebourne EA, Anderson RH. Morphological features of the levoatriocardinal (or pulmonary-to-systemic collateral) vein. *Pediatr Pathol* 1993; **13**: 751–761.

8. Lucas RV Jr, Woolfrey BF, Anderson RC, Lester RG, Edwards JE. Atresia of the common pulmonary vein. *Pediatr* 1962; **29**: 729–739.

9. Nakib A, Moller JH, Kanjuh VI, Edwards JE. Anomalies of the pulmonary veins. *Am J Cardiol* 1967; **20**: 77–90.

10. Bharati S, Lev M. Congenital anomalies of the pulmonary veins. *Cardiovascular Clinics* 1973; **5**: 23–41.

11. DeLisle G, Ando M, Calder AL, Zuberbuhler JR, Rochenmacher S, Alday LE, Mangino O, Van Praagh S, Van Praagh R. Total anomalous pulmonary venous connection: report of 93 autopsied cases with emphasis on diagnostic and surgical considerations. *Am Heart J* 1976; **91**: 99–122.

12. Neill CA, Ferencz C, Sabiston DC, Sheldon H. The familial occurrence of hypoplastic right lung with systemic arterial supply and venous drainage 'scimitar syndrome'. *Johns Hopkins Medical Journal* 1960; **107**: 1–15.

13. Chauvin M, Shah DC, Haisseguerre M, Marcellin L, Brechenmacher, C. The anatomic basis of connections between the coronary sinus musculature and the left atrium in humans. *Circulation* 2000; **101**: 647–652.

14. Brom AG. Narrowing of the aortic isthmus and enlargement of the mind. *J Thorac Cardiovasc Surg* 1965; **50**: 166–180.

15. Ho SY, Anderson RH. Coarctation, tubular hypoplasia and the ductus arteriosus: a histological study of 35 specimens. *Br Heart J* 1979; **41**: 268–274.

16. Elzenga NJ, Gittenberger-de-Groot AC. Localised coarctation of the aorta. An age dependent spectrum. *Br Heart J* 1983; **49**: 317–323.

17. Becker AE, Becker MJ, Edwards JE. Anomalies associated with coarctation of the aorta. Particular reference to infancy. *Circulation* 1970; **41**: 1067–1075.

18. Hamilton WF, Abbott ME. Coarctation of the aorta of the adult type: Part I. Complete obliteration of the descending arch at insertion of the ductus in a boy of fourteen; bicuspid aortic valve; impending rupture of the aorta; cerebral death. Part II. A statistical study and historical retrospect of 200 recorded cases, with autopsy, of stenosis or obliteration of the descending arch in subjects above the age of two years. *Am Heart J* 1928; **3**: 381–421.

19. Lerberg DB. Abbott's artery. *Ann Thorac Surg* 1982; **33**: 415–416.

20. Pierpont MEM, Zollikofer CL, Moller JH, Edwards JE. Interruption of the aortic arch with right descending aorta. *Pediatr Cardiol* 1982; **2**: 153–159.

21. Ho SY, Wilcox BR, Anderson RH, Lincoln JCR. Interrupted aortic arch-anatomical features of surgical significance. *Thorac Cardiovasc Surg* 1983; **31**: 199–205.

22. Barry A. Aortic arch derivatives in the human adult. *Anat Rec* 1951; **111**: 221–238.

23. Stewart JR, Kincaid OW, Edwards JE. *An Atlas of Vascular Rings and Related Malformations of the Aortic Arch System*. Springfield, Illinoi, Charles C. Thomas. 1964.

24. Pool PE, Vogel JHK, Blount SG Jr. Congenital unilateral absence of a pulmonary artery. The importance of flow in pulmonary hypertension. *Am J Cardiol* 1962; **10**: 706–732.

25. Contro S, Miller RA, White H, Potts WJ. Bronchial obstruction due to pulmonary artery anomalies. I. Vascular sling. *Circulation* 1958; **17**: 418–423.

26. Maier HC, Gould WJ. Agenesis of the lung with vascular compression of the tracheobronchial tree. *J Pediatr* 1953; **43**: 38–42.

27. Harrison MR, Hendren WH. Agenesis of the lung complicated by vascular compression and bronchomalacia. *J Pediatr Surg* 1975; **10**: 813–817.

28. Harrison MR, Heldt GP, Brasch RC, de Lorimier AA, Gregory GA. Resection of distal tracheal stenosis in a baby with

agenesis of the lung. *J Pediatr Surg* 1980; **15**: 938–943.

29. Gross RE. Surgical management of patent ductus arteriosus with summary of four surgically treated cases. *Ann Surg* 1939; **110**: 321–356.

30. Ali Kahn MA, Al Yousef S, Mullins CE, Sawyer W. Experiences with 205 procedures of transcatheter closure of ductus arteriosus in 182 patients, with special reference to residual shunts and long term follow-up. *J Thorac Cardiovasc Surg* 1992; **104**: 1721–1727.

31. Lloyd TR, Fedderly R, Mendelsohn AM, Sandhu SK, Beekman RH. Transcatheter occlusion of patent ductus arteriosus with Gianturco coils. *Circulation* 1993; **88 (part 1)**: 1414–1420.

32. Pontius RG, Danielson GK, Noonan JA, Judson JP. Illusions leading to surgical closure of the distal left pulmonary artery instead of the ductus arteriosus. *J Thorac Cardiovasc Surg* 1981; **82**: 107–113.

33. Mendel V, Luhmer J, Oelert H. Aneurysma des Ductus arteriosus bei einem Neugeborenen. *Herz* 1980; **5**: 320–323.

34. Wilcox BR, Peters RM. The surgery of patent ductus arteriosus: a clinical report of 14 years' experience without an operative death. *Ann Thorac Surg* 1967; **3**: 126–131.

35. Faulkner SL, Oldham RR, Atwood GF, Graham TP. Aortopulmonary window, ventricular septal defect and membranous pulmonary atresia with a diagnosis of truncus arteriosus. *Chest* 1974; **65**: 351–353.

36. Ogden JA. Congenital anomalies of the coronary arteries. *Am J Cardiol* 1970; **25**: 474–479.

37. Becker AE. Variations of the main coronary arteries. Edited by Becker AE, Losekoot T, Marcelletti C, Anderson RH. Edinburgh Churchill Livingstone. In *Pediatr Cardiol* 1983; **3**: 263–277.

38. Smith A, Arnold R, Anderson RH, Wilkinson JL, Qureshi SA, Gerlis LM, McKay R. Anomalous origin of the left coronary artery from the pulmonary trunk. Anatomic findings in relation to pathophysiology and surgical repair. *J Thorac Cardiovasc Surg* 1989; **98**: 16–24.

39. Takeuchi S, Imamura H, Katsumoto K, Hayashi I, Katohgi T, Yozu R, Ohkura M, Inoue T. New surgical method for repair of anomalous left coronary artery from the pulmonary artery. *J Thorac Cardiovasc Surg* 1979; **78**: 7–11.

40. Ishikawa T, Otsuka T, Suzuki T. Anomalous origin of the left main coronary artery from the non-coronary sinus of Valsalva. (Letter). *Pediatr Cardiol* 1990; **11**: 173–174.

41. Debich DE, Williams KE, Anderson RH. Congenital atresia of the orifice of the left coronary artery and its main stem. *Int J Cardiol* 1989; **22**: 398–404.

42. Kragel AH, Roberts WC. Anomalous origin of either right or left main coronary artery from the aorta with subsequent coursing between aorta and pulmonary trunk: analysis of 32 necropsy cases. *Am J Cardiol* 1988; **62**: 771–777.

10

Positional anomalies of the heart

The surgical problems posed by cardiac malformations may be considerably increased when the heart itself is in an abnormal position. This is, in part, due to the unusual anatomical perspective presented to the surgeon because of the malposition, and also to the abnormal locations of the cardiac chambers which may necessitate approaches other than those already discussed. Cardiac malposition itself, nonetheless, constitutes a diagnosis. Any normal or abnormal segmental combination can be found in a heart which is itself abnormally located. The heart may be normal, despite the malposition, but extremely complex anomalies are frequently present. Consequently, the very presence of an abnormal cardiac position emphasises the need for a full and detailed segmental analysis of the heart. All the rules enunciated in Chapter 6 apply when the heart is not in its anticipated position. In this chapter, we confine ourselves to a description of malpositioned hearts, giving a more detailed discussion for specific types of malposition. We conclude with a brief review of the surgical significance of isomerism of the atrial appendages, which is generally agreed to be one of the major harbingers of abnormal cardiac position.

THE ABNORMALLY POSITIONED HEART

When describing an abnormally located heart, it is necessary to take account of both its position within the chest and the direction of its apex. In the normal individual, the heart is positioned with its apex to the left, and with two-thirds of its bulk to the left of the midline. Mirror-imaged atrial arrangement is usually accompanied by mirror-imaged cardiac arrangement. The norm is then for the apex to point to the right, with the greater part of the cardiac mass in the right hemithorax. With isomerism of the atrial appendages and visceral heterotaxy, there is no norm. Thus, for all patients with isomerism, and for those with the usual or mirror-image atrial arrangements and abnormally positioned hearts, it is necessary to have a system simply to describe the abnormal cardiac position. In the past, formidable conventions have been constructed, using terms such as dextrocardia, dextroposition, dextrorotation, and pivotal dextrocardia[1]. In practice, the only requirement is a system which accounts for two major features: the position of the cardiac mass relative to the silhouette of the chest, and the direction of the cardiac apex. This is because position of the heart, and orientation of its apex, although usually congruent, is not invariably linked together. In the past, we have defined dextrocardia as the situation in which the heart is in the right chest, with the apex pointing to the right (Fig. 10.1). But what happens on the rare occasion when the heart is in the right chest, but its apex is pointing to the left? This situation is readily, and unambiguously, described as "heart in right chest, apex to left". Those who wish to give nominative definitions to the arrangement are free so to do, but the descriptive approach is entirely adequate, and much less liable to misconstruction. Thus, the heart is described as being mostly in the left chest, mostly in the right chest, or symmetrical. The apical orientation is to the left, to the right, or to the middle.

EXTERIORISATION OF THE HEART

The description given above, however, does not account for the most severe cardiac malposition, namely exteriorization of the heart, or so-called ectopia cordis. It had been said that the

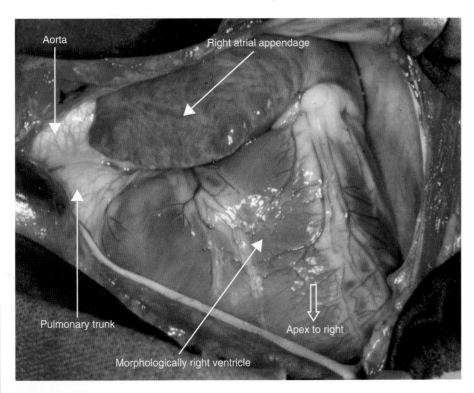

Aorta

Right atrial appendage

Pulmonary trunk

Apex to right

Morphologically right ventricle

Fig. 10.1 This operative view through a median sternotomy shows a patient with mirror-imaged arrangement of the organs. The heart is mostly in the right chest, with the apex pointing to the right (arrow).

heart can protrude from the thoracic cavity in cervical, thoracic, thoracoabdominal or abdominal positions. One review[2] has questioned the existence of the cervical and abdominal variants, arguing that all cases can be described as thoracic or thoracoabdominal. In the thoracic type, which is the most common, there is a sternal defect and absence of the parietal pericardium. The heart protrudes directly from the thorax[3]. Usually there is an associated

omphalocele, and the thoracic cavity is small.

In the thoracoabdominal type, the sternal defect is usually confluent with deficiencies of the abdominal wall and diaphragm, so the heart and various abdominal organs are displaced into an omphalocele. A variant of this abnormality is seen in patients with so-called Cantrell's syndrome[4]. These patients have a cleft lower sternum. The heart is beneath the skin in the upper epigastrium,

and is associated with an omphalocele (Fig. 10.2). Opening the skin demonstrates the heart to be low in the midline (Fig. 10.3), and extending toward the omphalocele through a diaphragmatic defect. These patients frequently have complex intracardiac defects, often including a diverticulum of the left ventricle. The heart illustrated in our patient (Fig. 10.4) had tetralogy of Fallot and isomerism of the right atrial appendages, but no diverticulum.

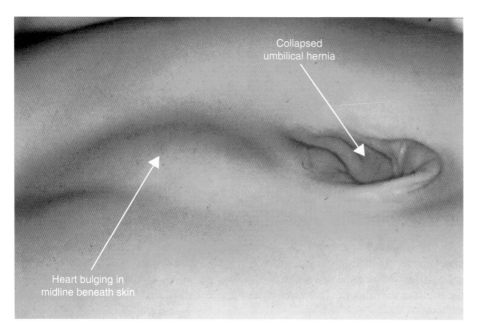

Collapsed umbilical hernia

Heart bulging in midline beneath skin

Fig. 10.2 This picture, taken from the right side of the epigastrium with the patient supine, shows the heart bulging through the skin because of a cleft in the lower sternum and diastasis of the rectus muscles. An associated abdominal hernia is collapsed.

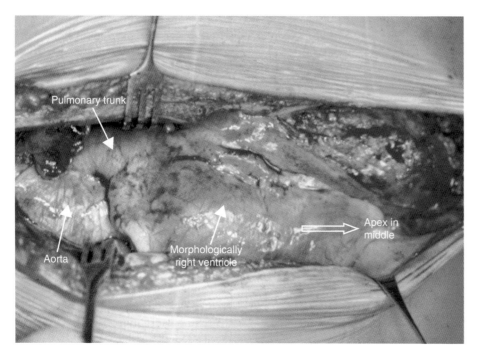

Pulmonary trunk

Aorta

Morphologically right ventricle

Apex in middle

Fig. 10.3 The skin and upper sternum has been opened in the patient shown in Fig. 10.2, revealing the heart to be positioned in the midline, with the apex pointing to the middle of the chest (arrow).

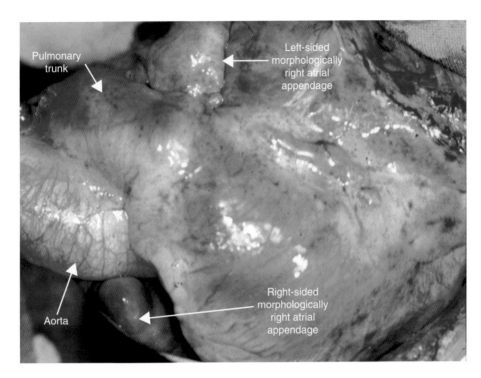

Pulmonary trunk

Left-sided morphologically right atrial appendage

Aorta

Right-sided morphologically right atrial appendage

Fig. 10.4 In the case shown in Figs. 10.2 and 10.3, inspection of the appendages shows them both to be broad and triangular. More detailed analysis confirmed the diagnosis of isomerism of the right atrial appendages.

RIGHT-SIDED HEART

Our descriptive system provides no information as to whether the abnormal location of the heart is the result of congenital malformation. The heart may be in the right chest secondary to a pulmonary defect, or because of gross enlargement of its right-sided chambers. In either case, the problems of surgical access are similar. Indeed, there is no reason for a patient with a lesion such as congenitally corrected transposition not to acquire a heart in the right chest because of pulmonary problems or right-sided hypertrophy.

There are certain lesions which immediately spring to mind when the heart is located in the right chest with the usual atrial arrangement, or when the heart is left-sided in patients with mirror-imaged atrial chambers. The most notable of these is congenitally corrected transposition. The potential complexity of this lesion simply emphasises that, in all patients with abnormally positioned hearts, it is essential that the surgeon be aware of the locations of the chambers within the malpositioned organ so that the operation can be planned appropriately.

CRISS-CROSS AND SUPERO-INFERIOR VENTRICLES

With the sophistication of modern diagnostic techniques, it is unlikely that the surgeon will be presented with a patient having an abnormally located heart without a full preoperative diagnosis. There are, nonetheless, particular arrangements of the cardiac chambers which can still give major difficulties in diagnosis, notably the so-called 'criss-cross hearts', and 'superoinferior ventricles'. In these anomalies, the ventricular relationships, or more rarely the ventricular topology, using the term 'topology' as defined in Chapter 6, are not as anticipated for given atrioventricular connections[5]. In a patient with congenitally corrected transposition and a 'criss-cross' arrangement, the morphologically right ventricle will be predominantly right-sided rather than in its anticipated left-sided position[6]. This is a consequence of rotation of the ventricular mass in its long axis (Fig. 10.5). In addition to these unusual relationships, there is the possibility that a catheter passed through the right atrioventricular valve in a heart with discordant atrioventricular connections and

'criss-cross' relationships may slip through a ventricular septal defect and opacify the right-sided morphologically right ventricle. This will give the spurious appearance of concordant atrioventricular connections[6].

The distribution of the coronary arteries is of considerable help in determining the position of the ventricles since, in congenitally corrected transposition, the anterior interventricular coronary artery arises from the right-sided coronary artery. Thus, in a heart which at first sight appears to represent simple transposition, finding the anterior interventricular artery arising from the right-sided coronary artery should alert the surgeon to the possible diagnosis of a discordant atrioventricular connections and congenitally corrected transposition.

Hearts with superoinferior ventricles present a similar situation to the 'criss-cross' arrangement, except that the heart is tilted along its long axis (Fig. 10.6). In some cases, it is rotated as well as tilted, so that both 'criss-cross' and superoinferior arrangements are present. Again, the interventricular coronary arteries are useful because they indicate the plane of the ventricular septum, serving as excellent guides to the position of the

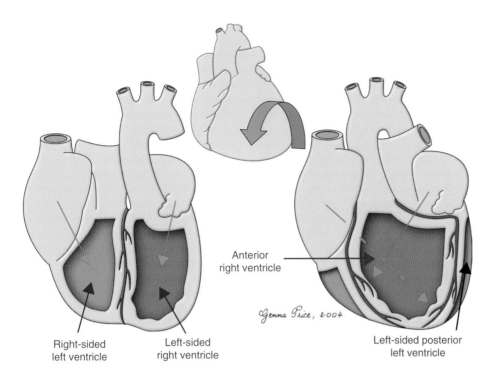

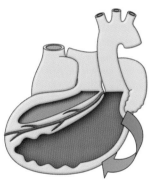

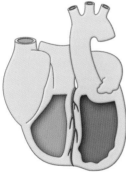

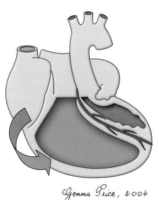

Anterior
right ventricle

Right-sided
left ventricle

Left-sided
right ventricle

Left-sided posterior
left ventricle

Gemma Price, 2004

Fig. 10.5 This cartoon, drawn in anatomic orientation, illustrates the rotational abnormality around the long axis (inset) that produces the so-called criss-cross abnormality. The left hand panel shows a heart with congenitally corrected transposition in the absence of rotation around the long axis. The morphologically left ventricle is right-sided. Subsequent to rotation (right hand panel), the morphologically right ventricle occupies a right-sided position, albeit still connected discordantly to the morphologically left atrium. The arrows in the right hand panel show the crossing atrioventricular valves, the dotted line depicting the posterior connection to the morphologically left ventricle, which has rotated to left-sided position.

Morphologically left ventricle
uppermost

Usual side-by-side
ventricles

Morphologically right ventricle
uppermost

Gemma Price, 2004

Fig. 10.6 This cartoon, drawn in anatomic orientation, shows the tilting along the long axis of the ventricular mass in a heart with congenitally corrected transposition, which usually has side-by-side ventricles (central panel). As seen, the tilting can produce the so-called "upstairs-downstairs" arrangement of the ventricles, or "superoinferior ventricles". Depending on the direction of tilting, either the morphologically left ventricle (left hand panel) or the morphologically right ventricle (right hand panel) can be positioned uppermost.

ventricular cavities. The distribution of the conduction tissue in these bizarre hearts, however, is governed by the connections between the chambers, and not by their position. These hearts are often further complicated by the presence of straddling and overriding atrioventricular valves. These abnormal relationships can be found with any combination of atrioventricular and ventriculo-arterial connections.

HEARTS WITH ISOMERIC ATRIAL APPENDAGES

The problems occurring in hearts with isomeric atrial appendages have already

been mentioned. Hearts with this arrangement are not only found in unusual positions, but are almost invariably associated with an abnormal arrangement of the thoracoabdominal organs, hence the popular rubric of visceral heterotaxy. It is still a widespread practice to classify these patients in terms of 'asplenia' and 'polysplenia'[7]. It is of greater value to base any system of categorisation on atrial morphology. Splenic morphology does not always correspond to the atrial anatomy. There is a greater correspondence between the anatomy of the appendages and what is expected of the 'splenic syndrome' than between these syndromes and splenic

morphology[8,9]. More important, it is of little consequence to the cardiac surgeon at the time of operation whether his patient has one spleen, multiple spleens, or no spleen at all. Use of the morphology of the appendages to define these anomalies concentrates the attention upon the heart, enabling the surgeon at operation to make immediately the diagnosis of isomerism, even if this had not been predicted by the preoperative studies.

The appendages are the best indicators of atrial morphology. They can easily be distinguished as being morphologically right or left (Fig. 10.7). The surgeon must always confirm that his patient possesses lateralised atrial appendages.

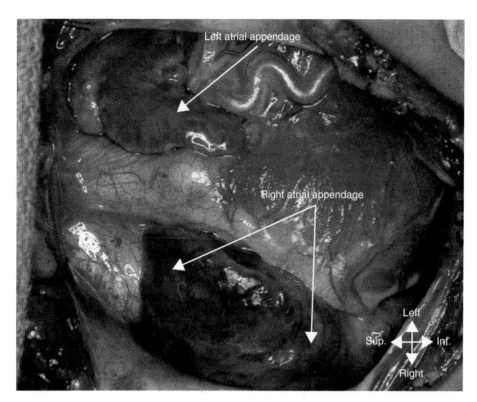

Fig. 10.7 This operative view, taken through a median sternotomy, shows the different morphology of the morphologically right as opposed to the morphologically left atrial appendages in a patient with usual atrial arrangement.

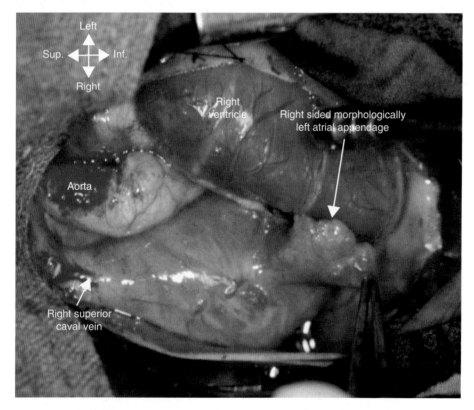

Fig. 10.8 This operative view, taken through a median sternotomy, shows that the appendage on the right side of the heart has left morphology. This patient had isomerism of the morphologically left atrial appendages.

Isomerism of the left (Fig. 10.8) or right (Fig. 10.9) appendages should immediately alert the surgeon to potential problems over and above those anticipated in the patient with usual atrial arrangement. In hearts with right isomerism, it is the rule to find complex intracardiac anomalies, usually with absence of the spleen. There is totally anomalous pulmonary venous connection even if the pulmonary veins are connected to the heart. Almost always there are major

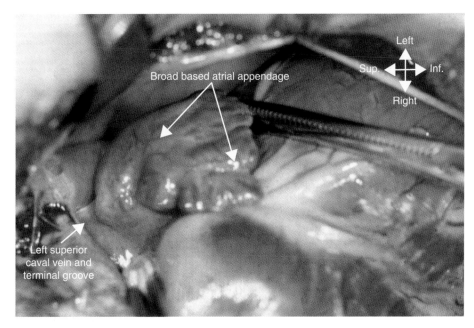

Fig. 10.9 In this patient, the left-sided atrial appendage is broad based, with a wide junction to the body of the atrium. Note that the left-sided superior caval vein joins to the atrial roof, and that there is a left-sided terminal groove. The right-sided appendage was also of right morphology. The patient has isomerism of the right atrial appendages.

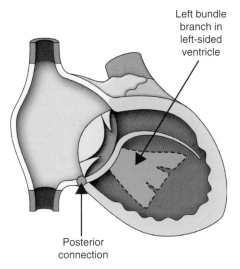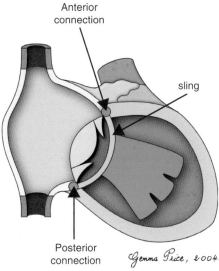

Fig. 10.10 This cartoon, drawn in anatomic orientation, shows the disposition of the axis of atrioventricular conduction tissue in hearts with isomerism of the atrial appendages, biventricular atrioventricular connections, and a common atrioventricular valve. The arrangement varies depending on whether there is right hand ventricular topology (left hand panel), when there is only a posterior connection of the ventricular conduction tissues, or left hand topology (right hand panel), when the ventricular conduction tissues are connected by both posterior and anterior atrioventricular nodes, giving the so-called "ventricular sling".

anomalies of systemic venous drainage. A common atrioventricular valve is usually present, often with univentricular atrioventricular connection. Pulmonary stenosis or atresia is frequently found, and there are bilateral sinus nodes. Although operative experience with these hearts is increasing, the various combinations of anomalies militate against successful outcomes. To be forewarned is of great value, so it should be remembered that the best preoperative guide to isomerism is either cross-sectional ultrasonography of the abdominal great vessels[10], or chest radiography to demonstrate bronchial morphology[11].

Although isomerism of the morphologically right appendages is almost always accompanied by severe intracardiac malformations, this is not necessarily the case with isomerism of the left appendages. Thus, the surgeon is more likely to be confronted with an undiagnosed case in the setting of left isomerism. It then becomes important to know that the sinus node is in an anomalous position. It is usually hypoplastic. If it can be found, it will be located close to the atrioventricular junction[12,13]. Interruption of the inferior caval vein, with return through the azygos venous system, is a frequent

accompaniment. In the more severely affected cases, there may be a common atrioventricular valve[14]. Pulmonary stenosis or atresia is not usually a feature, nor is the presence of univentricular atrioventricular connection, but there is frequently aortic coarctation.

Whatever the types of isomerism, when there is a common atrioventricular valve and each atrium is connected to its own ventricle, it is frequent to find a left hand pattern of ventricular topology. In this setting, the patient may well have been diagnosed as having congenitally corrected transposition. The presence of isomeric appendages, however, makes it highly likely that there will be a sling of ventricular conduction tissue joining dual atrioventricular nodes. This places the entire edge of the ventricular septum at risk should surgical correction be attempted. When isomerism of the appendages is found with biventricular atrioventricular connections and a right hand pattern of ventricular topology, the atrioventricular conduction axis should be expected in its usual posterior position (Fig. 10.10). This entire discussion emphasises the significance of full sequential segmental analysis of any patient presented for cardiac surgery.

References

1. Wilkinson JL, Acerete F. Terminological pitfalls in congenital heart disease. Reappraisal of some confusing terms, with an account of a simplified system of basic nomenclature. *Br Heart J* 1973; **35**: 1166–1177.

2. Van Praagh R, Weinberg PM, Matsuoka R, Van Praagh S. Malpositions of the heart. Edited by Adams FH, Emmanouilides. Baltimore: Williams & Wilkins. In *Moss's Heart Disease in Infants, Children and Adolescents* 1983; 422–458.

3. Byron F. Ectopia cordis. Report of a case with attempted operative correction. *J Thorac Surg* 1948; **17**: 717–722.

4. Cantrell JR, Haller JA, Ravitch MM. A syndrome of congenital defects involving the abdominal wall, sternum, diaphragm, pericardium and heart. *Surg Gynecol Obstet* 1958; **107**: 602–614.

5. Anderson RH, Smith A, Wilkinson JL. Disharmony between atrioventricular connections and segmental combinations – usual variants of "criss-cross" hearts. *J Am Coll Cardiol* 1987; **10**: 1274–1277.

6. Symons JC, Shinebourne EA, Joseph MC, Lincoln C, Ho SY, Anderson RH. Criss-cross heart with congenitally corrected transposition: report of a case with d-transposed aorta and ventricular preexcitation. *Eur J Cardiol* 1977; **5**: 493–505.

7. Stanger P, Rudolph AM, Edwards JE. Cardiac malpositions: an overview based on study of sixty-five necropsy specimens. *Circulation* 1977; **56**: 159–172.

8. Uemura H, Ho SY, Devine WA, Kilpatrick LL, Anderson RH. Atrial appendages and venoatrial connections in hearts with patients with visceral heterotaxy. *Ann Thorac Surg* 1995; **60**: 561–569.

9. Uemura H, Ho SY, Devine WA, Anderson RH. Analysis of visceral heterotaxy according to splenic status, appendage morphology, or both. *Am J Cardiol* 1995; **76**: 846–849.

10. Huhta JC, Smallhorn JF, Macartney FJ. Two dimensional echocardiographic diagnosis of situs. *Br Heart J* 1982; **48**: 97–108.

11. Deanfield J, Leanage R, Stroobant J, Chrispin AR, Taylor JFN, Macartney FJ. Use of high kilovoltage filtered beam radiographs for detection of bronchial situs in infants and young children. *Br Heart J* 1980; **44**: 577–583.

12. Dickinson DF, Wilkinson JL, Anderson KR, Smith A, Ho SY, Anderson RH. The cardiac conduction system in situs ambiguous. *Circulation* 1979; **59**: 879–885.

13. Ho SY, Seo J-W, Brown NA, Cook AC, Fagg NLK, Anderson RH. Morphology of the sinus node in human and mouse hearts with isomerism of the atrial appendages. *Br Heart J* 1995; **74**: 437–442.

14. Uemura H, Anderson RH, Ho SY, Devine WA, Neches WH, Smith A, Yagihara T, Kawashima Y. Left ventricular structures in atrioventricular septal defect associated with isomerism of the atrial appendages compared with similar features with usual atrial arrangement. *J Thorac Cardiovasc Surg* 1995; **110**: 445–452.

Index

Numbers in *italics* refer only to illustrations